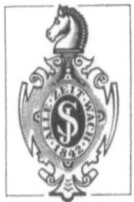

Walter A. Fuchs (Ed.)

Advances in CT

European Scientific User Conference SOMATOM PLUS
Zurich, March 1990

With 134 Figures and 29 Tables

Springer-Verlag Berlin Heidelberg New York
London Paris Tokyo Hong Kong

Professor Dr. med. WALTER A. FUCHS

Department of Medical Radiology
University Hospital Zürich
Rämistrasse 100, CH-8091 Zürich

ISBN-13: 978-3-642-95619-5   e-ISBN-13: 978-3-642-95617-1
DOI: 10.1007/978-3-642-95617-1

Library of Congress Cataloging-in-Publication Data
European Scientific User Conference SOMATOM PLUS (1990 : University Hospital
Zurich) Advances in CT / European Scientific User Conference SOMATOM PLUS,
March 1990 ; W. A. Fuchs (ed.). p. cm. ISBN 0-387-52561-0 (U. S. : alk. paper) 1. To-
mography-Congresses. I. Fuchs, W. A., 1929- . II. Title. [DNLM: 1. Tomography,
X-Ray Computed-trends-congresses. WN 160 E885a 1990] RC78.7.T6E92 1990
616.07'572-dc20 DNLM for Library of Congress 90-9781 CIP

© Springer-Verlag Berlin Heidelberg 1990
Softcover reprint of the hardcover 1st edition 1990

The use of general descriptive names, registered names, trademarks, etc. in this publication does not imply, even in the absence of a specific statement, that such names are
exempt from the relevant protective laws and regulations and therefore free for general
use.

Product Liability: The publisher can give no guarantee for information about drug
dosage and application thereof contained in this book. In every individual case the respective user must check its accuracy by consulting other pharmaceutical literature.

Typesetting, printing and binding: Appl, Wemding
2121/3145-543210 - Printed on acid-free paper

Preface

Though computed tomography has long been established in the field of radiological diagnosis, and the importance of this method has been described and discussed in numerous publications, the introduction of the SOMATOM PLUS computed tomography system in which the whole measuring system rotates continuously, provides the conditions necessary for the future technological and clinical development of this method.

In assessing this diagnostic advance, the exchange of ideas among users of the SOMATOM PLUS computed tomography system is of great importance. For this reason those radiologists who have already gained relevant experience in working with SOMATOM PLUS were invited to a User Conference in early March 1990. Reports and experiences concerning topics such as dynamic studies, artifact reduction using short scan times, thin-slice computed tomography, volume scanning, and three-dimensional reconstruction were presented, exchanged, and discussed. The aims of the conference were to demonstrate the increase in the range of applications of computed tomography which has been brought about by the SOMATOM PLUS, to exchange experiences, and to consider prospects for the future. More than 50 participants from nine European countries were present; 22 most interesting scientific papers were given, and these were followed by extensive discussions.

In order to share the experiences presented and discussed at the meeting with the members of the radiological community at large, it was decided to publish the proceedings of this most sucessful User Conference.

The scientific value of such a publication may be debatable. The contents of the various presentations published may be uneven and not too coherent. When editing manuscripts written in English, today's scientific language, by authors originating from various European countries, discrepancies in style and wording of course become apparent. Despite such possible shortcomings, the immediate publication of symposium proceedings certainly has an important role to play in the quick diffusion of scientific news within the medical and in particular the radiological community.

Acknowledgement is made of the excellent work of the secretarial and translating staff of the Department of Medical Radiology at University Hospital Zurich and of the superb and efficient editorial team at Springer-Verlag.

Zurich, March 1990   WALTER A. FUCHS

Contents

3D Reconstruction
Chairmen: H. Riemann, W. A. Fuchs

Dynamic Studies
Chairmen: J. v. Engelshoven, A. K. Dixon

Chairmen

Prof. Dr. med. E. BÜCHELER
Universitäts-Krankenhaus Eppendorf
Radiologische Universitätsklinik und Strahleninstitut
Martinistrasse 52, D-2000 Hamburg 20

Dr. med. A. K. DIXON
Departments of Radiology
Addenbrooke's Hospital and the University of Cambridge
Hills Road, GB-Cambridge CB2 2QQ

Prof. Dr. med. J. M. A. VAN ENGELSHOVEN
Academisch Ziekenhuis Maastricht
Sint Annadal 1, NL-6214 PA Maastricht

Prof. Dr. med. W. A. FUCHS
Department Medizinische Radiologie
Universitätsspital Zürich
Rämistrasse 100, CH-8091 Zürich

Prof. Dr. med. P. GERHARDT
Institut für Röntgendiagnostik
Klinikum rechts der Isar
Ismaninger Strasse 22, D-8000 München 80

Prof. Dr. med. P. VOCK
Institut für Diagnostische Radiologie
Universität Bern
Inselspital, CH-3010 Bern

Prof. Dr. med. H. E. RIEMANN
Abteilung für Allgemeine Röntgendiagnostik III
Klinikum der Johann-Wolfgang-Goethe-Universität
Frankfurt, Theodor-Stern-Kai 7, D-6000 Frankfurt 70

Prof. Dr. med. J. STRUYVEN
Hôpital Erasme, Service Radiologie
Route de Lennik 808, D-1070 Brussels

Participants

Dr. med. F. ASTINET
  Radiologische Klinik und Poliklinik
  Klinikum Rudolf Virchow
  Freie Universität Berlin
  Spandauer Damm 130, D-1000 Berlin 19

Priv.-Doz. Dr. med. W. BAUTZ
  Abteilung für Radiologische Diagnostik
  Radiologische Universitätsklinik
  Hoppe-Seyler-Strasse 3, D-7400 Tübingen 1

Dr. med. F. P. J. BILLET
  Radiologische Abteilung, Juliusspital
  Juliuspromenade 19, D-8700 Würzburg

Dr. med. A. K. DIXON
  Departments of Radiology
  Addenbrooke's Hospital and the University of Cambridge
  Hills Road, GB-Cambridge CB2 2QQ

Dr. med. K. ENGELHARD
  Röntgenabteilung
  Krankenhaus Martha-Maria
  Stadenstrasse 58, D-8500 Nürnberg 20

Dr. med. J. GAA
  Städtische Kliniken Darmstadt
  Akademisches Lehrkrankenhaus
  Johann-Wolfgang-Goethe-Universität Frankfurt
  Grafenstrasse 9, 6100 Darmstadt

Dr. P. A. GEVENOIS, MD.
  Department of Radiology
  Université Libre de Bruxelles
  Hôpital Erasme
  Route de Lennik 808, B-1070 Bruxelles

Dr. med. J. GMEINWIESER
  Abteilung für Radiologie
  Institut für Röntgendiagnostik
  Klinikum rechts der Isar
  Ismaninger Strasse 22, D-8000 München 80

Prof. Dr. med. M. HERBST
  Strahlentherapeutische Klinik und Poliklinik der
  Universität Erlangen-Nürnberg
  Universitätsstrasse 27, D-8520 Erlangen

Dr. med. J. HODLER
  Röntgendiagnostisches Zentralinstitut
  Universitätsspital
  Rämistrasse 100, CH-8091 Zürich

Dr. rer. nat. R. HUPKE
  Siemens Medical Systems Inc.
  186, Wood Avenue South
  Iselin, NJ 08830, USA

Dr. W. A. KALENDER, Ph. D.
  Bereich Medizin
  Siemens AG
  Henkestrasse 127, D-8520 Erlangen

Dr. M. OUDKERK, MD. PhD.
  Department of Diagnostic Radiology
  Dr. Daniel den Hoed Kliniek
  Groene Hilledijk 301
  NL-3075 EA Rotterdam

Prof. Dr. med. R. RIENMÜLLER
  Radiologische Klinik und Poliklinik
  Klinikum Grosshadern
  Ludwig-Maximilians-Universität München
  Marchioninistrasse 15, D-8000 München 70

Dr. med. H. RIGAUTS
  Department of Radiology
  University Hospitals K. U. Leuven
  Herestraat 49, B-3000 Leuven

Prof. Dr. med. P. VOCK
  Institut für Diagnostische Radiologie
  Universität Bern
  Inselspital, CH-3010 Bern

Dr. med. W. VOGEL
  Radiologie I
  Strahleninstitut der Städtischen Kliniken Darmstadt
  Grafenstrasse 9, D-6100 Darmstadt

Dr. med. C. ZWICKER
  Radiologische Klinik und Poliklinik
  Klinikum Rudolf Virchow
  Freie Universität Berlin
  Spandauer Damm 130, D-1000 Berlin 19

Image Quality,
Clinical Applications

Chairmen: E. Bücheler, P. Vock

The Advantages of Fast and Continuously-Rotating CT Systems

R. HUPKE

Summary

Slip ring systems in CT scanners make it possible to scan in quick succession with scan times less than one second. The sensitivity to motion artifacts is low, even when higher dose is required, because images can be produced with more than one rotation. The principles and advantages of this so called Multiscan Technique (MST) will be explained with phantom studies. In addition a clinical examination will be demonstrated. It can be shown that the consistent usage of MST not only reduces motion artifacts but also the whole examination time. The implementation and finally the limits of this method will be discussed in detail.

With some technical modifications of this Multiscan Technique it is also possible to reduce partial volume artifacts, which occure especially in the imaging of the posterior fossa. The technique involves contiguous thin axial sections which are averaged to create a composite image of larger slice thickness. The principles of this Volume Artifact Reduction program (VAR) are again demonstrated with phantom studies as well as patient examinations.

In conclusion, the continuously-rotating CT system SOMATOM PLUS shows superior improvements in image quality. In addition, such systems open up new fields of application and investigation for 3rd generation CT scanners. Finally it should be mentioned that this high-quality SOMATOM PLUS technique is the forerunner for a new dimension in CT: spiral scanning.

Introduction

Most of the actual 3rd generation CT scanners apply the stop-and-go principle. In this type of scanner, which utilizes a cable take-up assembly, minimal scan times are 2–3 seconds and minimal interscan times amount up to 10 seconds, this is related to the accelerating and decelerating of the large mass of the entire measuring system [Lee et al. 1989]. In contrast, the introduction of a 3rd generation CT scanner with a continuously rotating measuring system, the SOMATOM PLUS, provides the technical basis for rapid uninterrupted data acquisition. Routine measuring times of 0.7, 1 and 2 seconds result in sharp, artifact free images. In dynamic applications the continuously rotating measuring system offers zero interscan delay and opens up new horizons in Dynamic CT [Rigauts et al. 1990a, Bautz and Klier 1989].

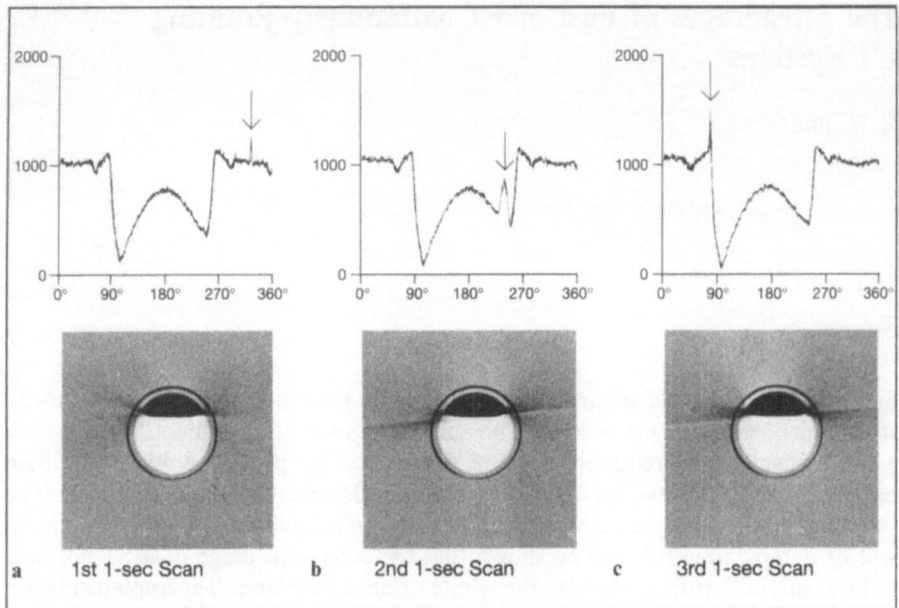

Fig. 1a-e. The principles of the Multiscan Technique (see text)

The aim of this contribution is to present an overview of various new scan modalities arising out of continuous rotation, together with some detailed explanations. These methods are demonstrated with phantom studies as well as with clinical examples.

Technical Review

SOMATOM PLUS is a completely new fast x-ray computer tomograph with continuous rotation of the whole measuring system. The time for one revolution is 1 second or 2 seconds. The energy transfer to the x-ray tube is realized by the use of high voltage slip rings. In practical operations, electric power up to 35 kW and voltage up to 137 kV can be transmitted [Alexander and Krumme 1988]. The self-collimating Quantillarc detector has 768 chambers. As a result of the Multifan principle, realized with the Flying Focal Spot x-ray tube, 1536 measurement channels per projection are available for uninterrupted data acquisition.

Multiscan Technique (MST)

With obese patients or examinations which require thin slice thicknesses e.g. studies of the adrenal gland, it is often requested to reduce the increased quantum

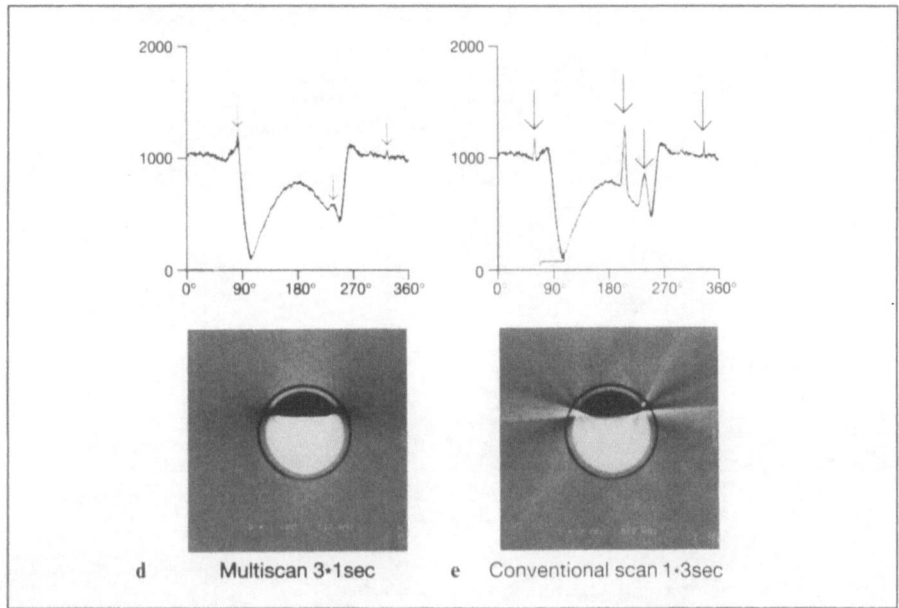

Fig. 1d, e

noise with the appropriate dose. Frequently this is achieved with higher tube load-ing. But this leads to longer tube cooling interruptions and to slower cycle times. To avoid this, it is necessary to raise the measuring time to 2 or more seconds, thus increasing the susceptibility to motion artifacts. Scanners such as the SOMATOM PLUS with fast and continuous rotation of the x-ray source introduce the opportu-nity to measure tomograms in rapid succession and to accumulate raw data mea-sured with N successive rotations of the gantry. Motion artifacts which may occur in one or more of the N rotations are reduced in the CT-image by reconstructing from the averaged data set, because each artifact is weighted by a factor of $1/N$ [Hupke and Pauli 1989].

This advantage of the so-called Multiscan Technique (MST) is illustrated in Fig. 1 by means of a phantom study. An opening was made in the center of a lucite phantom, in which a liquid surface could be moved by means of a well defined and reproducible pulse amplitude. The final tomogram of the 3*1-sec-MST was made with a dose corresponding to 510 mAs, that is, each of the three 1-sec rota-tions was performed with 170 mAs. Fig. 1a (top) shows a schematic of the profile from one 1-sec scan of the phantom measured for a single central channel. The abscissa is the projection angle in degrees and the ordinate shows the measured values in arbitary units. The arrow in the graph indicates the pulsatile motion of the contrast agent surface. If a CT image would be reconstructed from the com-plete raw data set, the result would be as shown at the image on the bottom of Fig. 1a. This tomogram shows a typical artifact resulting from contrast agent motion. Approximately the same situation can be seen in the second and third 1-sec scans (Fig. 1b, c).

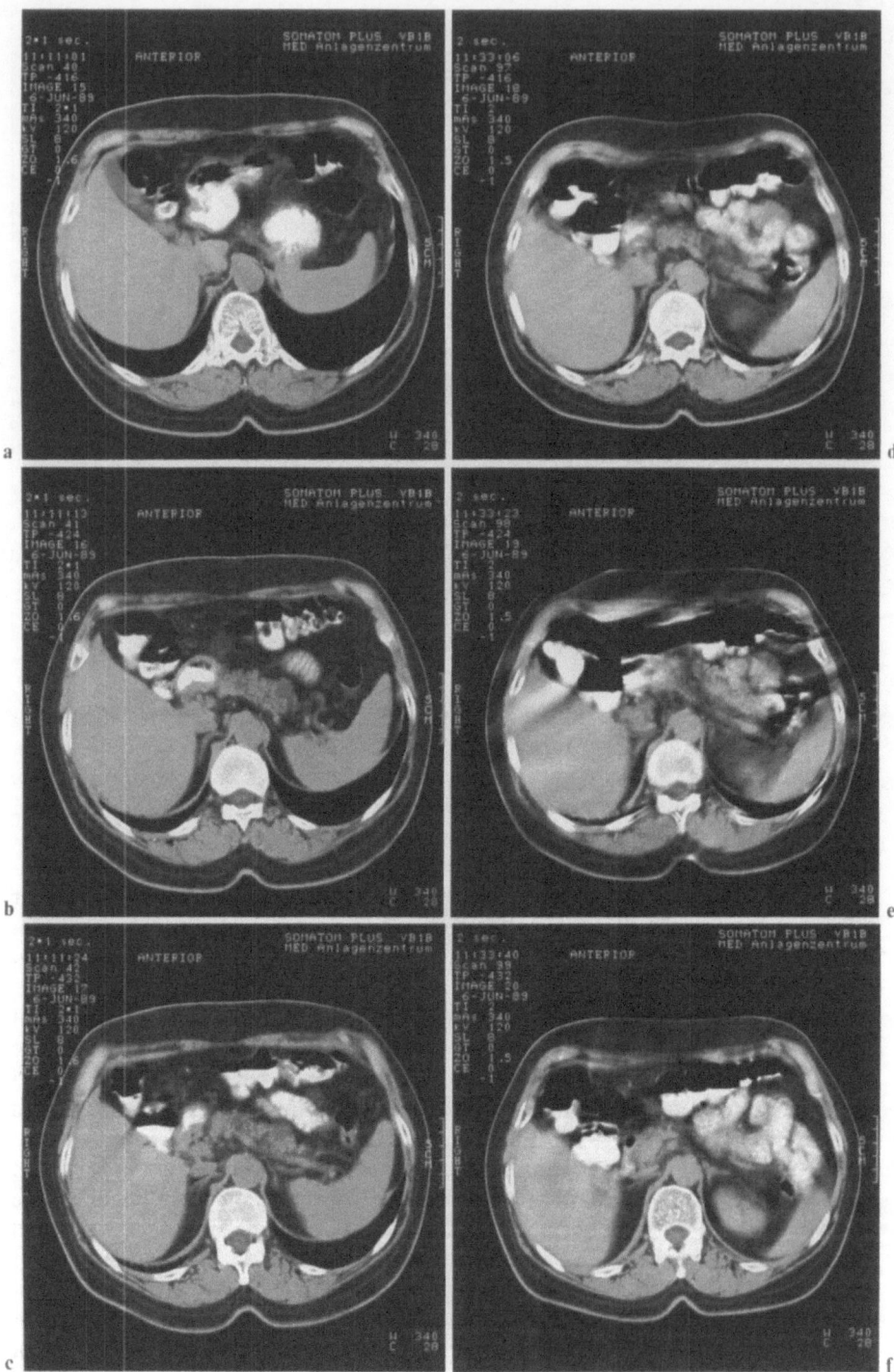

Fig. 2a–f. Comparison of 2*1-second (left) and 1*2-second modes (right)

In order to obtain the shortest computation time possible, the raw data sets, and not the CT images, are averaged. A comparison of the averaged profile (Fig. 1 d) and the single profiles (arrow) indicates a reduction of the artifacts by a factor of 3. The tomogram from the averaged raw data set of the 3*1-sec multiscan shows practically no artifacts. The comparison of the 3*1-sec multiscan (Fig. 1 d) with a conventional 1*3-sec scan (Fig. 1 e) with the same mAs-product shows impressively that the Multiscan Technique is superior to the standard method of 2 seconds scan time or longer in regions highly susceptible to motion artifacts.

For a given mAs product, the tube capacity increases with decreasing tube power. This is why the cycle time becomes shorter if the scan is performed using less power but with a longer measuring time. In contrast to the conventional technique, MST permits longer measuring times without any increase in the frequency or the intensity of motion artifacts. This advantage produces a significant gain in time, especially in the long screening examinations necessary when looking for metastases.

In order to demonstrate the clinical significance of MST a patient was first scanned after administering an oral contrast medium with MST-parameters 2*1-sec, 340 mAs, 8 mm and 8 mm table feed. An additional series with intravenous contrast medium was carried out with the conventional method (1*2-sec, 340 mAs, 8 by 8 mm). In Fig. 2 three successive scans of each series with the same table positions were chosen for comparison, without attempting to find exactly the same anatomical cuts. It is clearly seen in Fig. 2 (left) that MST is the method of choice if a longer measuring time is required in abdominal studies.

As long as the amplitude of the motion of the whole object is small compared to the size of the structures to be resolved, no blurring can be noticed in the MST-images. However, if one demands highest spatial resolution in body scans, the motion of the whole body has to be minimal during data acquisition. Only very short scan times will give images without motion artifacts.

In Fig. 3 the images show some studies of the fine structure in the lung produced with a 1 mm slice thickness and different scan times. It can be clearly seen that the image of the one second scan (Fig. 3 b) is much clearer than that of the 2*1-sec scan (Fig. 3 a). The same statement is valid if the conventional two second scan mode is taken. However, even a scan time of 1 second can be too long (Fig. 3 c): A double appearance of the fine structure (bronchus and vessels) due to cardiac motion can be observed. The same cut, reconstructed as a 0.7-sec scan (Fig. 3 d), does not show these artifacts any longer. For the detailed study of the lung interstitium, the equipment offers different additional scan modes (e. g. 1 mm, 0.7 sec) with ultra-high algorithms. These modes are part of the standard software, so there is no need of a special software package for high resolution CT (HRCT).

The console software is organized into pages from which the scan modality can be chosen. Apart from the acquisition parameters, different processing algorithms are available. In one page these algorithms vary over five steps of sharpness (ultra high to soft detail). In general these kernels are optimized to the considered anatomical region. For example, the kernel corresponding to "lung-high" has a characteristic which is totally different from that one in "shoulder-high". One reason is, that the highest spatial resolution is available only in the M*2-sec scanmode

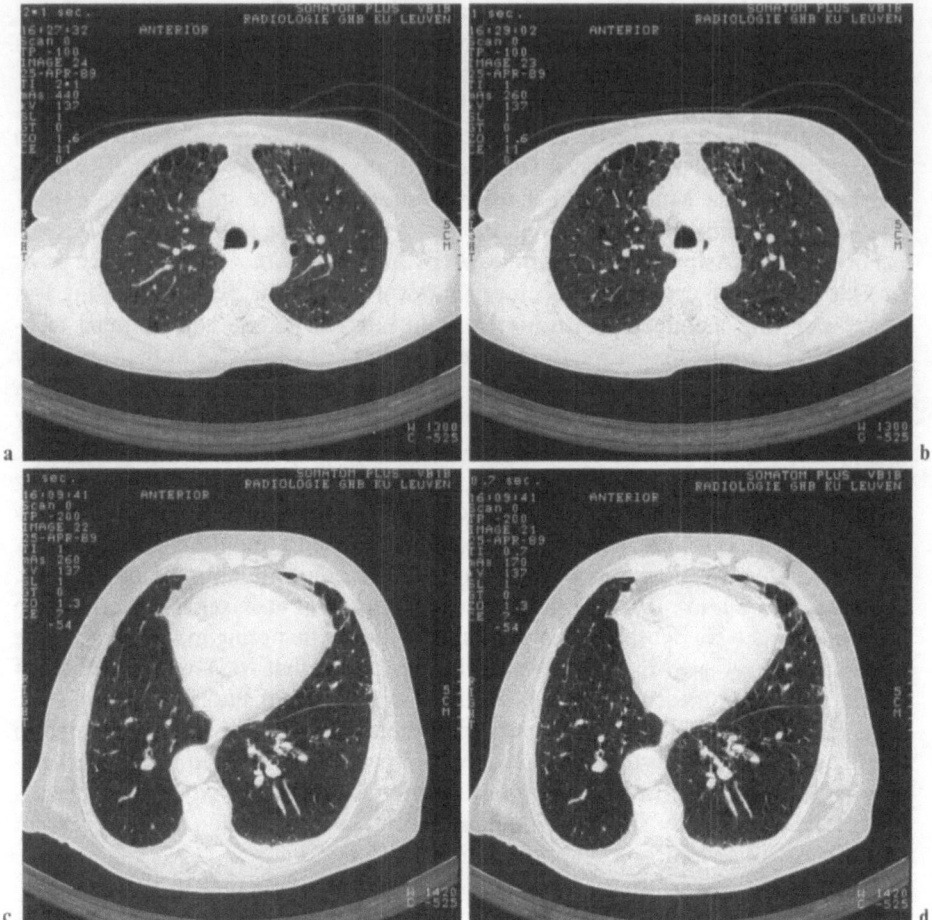

Fig. 3a-d. The limits of the MST (see text) lung studies, 1 mm slice thickness and different scan times

(M = 1,2,3). In addition, in this modes the sampling theorem is fulfilled, so no high-frequency artifacts are visible [Brooks et al. 1979]. The most prominent artifacts are those occuring along thin bony structures, such as the base of the skull. On the other hand it is not recommended to scan the lung for longer than one second, so the kernel in this mode has to have special features to get sharp artifact-free images [Glover and Eisner 1979, Yester and Barnes 1977]. The consistent use of this organ-specific protocols and kernels is very useful in clinical practice and offers the user the possibility to optimize the image presentation for the region under study.

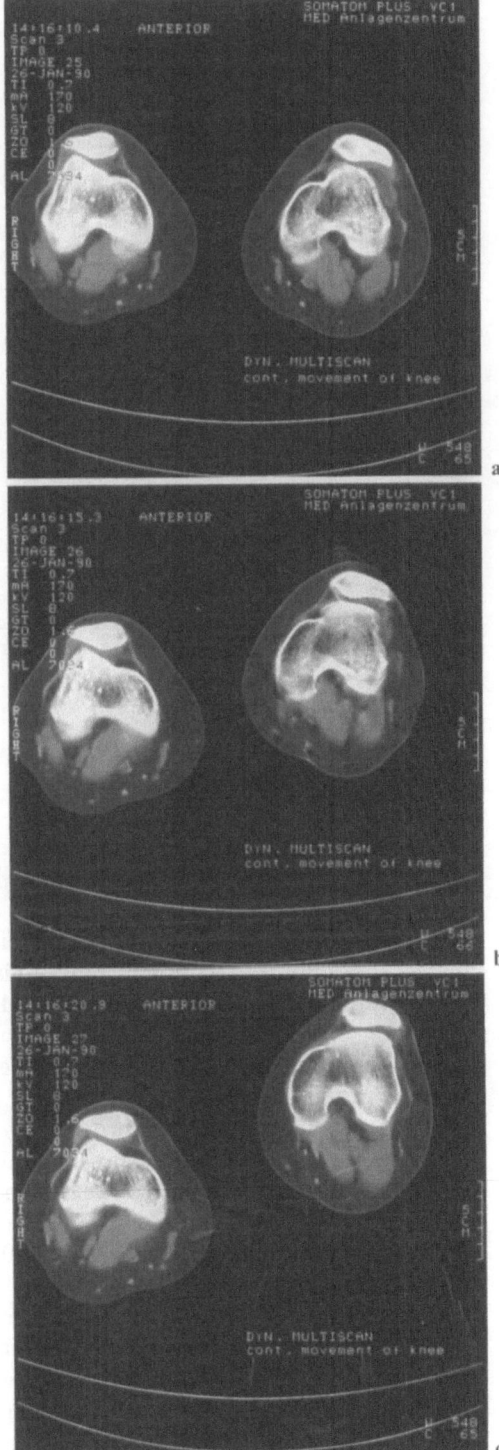

Fig. 4a-c. Dynamic Multiscan (12*1-sec) during movement (appr. 6 mm/sec) of the knee; these three images are picked out of a series of 17 images (reconstruction intervall 0.7 sec)

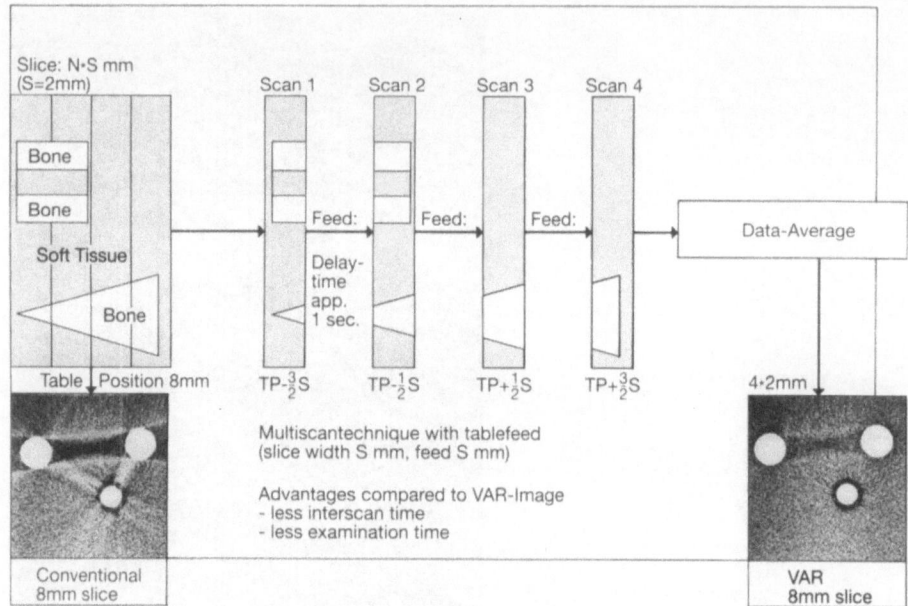

Fig. 5. A schematic prescription of VAR. A larger volume is divided into thin slices; the so measured data are averaged before image reconstruction

Dynamic Scanning Modes

The continuous rotation of the entire tube-detector system makes possible new dynamic examination techniques, e. g. such with zero interscan delay. With Dynamic Multiscan, a multirotational measurement of one slice is performed for up to 12 seconds. This mode allows the reconstruction of over 100 one-second images separated by only 0.1 seconds in time. This examination technique ensures the greatest possible resolution in time for fast dynamic processes, such as for the differentiation of arterial and venous processes. The Dynamic Serio mode allows scanning with freely selectable interscan intervals.

Moreover, the Dynamic Multiscan offers new fields even for unusual dynamic investigations, an example is shown in Fig. 4. While performing a Dynamic Multiscan (12*1-sec, 8 mm slice thickness, 170 mA) the patient was instructed to move her knee continuously during the measurement. As seen in Fig. 4 the mean movement of the knee was about 6 mm/sec. The orthopaedist was intersted in the dynamic behaviour of the patella. This first study demonstrates that the high speed data acquisition (one second per rotation) in combination with the split reconstruction (reconstruction window is 0.7 seconds) over the whole raw data set results in nearly artifact-free images of real dynamic processes. Because it is possible to reconstruct in small time intervalls a cine-mode display becomes very useful.

Dynamic Screening ensures the shortest possible cycle time with 5 seconds, including table advance and instantaneous image display. On the other hand, Dy-

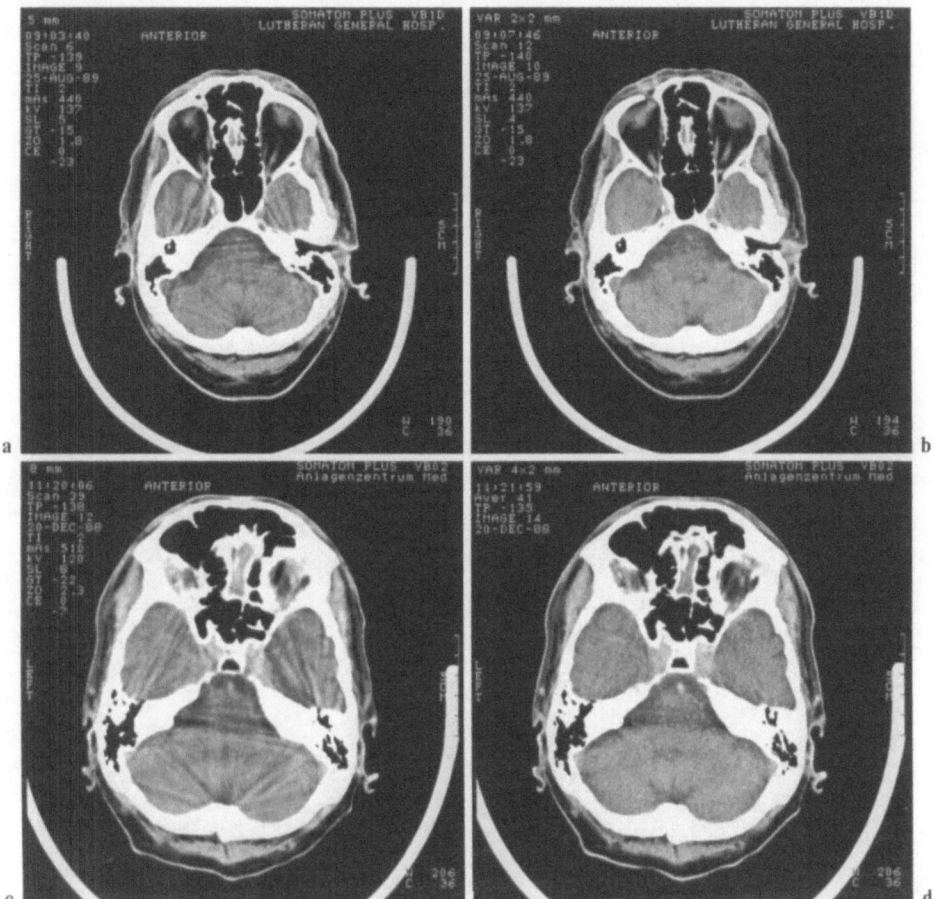

Fig. 6a-d. Clinical demonstration of the value of VAR (top: 5 mm; bottom: 8 mm). *Left:* conventional scanning. *Right:* the same anatomical regions now with VAR

namic Sequence with the shortest exposure series of 3 seconds presently allows the fastest examination of an anatomical region of the body, including table advance, for concurrent image reconstruction.

Volume Artifact Reduction

Since the advent of computed tomography, imaging of the posterior fossa has posed problems [Lee et al. 1989]. The proximity and density of the temporal bones give rise to the so-called partial volume artifact [Moström and Ytterbergh 1986, Radü et al. 1987]. Such artifacts are reduced by utilizing thin slices. However, this scan technique is not very economically in routine examinations. In order to ob-

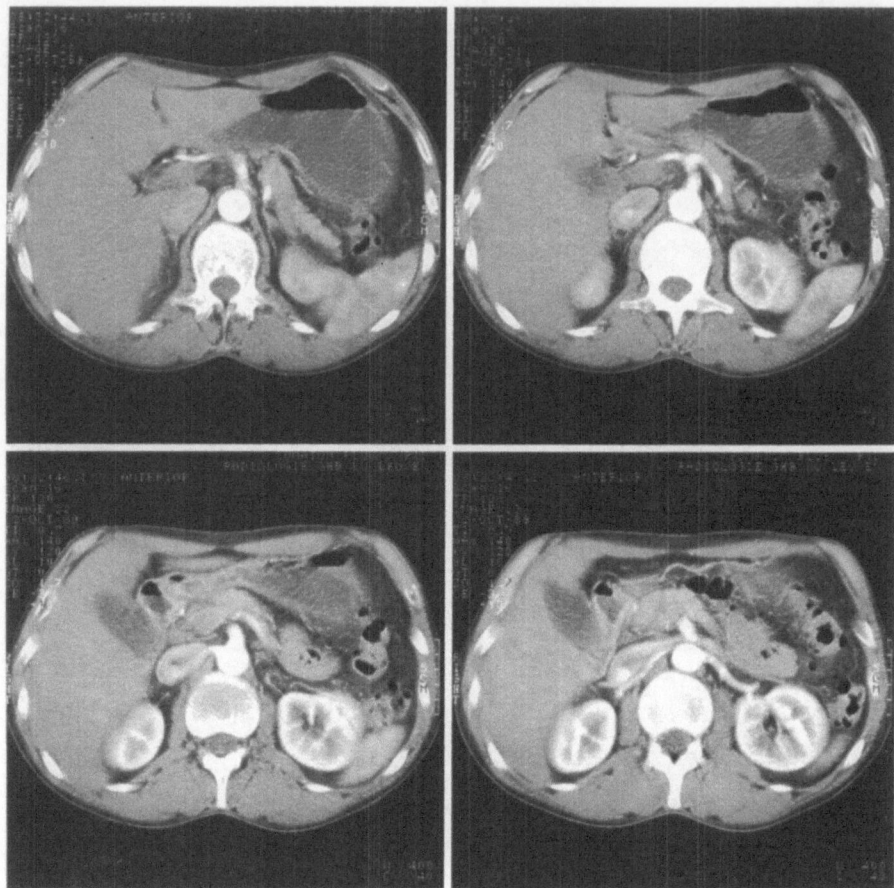

Fig. 7. Four consecutive images of spiral scanning with 8 mm slice width and 8 mm/sec table speed

tain artifact-free images of the posterior fossa as quickly as possible we have introduced a composite addition technique as a work in progress project.

The basic idea is to combine the Multiscan Technique as described above with a table feed between the single scans, carried out with thin slices, of one MST (Fig. 5). Then the raw data sets measured in M consecutive rotations are averaged. First of all, the measurement with thin slice thicknesses yields images with nearly no partial volume artifacts in each individual slice. If an artifact occurs in one slice (due to partial volume effects or to vascular pulsation), this artifact will be reduced by the factor $\frac{1}{M}$ according to the MST principle as shown in Fig. 1. In order to avoid aliasing artifacts scanning with M*2-sec is recommended. In addition, when scanning with higher tube voltage (137 kV), beamhardening artifacts are further reduced [Rührnschopf and Kalender 1981]. The softer the x-ray spectrum, the stronger the beamhardening effect. At the top of Fig. 6 a normal 5 mm slice (left)

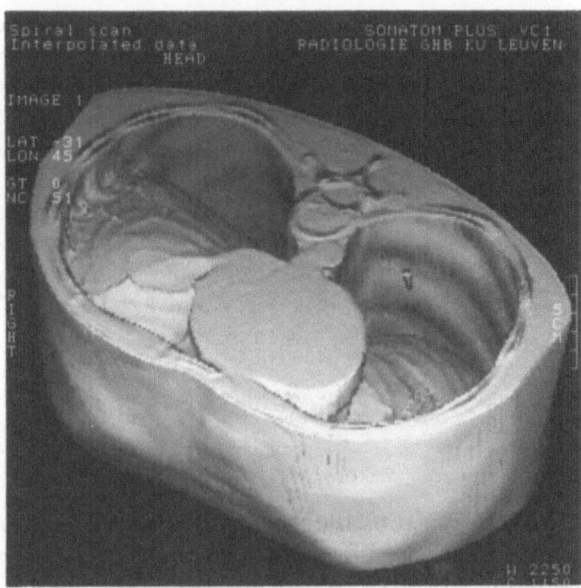

Fig. 8. 3 D-Image from a spiral scan. 10 mm slice width, 10 mm/sec table speed and 12*1-seconds scan time, reconstructed for a table incrementation of 2 mm

is compared to a 4 mm VAR slice (right) at nearly the same level. In the lower part of Fig. 6 a conventional (left) and a VAR 8 mm slice are shown.

The resulting images show a significant reduction of low frequency streak artifact from the temporal bones in the middle cranial fossa and from the internal occipital protuberance in the posterior fossa. Hounsfield artifacts are markedly reduced in the region of brainstem. Preliminary work indicates that this so called Volume Artifact Reduction (VAR) may also improve CT imaging of the spine, particularly in the lower cervical spine where shoulder artifacts often pose problems.

Spiral Scanning

The last logical step, to combine VAR with a continuous movement of the patient couch leads us to a totally new dimension in CT: the spiral (or volume) scanning. For this work in progress the Dynamic Multiscan is used, offering up to 12 consecutive 1 second scans, each at 170 mA. During the entire measuring time the table moves with constant speed, usually with one slice width per second. After raw date processing [Kalender et al. 1990, Rigauts et al. 1990 b] it is possible to reconstruct CT images for each start position (corresponding to table position) desired. The consistent usage of this method ensures the diagnosis of small lesions for example in the lung [Vock et al. 1989].

Another application of spiral scanning is 3 D respectively MPR. First of all the entire volume is measured in the shortest time possible, so patient motion is minimized. Data acquisition with a 10 mm slice thickness over 12 seconds scan time and at a table speed of 10 mm/sec makes it possible to interpolate raw data corresponding to a table feed down to 1 mm, and to reconstruct more than 100 overlapping CT images. Image interpolation in the patient direction, as required by 3 D-programs, in spiral scanning is shifted to an image reconstruction from of the measured raw data, so that slice artifacts are minimized.

Just to give a first impression of the image quality of spiral CT, some preliminary images are shown in Fig. 7 and Fig. 8 (3 D). This new method will be discussed in detail during this conference.

Conclusion

The continuously rotating SOMATOM PLUS CT-system shows superior improvements in image quality, even in scans of "difficult" patients such as new-born, elderly and intensive care patients, thanks to the short data acquisition time. In addition, this innovative equipment opens up new fields of application and investigation for 3rd generation scanners.

Finally it has been pointed out, this high-quality SOMATOM PLUS technique represents the forerunner for a new dimension in CT: spiral scanning.

Acknowledgment. For their support in providing clinical examples I would like to express my gratitude to Prof. Herbst, University of Erlangen (Fig. 1), Dr. Rigauts, University of Leuven, Belgium (Figs. 3, 7), Dr. Hirschfelder, University of Erlangen (Fig. 4) and Dr. Levy, Lutheran General Hospital, Chicago, USA (Fig. 6)

References

Alexander J, Krumme HJ (1988) SOMATOM PLUS: New perspectives in Computed Tomography. Electromedica 56: No 2, 50–56
Bautz W, Klier R (1989) SOMATOM PLUS: Clinical results of 3000 patient examinations. Electromedica 57: No 3
Brooks RA, Glover GH, Talbert AJ, Eisner RL, DiBianca FA (1979) Aliasing: A source of streaks in computer tomograms. Journal of Computer Assisted Tomography 3 (4): 511–518
Glover GH, Eisner RL (1979) Theoretical resolution of CT systems. Journal of Computer Assisted Tomography 3: 85–91
Hupke R, Pauli KH (1989) The advantages of producing CT images with multiple rotations of the radiation source per image. In: 17th International Congress of Radiology, p 980
Kalender WA, Seißler W, Klotz E, Vock P (1990) Single breathholding spiral volumetric computed tomography (SVCT) by continuous patient translation and scanner rotation. Submitted to Radiology 12/89
Lee SK, Sagel SS, Stanley R (1989) Computed body tomography with MRI correlations, second edition, Raven Press, New York
Moström U, Ytterbergh C (1986) Artifacts in computed tomography of the posterior fossa: A comperative phantom study. Journal of Computer Assisted Tomography 10 (4): 560–566

Radü EW, Kendall BE, Mosely IF (1987) Computertomographie des Kopfes. Thieme, Stuttgart, New York

Rigauts H, Marchal G, Baert AL, Hupke R (1990a) A six month clinical evaluation with the SOMATOM PLUS. Electromedica 58: No 1

Rigauts H, Marchal G, Baert AL, Hupke R, Kalender WA (1990b) First experiences with volume scanning. Submitted to Journal of Computer Assisted Tomography 11/89

Rührnschopf EP, Kalender WA (1981) Artifacts caused by nonlinear partial volume and spectral hardening effects in computerized tomography. Electromedica 2: 96-105

Vock P, Jung H, Kalender WA (1989) Single breathholding spiral volumetric CT of the lung. Radiology 1989a, 173(P): 400

Conventional and High-Resolution CT in Diagnosis of Occupational Lung Diseases: A Comparative Study – Preliminary Results

P. A. GEVENOIS, M. L. VAN SINOY, S. DEDEIRE, B. STALLENBERG, J. STRUYVEN

Summary

Twenty four asbestos and silica-exposed individuals were evaluated by means of conventional computed tomography (CT) and high-resolution computed tomography (HRCT). The aspects of asbestosis and silicosis and the diagnostic value of both methods were compared. The accuracy of each method was evaluated for the following abnormalities: nodules, masses, curvilinear subpleural lines, thickened interlobular lines, irregular interfaces, honeycombing, subpleural dependent density, parenchymal bands, ground-glass opacities, emphysema, subpleural blebs, rounded atelectasis, segmental or sub-segmental atelectasis, and hyaline and calcified pleural plaques. The diagnostic value of each technique is also estimated. HRCT is much more accurate in detecting curvilinear subpleural lines, thickened interlobular lines, irregular interfaces, honeycombing, ground-glass opacities and subpleural blebs. Conventional CT is dramatically more reliable for detection of small nodules. For the other abnormalities, our study was too limited by the relatively small number of cases to permit a definitive conclusion. We concluded on the basis of the preliminary report that both conventional and high-resolution computed tomography should be used in the examination of patient with occupational chest diseases.

Introduction

Chest radiographs are widely used to determine the presence and the extent of silicosis and asbestos-related lung and pleural disease. Conventional CT scanning is more sensitive than chest radiography for detection of pulmonary nodules [1], interstitial changes [2] and pleural disorders [3-5]. Neither routine chest radiography nor conventional CT can reliably detect early parenchymal lung fibrosis. High resolution CT (HRCT) scanning, performed with the optimal approach [6] affords much greater spatial resolution than conventional CT. High resolution CT of silicosis [7] and asbestosis [8, 9] are well described. The purpose of this study is to compare the accuracy of both, conventional and high resolution CT in the detection of occupational disease of the chest. In asbestos-related disorders, Lynch et al. have evaluated the usefulness of both techniques in focal lung masses [10], as have Aberle et al. for the detection of pleural abnormalities [8].

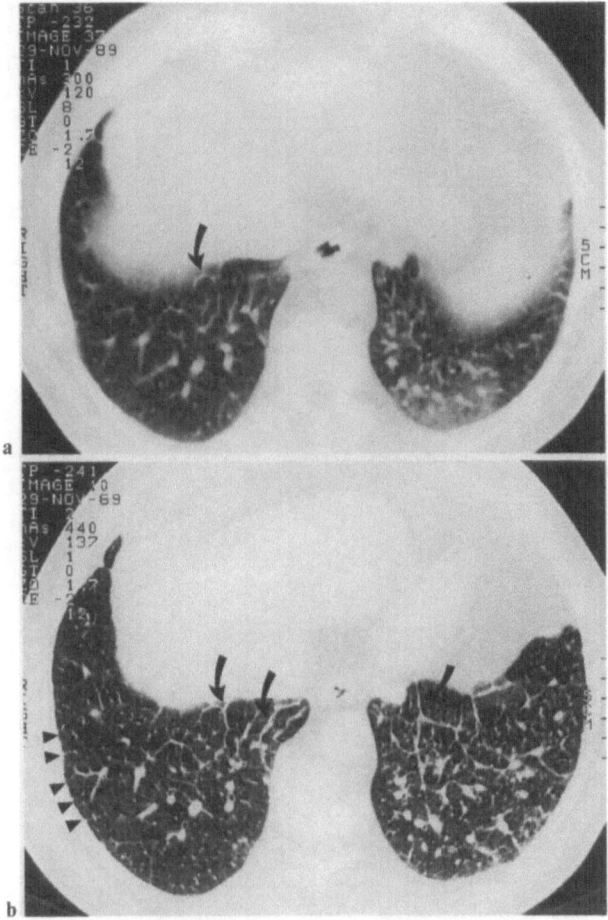

Fig. 1a, b. Conventional CT (a) and HRCT (b): bilateral interstitial short lines in subpleural lung (arrowheads) that contact pleura peripherally. This sign is only visualized in HRCT. Thickened septa marginate subpleural pulmonary lobule (arrows) are more evaluable on HRCT than on conventional CT

Materials and Methods

Population

Routine and high resolution CT were performed in 24 patients with suspected pneumoconiosis or asbestosis on the basis of a history of occupational exposure to dust for at least 10 years, and in whom the chest radiograph was not conclusive for occupational disease. The aim of the CT evaluation was to assess or to reject the diagnosis of occupational lung disease. All patients were men, with an average age of 59 years (range, 47-72 years).

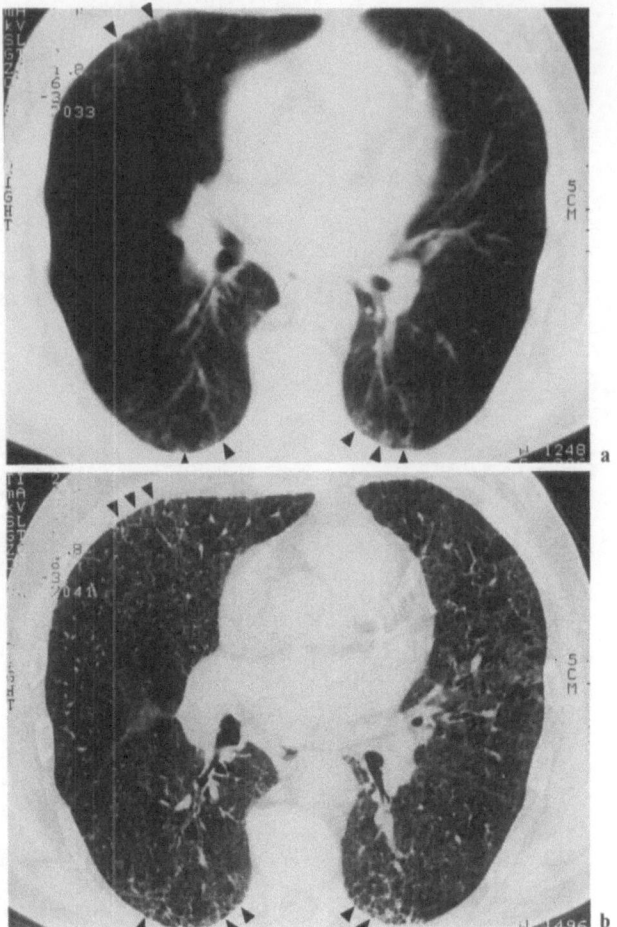

Fig. 2a, b. Conventional CT (**a**) and HRCT (**b**): Focal subpleural honeycombing and interlobular thickening (arrowheads) are better evaluable in HRCT than on conventional CT

Methods

The high resolution CT scans were obtained with a Siemens (Erlangen, West Germany) SOMATOM PLUS scanner at 3 cm intervals with 1.0-mm collimation and a bone-detail algorithm (ultra-high) from the apex of the lungs to the diaphragm during maintenance of maximal inspiration. To minimize the noise introduced by the use of thin collimation and a high spatial frequency algorithm, increased technical factors were used, including 137 kVp, 220 mA, and 2-second acquisition time. Patients were examined in the supine and prone position. Secondly routine CT was performed, consisting of contiguous scans 10 mm thick, extending from the lung apices to below the costophrenic angles. Routine techniques were used with image reconstruction, with use of a standard soft-tissue algorithm. All scans were imaged on separate window settings for mediastinal and lung details.

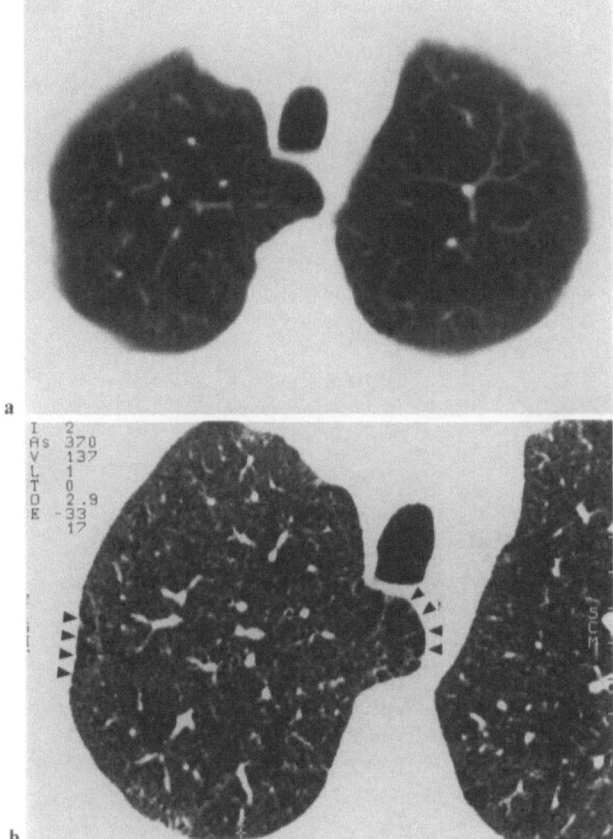

Fig. 3a, b. Conventional CT (a) and HRCT (b): Low attenuation area are evaluable on both techniques but subpleural blebs are more easily delineate on HRCT (arrowheads)

Analysis

All scans were examined prospectively by one observer and evaluated subsequently by a consensus of two reviewers. A probability score for the presence of asbestos or silica-related lung or pleural disorders was established by analyzing the conventional and high resolution CT for the presence of the following signs. The probability scores ranged from 0 (normal-appearing lung parenchyma or pleura), to 2 (strong probability of lung or pleural disease). An intermediate score ($=1$) was given for doubtful lesions or those seen retrospectively.

1. *Nodules:* small punctate opacities (Fig. 6).
2. *Masses*
3. *Curvilinear subpleural lines:* A linear density within 1 cm of the pleura and parallel to the inner chest wall has been described in patients with asbestosis [8, 11].
4. *Thickened interlobular lines:* These were single or branching lines 1–2 cm in length, seen in the subpleural parenchyma, extending toward the visceral pleu-

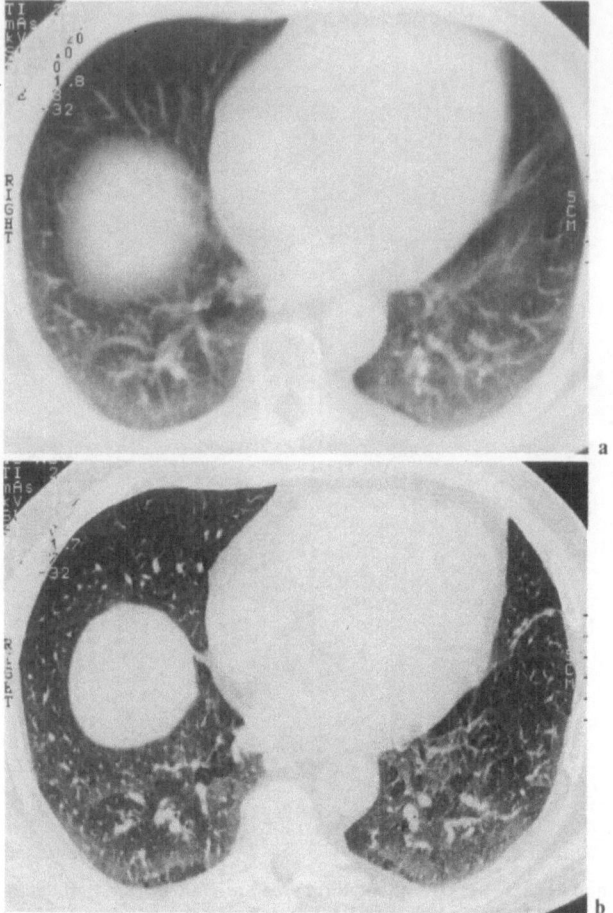

Fig. 4a, b. Conventional CT (a) and HRCT (b): Ground-glass opacities are more easily appreciated on HRCT than on conventional CT

ral surface [8]. These lines correspond to the interlobular septa containing venules and lymphatics (Fig. 1).

5. *Irregular interfaces:* Easily detected on peripheral and mediastinal pleura and occurring equally along fissures, vessels and bronchi.

6. *Honeycombing:* Area of lung containing small, cystlike spaces less than 1 cm in diameter with thick walls, most commonly seen in the subpleural regions of the lung [8, 9] (Fig. 2).

7. *Subpleural dependent density:* A band 2–30 mm thick of poorly marginated, increased lung density paralleling the dependent pleura and obscuring the underlying lung morphology [8, 9].

8. *Parenchymal bands:* Linear, nontapering densities 2–5 cm in length extending through the lung to contact the pleural surface. These lines often terminated at sites of thickened pleura. Their appearance does not vary with patient position [8, 9] (Fig. 5).

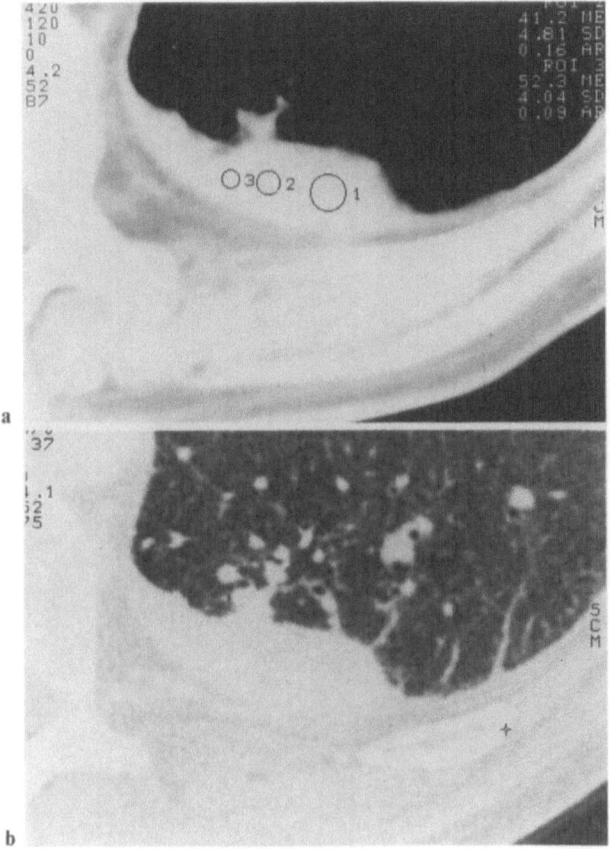

Fig. 5a, b. Conventional CT (a) and HRCT (b): Parenchymal bands are better depicted on HRCT

9. *Ground glass opacities:* Slightly hyperattenuated areas in which vessels and bronchi remain visible (Fig. 4).
10. *Emphysema:* Nonperipheral, small areas of low attenuation similar to those seen in centrilobular emphysema [7].
11. *Subpleural blebs* (Fig. 3)
12. *Rounded atelectasis:* Mass related to a pleural abnormality, with volume loss in the surrounding lung, partial interposition of lung between pleura and mass and a "comet tail" of vessels and bronchi sweeping into the mass [12]. Air bronchograms may occur [8].
13. *Segmental or subsegmental atelectasis*
14. *Hyaline pleural plaques*
15. *Calcified pleural plaques*

The diagnostic value of the routine and the high resolution technique was evaluated respectively (from 0 to 2) in each case.

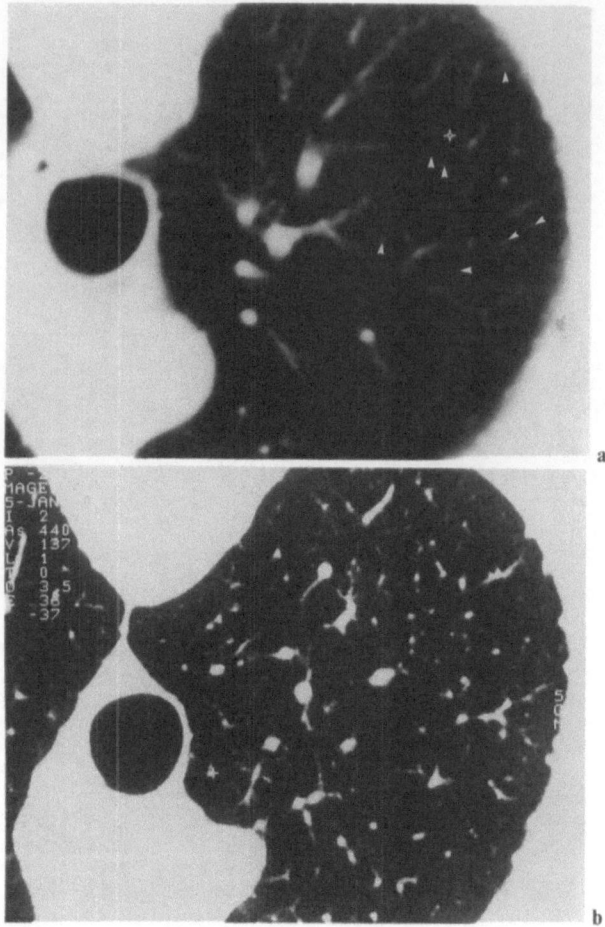

Fig. 6a, b. Conventional CT (a) and HRCT (b): small nodules are easily missed between HRCT sections and are difficult to distinguish from blood vessels

Results

Asbestosis and silicosis were suspected on the base of a history of an occupational exposure in 10 and 14 patients respectively. Two additional patients were suspected of having both diseases.

The average score of detectability of each sign, tabulated from 0 to 2 (see above), is summarized in Table 1. The two patients with both diseases are excluded from the columns of silicosis and asbestosis but are included in the total.

Curvilinear subpleural lines are seen only with HRCT. Thickened interlobular lines, irregular interfaces, honeycombing, ground-glass opacities, and subpleural blebs are definitely better appreciated with HRCT. Masses, parenchymal bands, emphysema, atelectasis and pleural plaques are observed equally well with both methods. Subpleural dependent opacities are slightly better defined on routine CT

Table 1

	Total		Silicosis		Asbestosis	
	CT	HRCT	CT	HRCT	CT	HRCT
Nodules	0.92	0.54	1.42	0.57	0.50	0.37
Masses	0.42	0.42	0.57	0.57	0.25	0.25
Curvilinear subpleural lines	0.00	0.17	0.00	0.00	0.00	0.25
Thickened interlobular lines	0.29	1.42	0.43	1.14	0.13	0.75
Irregular interfaces	0.25	0.38	0.38	0.50	0.00	0.00
Honeycombing	0.04	0.17	0.07	0.14	0.00	0.25
Subpleural dependent density	0.50	0.38	0.43	0.29	0.50	0.50
Parenchymal bands	0.17	0.17	0.00	0.00	0.50	0.50
Ground-glass opacities	0.13	0.25	0.07	0.14	0.25	0.50
Emphysema	0.46	0.50	0.43	0.43	0.63	0.75
Subpleural blebs	0.26	0.96	0.07	0.71	0.43	1.43
Rounded atelectasis	0.25	0.21	0.00	0.00	0.50	0.50
Segmental or subsegmental atelectasis	0.33	0.25	0.14	0.14	0.50	0.25
Hyaline pleural plaques	0.83	0.75	0.28	0.36	1.50	1.25
Calcified pleural plaques	0.42	0.33	0.00	0.00	0.75	0.75

Table 2

	Total		Silicosis		Asbestosis	
	CT	HRCT	CT	HRCT	CT	HRCT
Diagnostic value	1.00	1.75	2.00	1.79	1.00	1.63

than on HRCT, and nodules are much easier to evaluate on conventional CT than on HRCT.

The diagnostic value of both methods, routine and HR computed tomography are compared in Table 2.

Discussion

Conventional CT has been suggested for evaluating both pleural and parenchymal changes from asbestos and silica exposure [4, 5, 13–15]. These studies found that conventional CT sections of at least 10 mm thickness were significantly more sensitive than chest radiographs in detecting pleural thickening. The greater sensitivity of CT was attributed to the fact that pleural thickening was most common in paravertebral and posterobasal locations [4]. In addition, CT identified parenchymal fibrosis in 33% of the subjects, whereas radiographs were interpreted as abnormal in only 17%. More recently, Begin et al. [16] analyzed the usefulness of conventional CT scans relative to posteroanterior and four-view radiographs of the chest for detecting asbestos-related pleuroparenchymal fibrosis and they found that the three methods yielded comparable results. Recently, several reports have emphasized the role of HRCT in characterization of benign asbestos-related diseases [9, 10] and concluded that HRCT can complement the evaluation of asbestos-exposed subjects when other criteria for parenchymal fibrosis are equivocal or absent [9]. To the best of our knowledge, no studies report the comparative accuracy of both conventional and high-resolution CT in detecting and characterizating of silicosis. Akira et al. [7] described high-resolution aspects of radiographic type p pneumoconiosis and concluded that addition of HRCT to chest radiography is useful in achieving more accurate categorization of the lesions.

In our studies, HRCT is superior to 1-cm-collimation CT in demonstrating curvilinear subpleural lines, thickened interlobular lines, irregular interfaces, honeycombing, ground glass opacities and subpleural blebs. Müller and Munk respectively demonstrated the superiority of HRCT in outlining small cystic areas of honeycombing [17], in the assessment of disease activity in idiopathic pulmonary fibrosis [18] and in demonstrating polygonal lines in lymphatic spread of tumor [19].

We disagree with Aberle [9] when they concluded that asbestos-related pleural changes are observed more frequently on HRCT than on conventional CT. In our experience conventional CT was more reliable in detecting hyaline pleural plaques. This feature can be explained by the fact that contrast resolution between hyaline pleural plaques and subpleural tissue is worse with the bone algorithm used in HRCT than the soft-tissue algorithm used in conventional CT. When the pleural plaques are calcified, both techniques have the same confidence score; the contrast between calcium and soft subpleural tissue is spontaneously high.

We agree with Mathieson [20] on the fact that small nodules can be easily missed between high-resolution CT sections and, when present, are difficult to distinguish from blood vessels.

The diagnostic value of each method for asbestosis and silicosis is different. In silicosis, conventional CT is more reliable than HRCT. In this disease, the predominant role of CT is detection of small nodules, especially when the chest radiograph is questionable or normal as in our studies. In asbestosis, HRCT is more reliable than conventional CT because of its high capability for detecting fine interstitial changes.

The results of this study demonstrate that assessment of parenchymal interstitial lesions is definitely more accurate with HRCT, but since small nodule detection is optimal with conventional CT, we advocate that both techniques be used in the examination of patients with occupational chest diseases.

References

1. Coddington R, Mera SL, Goddard PR, Bradfield JWB (1982) Pathological evaluation of computed tomography images of lungs. J Clin Path 35: 536–540
2. Naidich DP, Zerhouni EA, Siegelman SS (1984) Computed tomography of the thorax. Raven, New York, pp 201–206
3. Friedman AC, Fiel SB, Fisher MS, Radecki PD, Lev-Toaff AS, Caroline DF (1988) Asbestos-related pleural disease and asbestosis: A comparison of CT and chest radiography. AJR 150: 269–275

4. Katz D, Kreel L (1979) Computed tomography in pulmonary asbestosis. Clin Radiol 30: 207–213
5. Kreel L (1976) Computed tomography in the evaluation of pulmonary asbestosis: Preliminary experiences with the EMI general purpose scanner. Acta Radiol (Diagn) (Stockh) 17: 405–412
6. Mayo RJ, Webb WR, Gould R, Stein MG, Bass I, Gamsu G, Goldberg HI (1987) High-resolution CT of the lungs: an optimal approach. Radiology 163: 507–510
7. Akira M, Higashihara T, Yokoyama K, Yamamoto S, Kita N, Morimoto S, Ikezoe J, Kozuka T (1989) Radiographic type p pneumoconiosis: high-resolution CT. Radiology 171: 117–123
8. Aberle DR, Gamsu G, Sue Ray C, Feuerstein IM (1988) Asbestos-related pleural and parenchymal fibrosis: detection with high-resolution CT. Radiology 166: 729–734
9. Aberle DR, Gamsu G, Sue Ray C (1988) High-resolution CT of benign asbestos-related diseases: clinical and radiographic correlation. AJR 151: 883–891
10. Lynch DA, Gamsu G, Ray CS, Aberle DR (1988) Asbestos-related focal lung masses; manifestation on conventional and high-resolution CT Scans. Radiology 169: 603–607
11. Yoshimura H, Hatakeyama M, Otsuji H, Maeda M, Ohishi H, Uchida H, Kasuga H, Katada H, Narita N, Mikami R, Konishi Y (1986) Pulmonary asbestosis: CT study of subpleural curvilinear shadow. Radiology 158: 653–658
12. Doyle TC, Lawler GA (1984) CT of rounded atelectasis of the lung. AJR 143: 225–228
13. Sperber M, Mohan KK (1984) Computed tomography: a reliable diagnostic modality in pulmonary asbestosis. Comput Radiol 8: 125–132
14. Bergin CJ, Müller NL, Vedal S, Chan-Yeung M (1986) CT in silicosis: correlation with plain films and pulmonary function tests. AJR 146: 477–483
15. Begin R, Bergeron D, Samson L, Bocto M, Cantin A (1987) CT assessment of silicosis in exposed workers. AJR 148: 509–514
16. Begin R, Boctor M, Bergeron D et al. (1984) Radiographic assessment of pleuropulmonary disease in asbestos workers: posteroanterior, four view films, and computed tomograms of the thorax. Br J Ind Med 41: 373–383
17. Müller NL, Miller RR, Webb WR, Evans KG, Ostrow DN (1986) Fibrosing alveolitis: CT-pathologic correlation. Radiology 160: 585–588
18. Müller NL, Staples CA, Miller RR, Vedal S, Thurlbeck WM, Ostrow DN (1987) Disease activity in idiopathic pulmonary fibrosis: CT and pathologic correlation. Radiology 165: 731–734
19. Munk PL, Müller NL, Miller RR, Ostrow DN (1988) Pulmonary lymphangitic carcinomatosis: CT and pathologic findings. Radiology 166: 705–709
20. Mathieson JR, Mayo JR, Staples CA, Müller NL (1989) Chronic diffuse infiltrative lung disease: comparison of diagnostic accuracy of CT and chest radiography. Radiology 171: 111–116

Detection of Hilar Lymphadenopathy with CCT (Continuous Rotating CT)

M. OUDKERK, S. MALI, S. TJIAM, W. A. KALENDER

Introduction

Enlargement of hilar lymphnodes may be seen in many benign and malignant diseases (Table 1), such as in acute and chronic infectious diseases of the lungs, heart and mediastinum as well as in neoplastic diseases of the lung, thyroid, stomach, pancreas, colon, breast etc. (Table 2). Neoplastic disease of the lung is the most common cause of regional metastases in the hilar lymphnodes with or without enlargement.

The prognosis of pulmonary carcinoma sharply decreases in proportion to the presence and extent of hilar lymphnode metastases (Table 3). Since the demonstration of hilar lymphnode involvement, at least in the contra-lateral nodes, may be a contra-indication to definitive surgery, evaluation of the lung hili is important in all patients with proven pulmonary carcinoma (Table 4).

Without biopsy, the principal criterion upon which evidence of metastases is based is nodal enlargement. As a rule of thumb, lymphnodes in the abdomen are considered normal if the diameter is 1 cm or less. Those of 1,5 cm or greater are considered to be pathological. This rule has also been applied to the mediastinum, but from our own experience we doubt its validity. We think, instead, that in any patient with proven pulmonary carcinoma in whom there is any suspicion of mediastinal metastases, pathological examination should be carried out by means of mediastinoscopy or needle aspiration under bronchoscopy. However, hilar lymphnode involvement is even more critical. Ekholm et al. demonstrated in a patient series for pre-operative staging of pulmonary carcinoma malignant infiltration in more than 35% of patients with hilar lymphnodes less than 1 cm diameter [1].

In the same series, malignant infiltration was found in only 12% of patients with lymphnodes greater than 1 cm. Therefore imaging techniques can play no other role than assessing the presence or absence of nodal enlargement. CT-guided transthoracic needle aspiration biopsy (TTNA) is probably the next best diagnostic procedure in patients with proven hilar enlargement giving far better results than transbronchial biopsy [2]. Hilar metastases of lung carcinoma are not directly correlated to node size or node enlargement. Therefore detection of even very small hilar lymphnodes can be useful in the staging procedure for patients with regional metastases of pulmonary carcinoma or distant metastases of other neoplastic diseases.

ıble 1

	N-Regional Lymph Nodes		N-Regional Lymph Nodes
0	No demonstrable metastasis to regional lymph nodes.	N0	No demonstrable metastasis to regional lymph nodes.
1	Metastasis to lymph nodes in the ipsilateral hilar region (including direct extension).	N1	Metastasis to lymph nodes in the peribronchial or the ipsilateral hilar region, or both (including direct extension).
2	Metastasis to lymph nodes in the mediastinum.	N2	Metastasis to ipsilateral mediastinal lymph nodes and subcarinal lymph nodes.
		N3	Metastasis to contralateral mediastinal lymph nodes, contralateral hilar lymph nodes, ipsilateral or contralateral scalene or supraclavicular lymph nodes.

ıble 2. Diseases associated with (hilar) lymph node enlargement

I *Infectious diseases*
  A Viral infections: infectious hepatitis, infectious mononucleosis syndromes (cytomegalovirus, EB virus), AIDS, rubella, varicella-herpes zoster, vaccinia
  B Bacterial infections: streptococci, staphylococci, salmonella, brucella, Francisella tularensis, *Listeria monocytogenes, Pasteurella pestis, Hemophilus ducreyi,* cat-scratch disease
  C Fungal infections: coccidioidomycosis, histoplasmosis
  D Chlamydial infections: Lymphogranuloma venereum, trachoma
  E Mycobacterial infections: tuberculosis, leprosy
  F Parasitic infections: trypanosomiasis, microfilariasis, toxoplasmosis
  G Spirochetal diseases: syphilis, yaws, endemic syphilis (bejel), leptospirosis

'I *Immunologic diseases*
  A Rheumatoid arthritis
  B Systemic lupus erythematosus
  C Dermatomyositis
  D Serum sickness
  E Drug reactions – diphenylhydantoin, hydralazine, allopurinol
  F Angioimmunoblastic lymphadenopathy

'I *Malignant diseases*
  A Hematologic: Hodgkin's lymphoma, acute and chronic T-, B-, myeloid, and monocytoid cell leukemias and lymphomas, malignant histiocytosis
  B Metastatic tumors to lymph nodes: melanoma, Kaposi's sarcoma, neuroblastoma, seminoma, tumors of lung, breast, prostate, kidney, head and neck, gastrointestinal tract

V *Endocrine diseases:* hyperthyroidism

V *Lipid storage diseases:* Gaucher's and Niemann-Pick diseases

'I *Miscellaneous diseases* and diseases of unknown cause
  A Giant follicular lymph node hyperplasia
  B Sinus histiocytosis
  C Dermatopathic lymphadenitis
  D Sarcoidosis
  E Amyloidosis
  F Mucocutaneous lymph node syndrome
  G Lymphomatoid granulomatosis
  H Multifocal Langerhans cell (eosinophilic) granulomatosis

Table 3

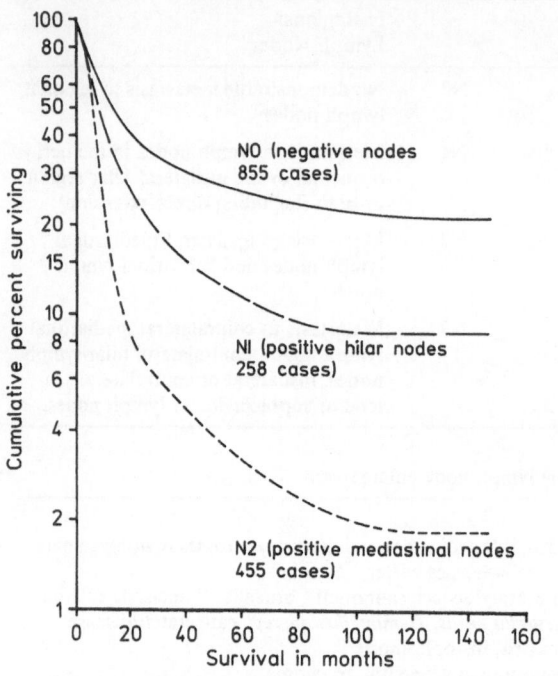

Prognosis in Patients with Lung Cancer: N Factor. Survival in lung cancer stratified by the extent of the regional lymph node involvement (N factor), excluding undifferentiated small cell carcinoma; 1568 cases. (From Mountain CF, Carr DT, Anderson WAD, Am J Roentgenol *120:* 130, 1974.)

Table 4. Frequency of radiographic presenting signs (%)[a]

	All types of lung cancer	Epider-moid	Adeno-carcinoma	Large cell undifferentiated	Small cell undifferentiated
Peripheral opacity	49	31	74	65	32
Atelectasis	21	37	10	13	18
Consolidation	21	20	15	25	24
Hilar enlargement	42	40	18	32	78
Mediastinal enlargement	6	2	3	10	13
Multiple abnormalities	42	36	30	42	62

[a] Data adapted from Byrd et al. (1968): *Mayo Clinic Proc* 43: 327. Byrd et al. (1968): *Mayo Clinic Proc* 43: 337. Lehar et al. (1967): *Am Rev Resp Dis* 96: 245. Byrd et al. (1968): *Mayo Clinic Proc* 43: 333

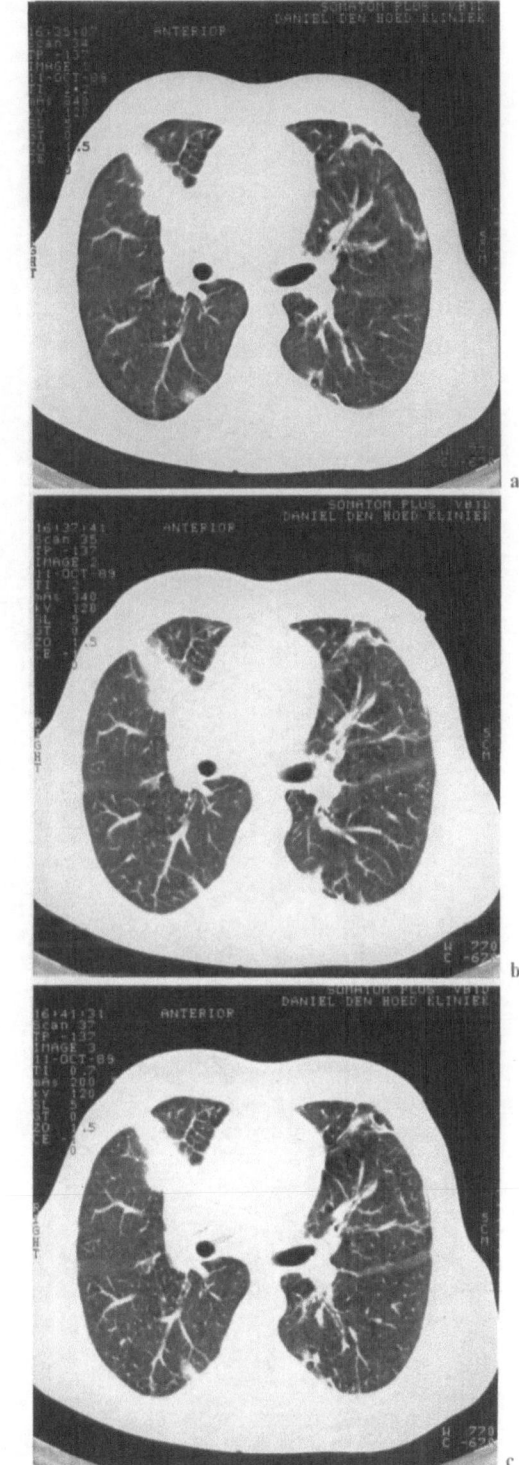

Fig. 1a–c. Comparison between
4 (2*2) sec. (a), 2 sec. (b) and 0.7 sec. (c)
scans. Note the sharpness and detail of
the lung-parenchyma at shortest scan
time

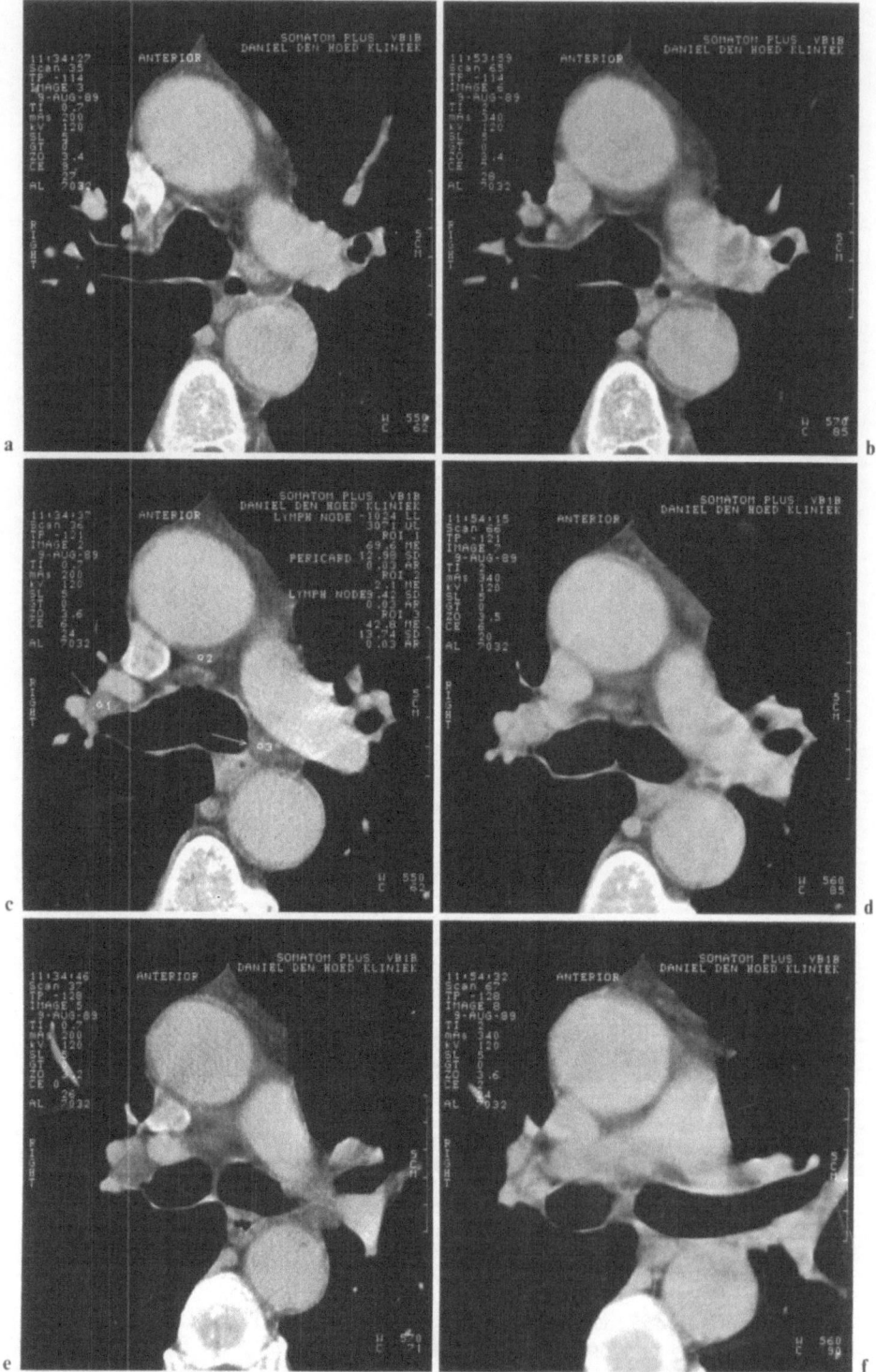

Hilar Lymph Node Detection

Plain film examination only reveals relatively large hilar masses. Multi-directional (MD) tomography is invaluable in the study of the hilar regions of the lung in the assessment of node enlargement, although several authors have suggested that (55 degree oblique) MD tomography is equivalent to CT in this determination [3–11]. These (comparative) studies are all outdated because of the rapid rate of development of CT equipment. In the literature no comparative data comparing 55 degree oblique multi-directional tomography and CT exists with respect to CT equipment less than five years old. This, together with the fact that high performance MD tomography equipment is no longer produced, makes it unlikely for new studies to be expected. Probably its use has declined in practice due to CT superiority, which has made its production unprofitable. Therefore, during the last few years, hilar pathology studies have concentrated on the comparison between conventional CT and MRI [12, 13]. In the most recent study MRI is regarded as slightly inferior to conventional CT in the diagnosis of mediastinal and hilar lymphadenopathy [14]. In the same study, however, MR is regarded as being superior to conventional CT in diagnosing tumor invasion to the heart and great vessels, and in the superior region at the thoracic inlet.

From a clinical point of view, it appears that in the case of a negative conventional CT examination for hilar (and mediastinal) lymph node involvement of a lung carcinoma 57% of surgeons see entirely no need for surgical staging [15]. In conclusion it can be stated that the specificity of CT for the detection of hilar lymph node involvement will never be adequate without cytology/biopsy (TTNA). However, it is very important to improve the sensitivity of CT in the detection of hilar lymph node involvement to exclude the presence of metastases with more certainty.

Continuous Rotating Computed Tomography

The spatial and low contrast resolution of modern CT equipment are of high standard. The detection of hilar lymph nodes with a densitiy of ± 60 HU and a diameter of 3 mm should easily be possible and also discrimination from structures with a density difference of more than 50 HU, such as fat or contrast enhanced vessels. This resolution is easily achieved in the mediastinum, but not in the lung hilus. Our hypothetical explanation was motion. Heart, great vessels and lung hilus should be considered as one large pulsating mass. These pulsations cause severe problems: spatial resolution is impaired; peripheral hilar structures are not reproducibly imaged moving in and out of the slice during data sampling. Image

---

Fig. 2 a–f. Comparison between 0.7 sec. (**a, c, e**) and 2 sec. (**b, d, f**) scans in adjacent slices with 7 mm. interval. Two hilar lymphnodes are seen at 0.7 sec. in scan **c**. Note that both lymphnodes are not visualized at 2 sec. scanning

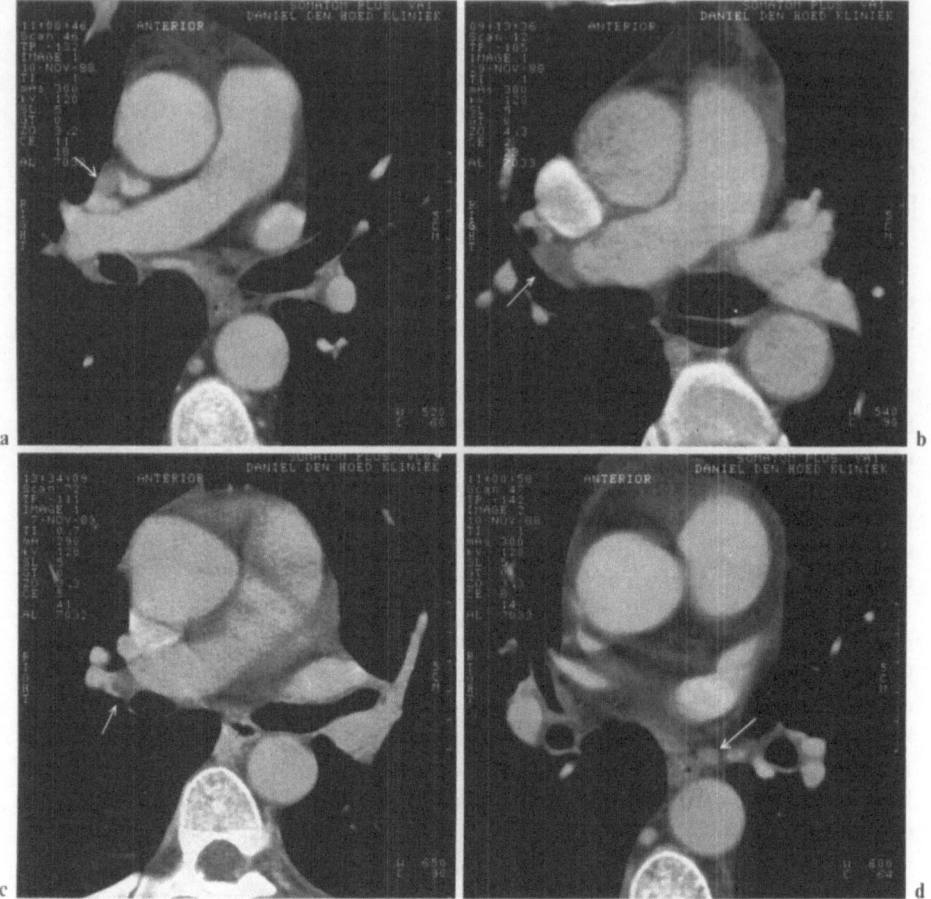

Fig. 3a–d. Hilar lympnodes with a diameter smaller than 1 cm

quality is further impaired by motion artefacts. Cardiac gating has already been proven to be helpful in hilar lymph node detection with MR [16]. This method is nicely applicable in MR but not so in CT.

One of the best and oldest ways to cope with motion in imaging is to reduce exposure time. With the production of a continuous rotating CT (CCT), this goal became possible. With the installation of CCT in our Cancer Centre at Rotterdam we started to make a comparison between subsecond, one second and two second scanning for the detection of hilar lymph node pathology.

After obtaining informed consent, repeated scans with different scan times were taken with each patient to optimize comparability. Figure 1 shows four different scan times at the same midthoracic level. There is a striking difference in image quality between 3, 2, 1 and 0.7 second scans. Three and two second scans are clearly of inferior image quality. Between 1 and 0.7 second scans there is little difference in severity of artefacts in the mediastinum. For more peripheral hilar struc-

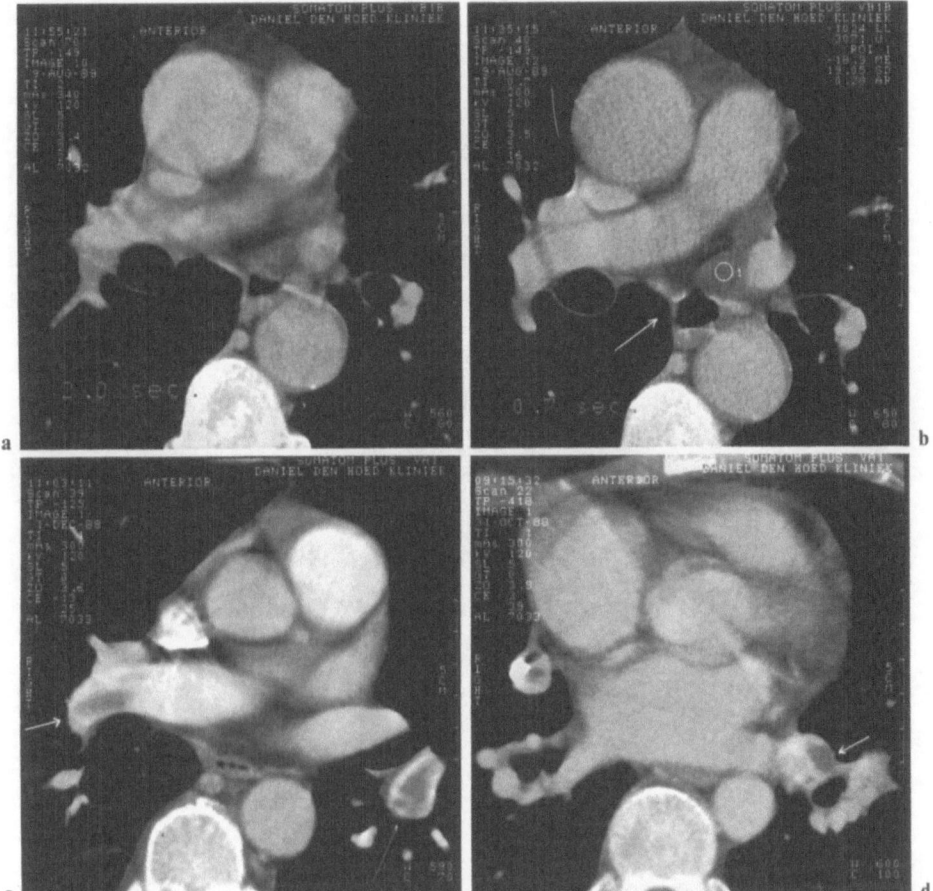

Fig. 4a-d. At 2 sec. scan suspicion of left hilar lymphadenopathy existed (**a**). At 0.7 scan lymphadenopathy could be excluded. Structure was proven to be pericardial fold (**b**). **c** NHL patient with NED. Submitted with fever and left hilar enlargement on chest X-ray. On suspicion of lymphadenopathy in recurrent NHL CCT evaluation of hili and mediastinum was performed. CCT proved bilateral lungemboli. **d** Patient suspected of left hilar lymphadenopathy on chest X-ray. CCT proved (tumor) thrombus in left lower pulmonary vein

tures and for the lung, however, we found 0.7 second scans to be better in reproducibility and morphological differentiation.

For the hilar protocol, 0.7 and 2 second scans were used with 7 mm spacing, 5 mm slice thickness and 200 mAs. As contrast medium, Isopaque cerebral in a 1:1 solution (Nycomed) was administred as iv. infusion with a volume of 100 ml, a flow rate of 0.65 ml/s under a 150 PSI pressure limit, programmed with a Liebel Flarsheim Angiomat CT injector system.

The 0.7 and 1.0 second scan protocols are standard and have been performed in more than 1000 patients. The comparison between 0.7 and 2.0 second scan was performed in a series of 50 patients. The image quality of the hilar region was

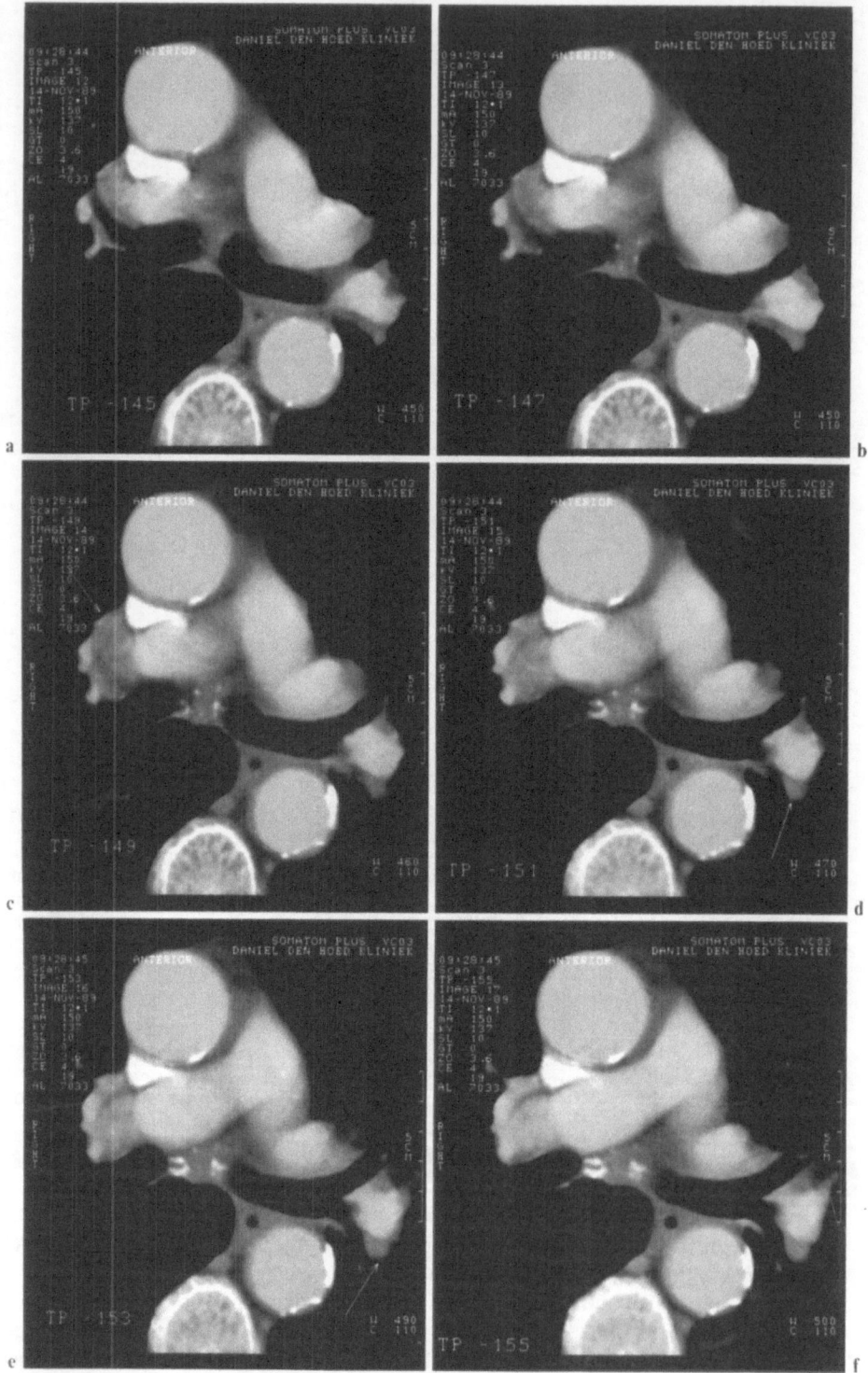

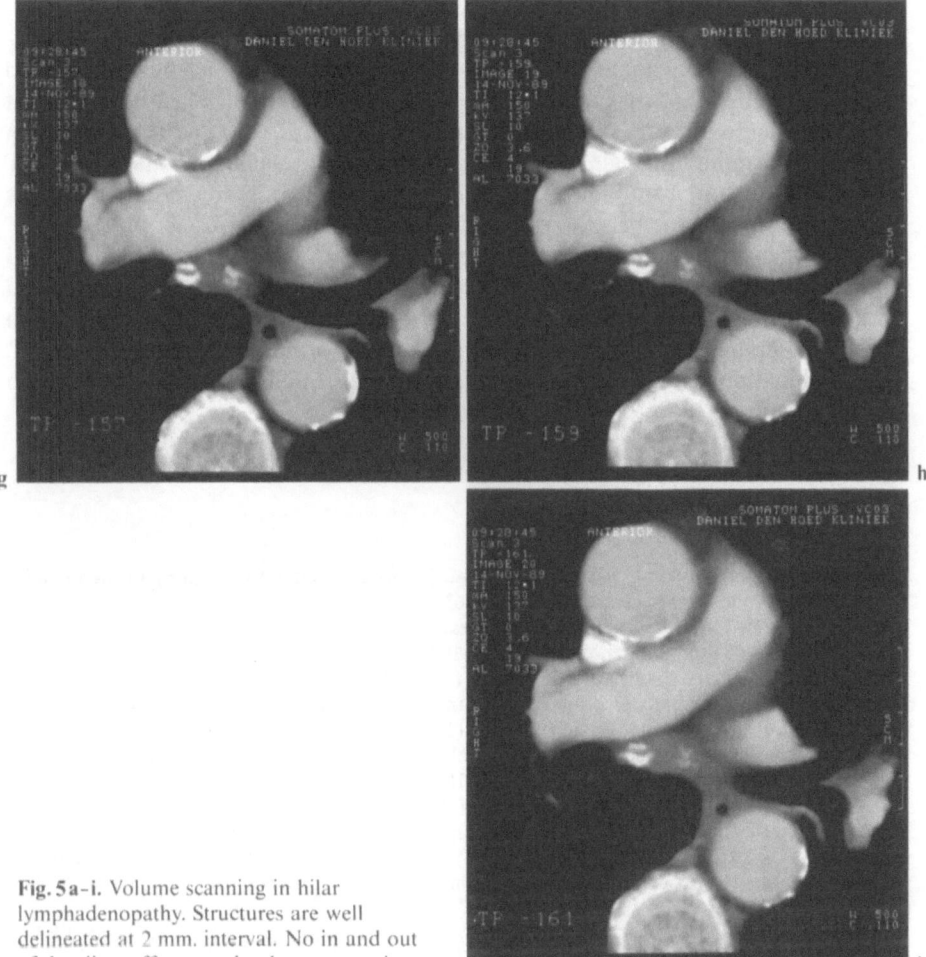

Fig. 5a–i. Volume scanning in hilar
lymphadenopathy. Structures are well
delineated at 2 mm. interval. No in and out
of the slices effects can be demonstrated

markedly improved for 0.7 and 1.0 second scan times in almost all cases. Only in
three patients did the 2 second scans give comparable or slightly better results,
probably due to a slow heart frequency. Voluntary and involuntary patient motion
is only roughly predictable. Therefore, there is no guarantee that shorter scan
times gave better results in every case. However, in the large number of other
direct comparisons we found a significantly improved image quality for the shorter scan times (Fig. 2). It should be noted that perception can mislead the interpret-
er. Smoothness is often regarded as synonymous to image quality, but images
which look more granular can contain a lot more information, both in terms of
border sharpness and tissue differentiation. At shorter scan times we found better
morphological differentiation. Also multiple hilar lymph nodes were found with
diameters smaller than 1 cm in lung cancer patients (Fig. 3).

The high image quality of hilar structures proved to be extremely helpful in differential diagnosis of several cases (Fig. 4).

Volume scanning (VCT) was also applied for the detection of hilar lymphadenopathy in 15 patients (Fig. 5). Until now no major advantages could be demonstrated as far as image quality is concerned. In theory, VCT in a single breathhold
should guarantee that no pathology is missed due to motion out of the slice. It
allows optimal utilization of contrast administration; is easier on the patient than
successive scanning of single slices and should have the same advantages as CCT
with regard to short scan times. Images look smoother compared with single slice
scanning, however, one gets the impression of less detailed information.

In conclusion, shorter scan times improve spatial and contrast resolution and
diminish severity and frequency of motion artefacts. Diagnosis of hilar lymph
node enlargement is significantly improved in 1.0 and 0.7 second scanning with
CCT as compared to 2 seconds and more as is performed with conventional CT.
The combination of high temporal and high spatial resolution permits delineation
of hilar lymph nodes of diameters less than 1 cm.

References

1. Ekholm S, Albrechtsson U, Kugelberg J, et al. (1980) Computed tomography in preoperative
   staging of bronchogenic carcinoma. CT 4: 763
2. Sider L, Davis TM Jr (1987 Jul) Hilar masses: Evaluation with CT-guided biopsy after negative bronchoscopic examination. Radiology 164 (1), p 107–109
3. Shevland JE, Chiu LC, Schapiro RL, et al. (1978) The role of conventional tomography in
   assessing the resectability of primary lung cancer: A preliminary report. CT 2: 1
4. Osborne DR, Korobkin M, Ravin CE, et al. (1982) Comparison of plain radiography, conventional tomography, and computed tomography in detecting intrathoracic lymph node metastases from lung carcinoma. Radiology 142: 157
5. Mintzer RA, Malave SR, Neiman HL, et al. (1979) Computed vs. conventional tomography in
   evaluation of primary and secondary pulmonary neoplasms. Radiology 132: 653
6. Khan A, Gersten KC, Garvey J, et al. (1985) Oblique hilar tomography, computed tomography, and mediastinoscopy for prethoracotomy staging of bronchogenic carcinoma. Radiology 156: 295
7. Webb RW, Gamsu G, Speckman JM (1983) Computed tomography of the pulmonary hilum
   in patients with bronchogenic carcinoma. CT 7: 219
8. Brown LR, DeRemee RA (1976) 55 degree oblique hilar tomography. Mayo Clin Proc 51: 89
9. Glazer GM, Gross BH, Aisan AM, et al. (1985) Imaging of the hilum: a prospective comparative study in patients with lung cancer. AJR 145: 245
10. Heitzman ER (1986) The role of computed tomography in the diagnosis and management of
    lung cancer. Chest 89 (suppl): 237 S
11. Genereux GP (1983) Conventional tomographic hilar anatomy emphasizing the pulmonary
    veins. AJR 141: 1241
12. Musset D, Grenier P, Carette MF, et al. (1986) Primary lung cancer staging: Prospective com-
    parative study of MR imaging with CT. Radiology 160: 607
13. Poon PY, Bronskill MJ, Henkelman RM, et al. (1987) Mediastinal lymph node metastases
    from bronchogenic carcinoma: Detection with MR imaging and CT. Radiology 162: 651
14. Kono M, Sako M, Adachi S, Hirota S, Shimizu T, Tanaka K, Yamasaki K, Kusumoto M,
    Sakai E (1989) MR imaging in the assessment of lung cancer patients: primary lung cancer
    staging, evaluation of therapeutic effect and diagnosis of recurrent tumor. Nippon Igaku
    Hoshasen Gakkai Zasshi. Jul 25, 49 (7), p 831–840
15. Epstein DM, Stephenson LW, Gefter WB, et al. (1986) Value of CT in the preoperative assess-
    ment of lung cancer: a survey of thoracic surgeons. Radiology 161: 423
16. Westcott JL, Henschke CI, Bermen Y (1985) MR imaging of the hilum and mediastinum:
    effects of cardiac gating. J Comput Assist Tomogr. Nov–Dec. 9 (6), p 1073–1078

New Directions in CT Diagnosis of the Pancreas

W. Bautz, M. Skalej, Chr. Thomas, W. A. Kalender, C. D. Claussen

Summary

The short scan times of the SOMATOM PLUS greatly reduce motion artifacts. In conjunction with high spatial resolution, the minimization of artifacts improves detailed diagnosis of the pancreas as compared to CT devices operating with the start-stop method. Short scan times and cycle times reduce examination time and the amount of contrast medium needed. The rotating measurement system of the SOMATOM PLUS, which enables continuous data acquisition of up to 12 seconds, provided the basis for developing the so-called Spiral-CT. This technology will be used primarily for examinations of the abdomen and thorax. Spiral-CT and cine evaluation technology present us with two important new methods for diagnosing diseases of the pancreas.

Introduction

Sonography, computer tomography (CT) and endoscopic retrograde pancreatico-cholangiography (ERCP) are the leading imaging methods for diagnosing pancreatic diseases (Table 1). As compared to sonography, considered to be the basic diagnostic device for pancreas examinations, computer tomography provides the advantage of cross-sectional imaging and image quality barely affected by bowel gas. The articles published to date on diagnostic procedures for pancreatic disease confirm that the results obtained with CT surpass those achieved with sonography. Computer tomography, in turn, is surpassed by ERCP in the diagnosis of changes

Table 1. Pancreatic diseases: Diagnostic imaging devices

Survey radiograph of the abdomen
Gastro-intestinal tract passage
Cholangiography
Arteriography
Sonography
Computer tomography
ERCP
Magnetic Resonance Imaging

in the pancreatic duct. ERCP, which is rather stressful for the patient, is used either as a pre-operative or as an additional diagnostic confirmation after the patient has been examined with CT or sonography.

Computer tomography occupies a central position in the spectrum of diagnostic imaging devices for pancreatic examination. The accuracy of this method has been further enhanced by the development of continuous rotation scanners [Bautz, Klier 1989]. The SOMATOM PLUS provides scanning times in the sub-second range at short cycle times. The multi-fan measurement system and the 1024 × 1024 display matrix ensure spatial resolution which surpasses that of CT systems operating with the start-stop method. The continuous rotation measurement system constitutes the prerequisite for developing new scanning techniques which advance diagnostic accuracy in pancreatic examinations. As compared to previous CT generations, the SOMATOM PLUS offers the following advantages:

- Minimization of motion artifacts (caused by involuntary patient movement, vessel pulsation, and colon peristalsis).
- Improved Spatial Resolution and Detailed Diagnosis
- Shorter examination times due to short cycle times, and, as a result, new perspectives for examinations using contrast agents.

In what follows, this article examines the practical realization of these expectations and the effect of the new scan and evaluation methods such as spiral-CT and cine mode on the strategies used in CT examinations of the pancreas.

Plain Examination of the Pancreas

When examining the pancreas with CT, plain scans are performed after the contrast agent for the colon has been administered orally. These scans are used to determine the position, the size, the shape and the contours of the organ, as well as the parenchymal density and the collateral phenomena for pancreatic diseases (changes in the peri and parapancreatic space, liver parenchyma defects, gall stones, retention of bile, size of spleen, etc.).

The improvement in image quality becomes quite noticeable when comparing the results obtained with the SOMATOM PLUS to those obtained with the SOMATOM DR3. We quantified the image quality by using ROC analysis (ROC – Receiver Operator Characteristics). To this end, 2 × 50 CT examinations of the pancreas of patients with confirmed diagnosis were used. The images were generated with the SOMATOM DR3 and SOMATOM PLUS; the image quality obtained for the three sections of the pancreas was evaluated by three experienced radiologists. All examinations were performed in the automatic scan mode with the parameters listed in Table 2. A rating system ranging from 1 through 6 was used to evaluate image quality (from hard copy). Images which allowed the radiologist to rule out pathological changes were given the highest rating (1), and images which did not allow for diagnostic interpretation were given the lowest rating (6).

Table 2. CT scan parameters for the pancreas

SOMATOM	DR3	PLUS
Slice thickness (mm)	8 (4)	10
Slice distance (mm)	8 (4)	10
Scan time (s)	5	1
Cycle time (l/min)	3	6
kV	125	120
mAs	350	210
Average examination time (min)	5	2

The results of this evaluation are shown in Table 3. We were able to show that the image quality of the SOMATOM PLUS is considerably higher than that of the SOMATOM DR3. This improvement in image quality allows for greater diagnostic accuracy. In addition, a more consistent image quality was obtained with the SOMATOM PLUS than with the SOMATOM DR3.

When analyzing the unsatisfactory image quality obtained with the SOMATOM DR3, motion artifacts were established as the leading cause for image degradation. For example, during scan times of 5 seconds, colon peristalsis and aortic pulsations transmitted to the duodenum and jejunum generate considerable artifacts in the area of the pancreas.

Despite higher image noise, detail recognition is improved with the SOMATOM PLUS. However, image noise becomes more problematic when using the thin slice technique and scan times of 1 second. In this case, the SOMATOM DR3 offers greater advantages with, e. g., a 4 mm slice thickness. In our experience, oblique patient positioning frequently used in the past (better filling of the duodenum) may be omitted in most cases when performing examinations with the SOMATOM PLUS. As compared to the DR3, the use of the SOMATOM PLUS reduces the measurement time for examinations of the pancreas by 50%. This difference in measurement time can be explained, on the one hand, by the larger slice thickness of 10 mm for contiguous slices as compared to the 8 mm thickness for the SOMATOM DR3, and, on the other, by the much higher scan frequency shown in Table 2.

Contrast Medium Studies of the Pancreas

The pancreas is a highly vascularized organ. Through intravenous injection of contrast medium (CM), the contrast of the parenchyma of the pancreas is enhanced in comparison to pathological changes in the pancreas and its surrounding tissue. The result is increased detail recognition. The peripancreatic vessels are better delineated and their blood flow is evaluated. CM examinations of the pancreas are indicated i) when the CT reference scan does not show any pathology despite a tentative diagnosis of pancreatic disease, ii) when determining the degree

Table 3. SOMATOM DR3 vs. PLUS image quality (pancreas, nativ)

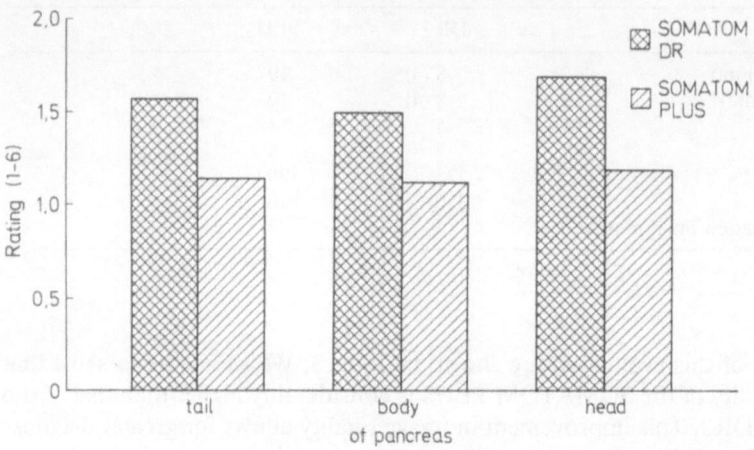

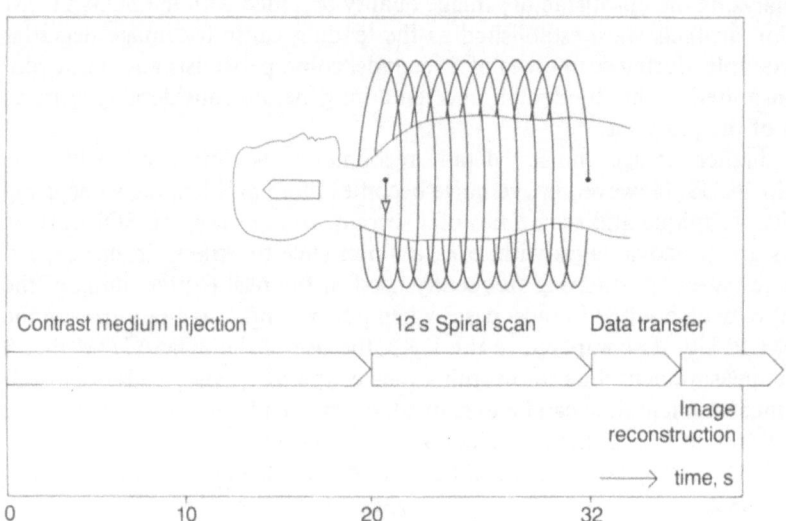

Fig. 1. Timing of spiral CT studies of the pancreas

of acute pancreatitis, iii) when diagnosing pancreatic carcinoma extension, iiii) when quantifying the space occupied by the pancreas (active endocrine tumors). CM examinations are performed after completion of the plain scan.

To date, contrast agents are either applied as a bolus (50 ml) with subsequent infusion (50–100 ml) or as a so-called fractionated bolus. We prefer the fractionated bolus method. After administering 50 ml CM, an additional 30 ml CM is manually injected intravenously after 3–4 scans. This allows for high contrast concentration in the pancreatic vessels. Dynamic CT proved suitable for determining the vital parenchyma in the presence of necrotizing pancreatitis (Fig. 6) or for locating active endocrine tumors [Rossi et al. 1985]. It may be necessary to scan several planes to acquire the entire organ. In the case of confirmed pathologies, the entire epigastrium or the entire abdomen should be examined after the CM examination to facilitate detection of diagnostically valuable collateral phenomena such as metastases of the liver. Spiral-CT opens up new perspectives after the contrast agent has been administered as a bolus.

The shorter scan and interscan times of the SOMATOM PLUS allow a 30–50% reduction in contrast agent as compared to pancreatic examinations with the SOMATOM DR3. The enhancement of the pancreas is improved and the image quality of the slice series is more consistent. The results have considerably improved spatial resolution and detail recognition. In our experience, the ductus pancreaticus with a lumen diameter of 2–4 mm is visible in a normal pancreas in approximately 50% of all examinations.

New Directions in CT Diagnosis of the Pancreas: Spiral-CT and Cine Mode

The rotating measurement system of the SOMATOM PLUS enables continuous scanning of a section of the body during a single breathhold (so-called volume scanning with Spiral-CT). The hardware and software have to be upgraded accordingly.

When using Spiral-CT [Kalender et al. 1989], the table is moved slowly at an accurately controlled speed (stepper motor) while the measurement system is rotating. Measurement times are limited by the output of the x-ray tube and the capacity of the image memory. At present, data acquisition of up to 12 s is possible. This means that 120 mm are acquired with a table feed of 10 mm/s. After the measurement, scans are reconstructed from the original data file with a newly developed algorithm ("spiral"). The scans are free from motion artifacts in spite of the table feed [Kalender et al. 1989]. The slice profile of the reconstructed computer tomograms is wider than the nominal value by a factor of 1.3; this means that a slice thickness of 10 mm represents an effective slice thickness of 13 mm.

The advantages of Spiral-CT are continuous acquisition of the entire measurement volume in a single breathhold. The problems experienced with poorly reproducible inspiration phases during successive scan series are completely eliminated. The reconstructed images display the complete organ in either overlapping slices

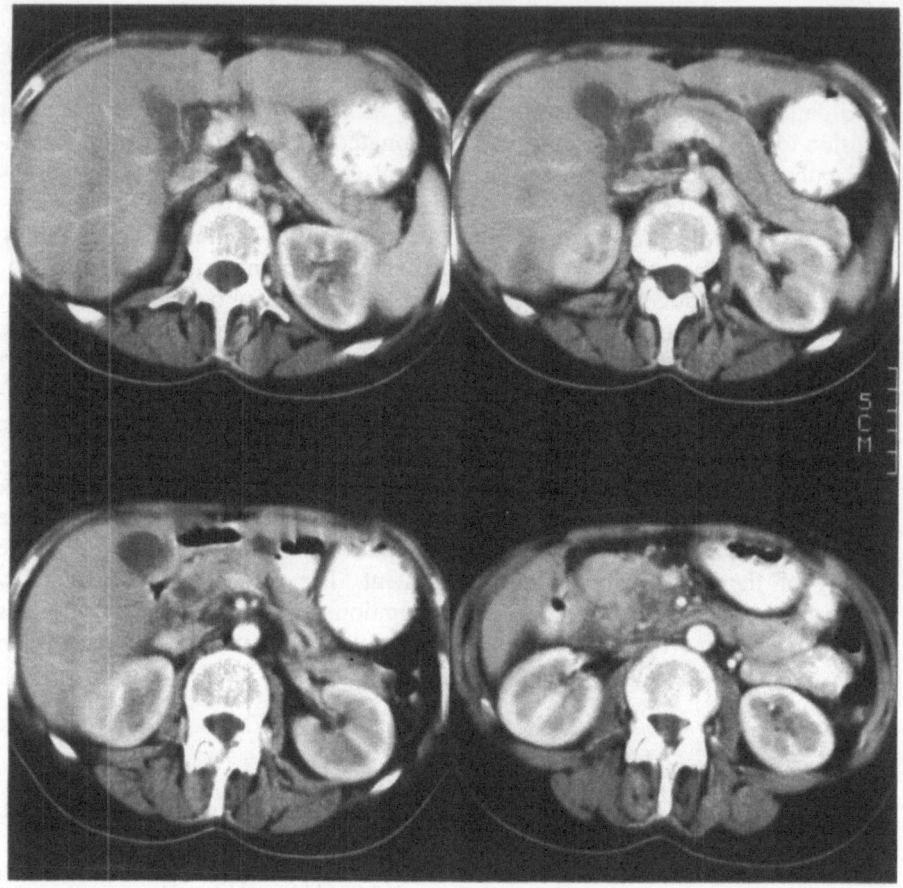

Fig. 2a, b. Spiral-CT (carcinoma in the head of the pancreas). **a** Computer tomograms directly reconstructed from the data set of Spiral-CT. Motion artifacts caused by table feed

or as adjacent slices. When reconstructing overlapping slices, partial volume effects no longer obscure diagnostic interpretation. Spiral-CT opens new perspectives for CM examinations. Also, contrast enhancement of smaller volumes is greatly improved due to the short scan time.

Spiral-CT is highly suitable for diagnostic procedures in pancreatic disease, because the organ does not extend by more than 6–8 cm in the longitudinal body axis. In most cases the entire organ including pathological changes may be acquired with a spiral scan of 120 mm. Maximum enhancement of a healthy pancreas may be measured 15–20 seconds after the contrast agent has been injected [Clausen et al. 1983]. This factor has to be included in the examination (Fig. 1). A power injection of 100 ml CM is administered 20 seconds prior to enabling the Spiral-CT mode. The injection is completed when measurement begins. Spiral-CT is performed over a period of 12 seconds with a table feed of 10 mm/s.

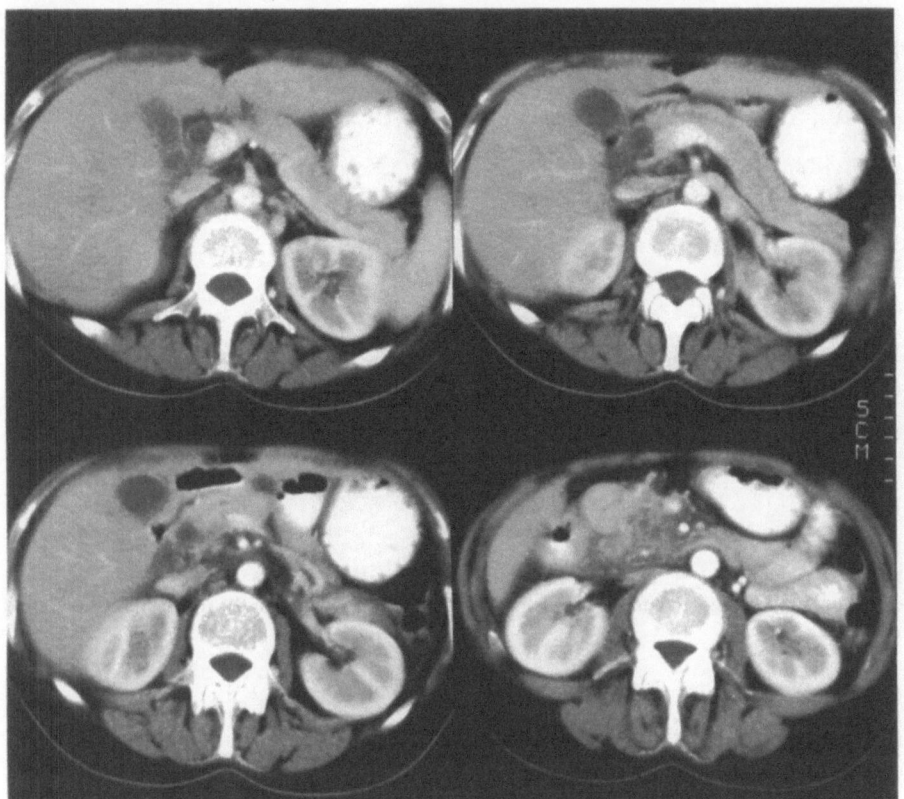

Fig. 2b. Artifact-free computer tomograms computed with algorithm "spiral"

After the measurement, the data of 12 computer tomograms degraded by artifacts (table feed) are computed from the raw data set. The subsequently reconstructed images (Fig. 2a) are used to verify the acquired volume. Computation requires approximately 10 minutes. During post-processing, the data of artifact-free computer tomograms are computed with the newly developed "spiral" algorithm (Fig. 2b). Freely-selectable intermediate slices are subsequently reconstructed through interpolation. To date, the capacity of the image memory allows for reconstruction of computer tomograms with a nominal slice thickness of 10 mm offset by a minimum of 1 mm. Reconstruction may require up to 1 hour with the currently available lab version.

The computer tomograms are individually analyzed and read into the "cine" program. This program allows for high-speed display of CT image series (3–8 images/s) with smooth transitions so that a moving image is displayed on the monitor. The combination of spiral-CT and image display in cine mode seems to be an ideal one. The human eye detects pathological changes more quickly in a moving image than in a static image. Additional examinations will show whether

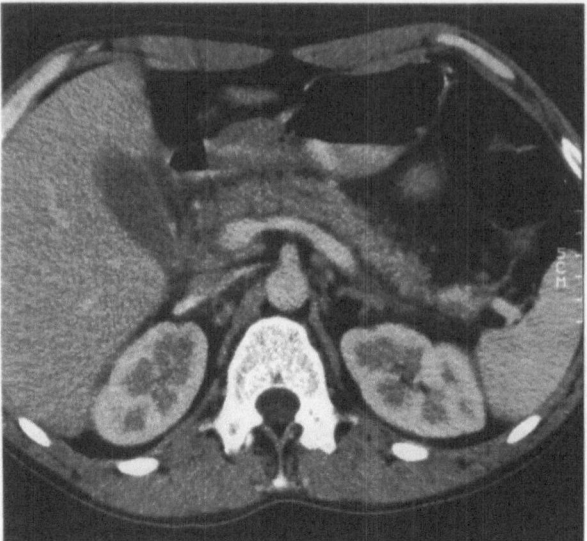

Fig. 3. Sero-exudative pancreatitis. Peripancreatic discrete exudative changes. Pancreas is not extended and the organ contours are easily distinguishable. Sections of the ductus pancreatitis are visible

the combination Spiral CT/cine mode increases the accuracy of diagnostic procedures in pancreatic disease.

Clinical Application

Computer tomography plays an important role in the primary diagnosis of acute pancreatitis, treatment monitoring, and subsequent therapeutic application. An enlarged organ is symptomatic of edematous pancreatitis; an increased homogeneous enhancement after intravenous application of contrast agent is indicative of inflammation. Peripancreatic exudate or fat necroses are symptomatic of sero-exudative pancreatitis, which may be more easily distinguished from the pancreas after administering the contrast agent. Sero-exudative pancreatitis may be diagnosed in the early stages with the SOMATOM PLUS (Fig. 3). In the case of hemorrhagic-necrotizing and abscess-forming types of acute pancreatitis, the region of the necrosis does not absorb the contrast agent. This allows the physician to estimate the percentage of vital tissue and/or the extent of necrosis (Fig. 4). CT is not suited for differentiating between hemorrhagic-necrotizing and abscess-forming pancreatitis. Its suitability lies in distinguishing between sero-exudative and necrotizing tissue and in detecting collateral phenomena such as the presence of pseudocysts, peripancreatic edema, and inflamed infiltrations of the peritoneum (mesenterium, mesocolon, bands of necrosis, pleural effusion or cholestasis).

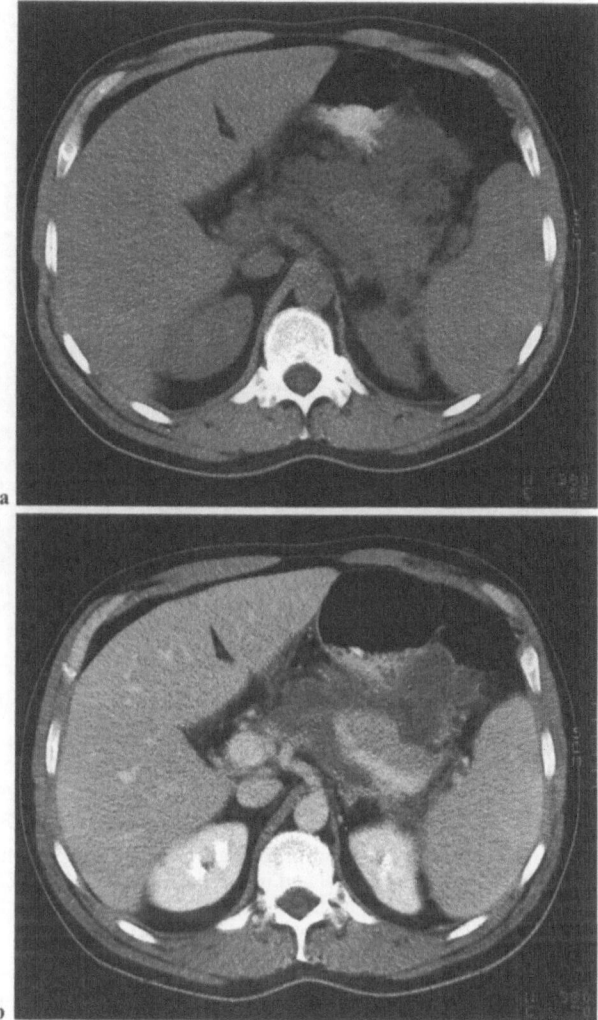

Fig. 4a, b. Necrotizing pancreatitis with extensive bands of necrosis. **a** Plain scan: vital pancreatic parenchyma. It is not possible to differentiate between necroses and vessels. **b** CM-CT (dynamic CT): perfused parenchyma in tail of the pancreas. Parenchyma absorbs contrast agent. Distinction between parenchyma, necrosis and dorsal V. lienalis

Detailed diagnosis of chronic pancreatitis is also improved by the use of the SOMATOM PLUS. Irregular scarring of the parenchyma, frequent calcification, focal tissue necrosis and pseudocysts are indicative of chronic pancreatitis. To date, pseudocysts had to measure at least 1 cm in diameter to be detected with computer tomography. In our experience, the SOMATOM PLUS provides proof of cystic changes in the millimeter range after administering the contrast agent.

Seventy-five percent of all pancreatic carcinomas are located in the head of the pancreas. In 90% of the cases, the epithelium of the pancreatic duct is the primary

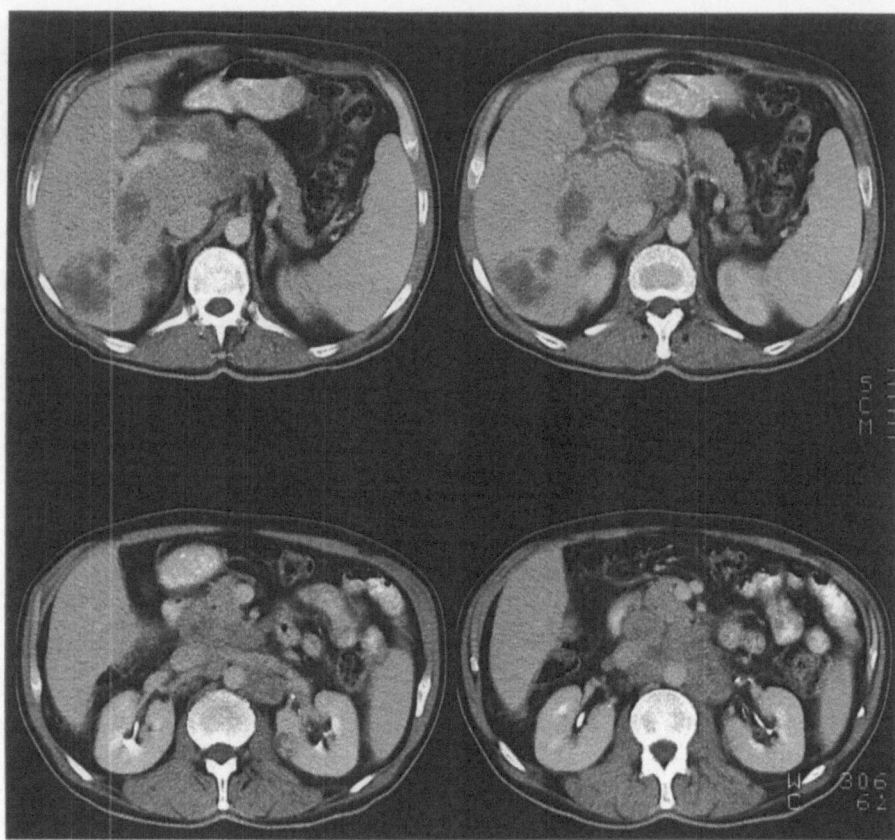

Fig. 5. Carcinoma in the head of the pancreas. Multiple lymph node metastases in the porta of the liver, paraaortal, paracaval and in the mesenteric root. Metastases of the liver. Good display of vessels. Angiomyolipoma in the left kidney

site [Kloeppel 1986]. In the past, these tumors could be diagnosed with CT only after the respective organ showed sufficient enlargement. Chronic pancreatitis shows similar changes in organ size so that only collateral phenomena such as metastases of the liver confirm the presence of pancreatic carcinoma. The objective of all diagnostic procedures is to detect pancreatic tumors in their early stages, because the size of the tumor determines prognosis. Patients suffering from a peri-ampullar carcinoma in the head of the pancreas can be operated upon in the early stages of this disease, because symptoms (cholestasis) appear rather quickly. Statistically, these patients have a 40% chance of surviving an additional five years as compared to the usual 10% chance for patients suffering from pancreatic carcinoma [Gmelin et al. 1988].

The sensitivity of the method in proving pancreatic disease will be further improved through dynamic CT [Lammer et al. 1984] and, most probably, through the use of Spiral-CT. After CM application, small pancreatic carcinomas are hypodense as compared to normal pancreatic tissue. By administering contrast agents, infiltrations, especially in the V. lienalis, V. mesenterica, and V. portae are confirmed. This confirmation is decisive in the indication and planning of surgery. In this case, Spiral-CT in combination with the cine mode surpasses dynamic CT performed in a single plane. It is frequently quite difficult to differentiate pancreatic metastases from pancreatic carcinomas with the support of CT. To date, this type of differentiation was successful in not more than 44% of all cases [Zeman et al. 1985]. In our experience, improvement will occur when using the examination method described in this article.

Computer tomography is also a contributing factor in determining the type of pancreatic tumor such as microcystic adenoma, macrocystic adenoma and active endocrine tumors. Active endocrine tumors of the pancreas (insulinoma and gastrinoma) are usually small and heavily vascularized tumors. In the past, they were diagnosed by using the fractionated bolus method or dynamic CT in several planes. The large amount of contrast agent required for this examination [Rossi et al. 1985] can be reduced due to the improved image quality obtained with the SOMATOM PLUS and Spiral-CT.

In our opinion, Spiral-CT is the technology of the future which can be developed into a new scanner generation. At present, this technology, which provides us with a wide range of applications in addition to its use in diagnosing pancreatic disease, is improving the performance of diagnostic CT devices.

References

Anacker H, Weiss HD, Kramann B (1977) Endoscopic retrograde pancreaticocholangiography (ERCP). Springer, Heidelberg New York

Bautz W, Klier R (1989) SOMATOM PLUS: Clinical results of 3000 patient examinations. Electromedica 57: 82-87

Claussen CD, Lochner B (1983) Pankreasdiagnostik durch Einsatz der dynamischen Computertomographie (Serien-CT). Fortschr Röntgenstr 139: 389-393

Gmelin E, Ollrogge C, Trötschel H (1988) Pankreasdiagnostik II: Aktueller Stand der CT und Wertung bildgebender Verfahren. In: Claussen C, Felix R (Hrsg) Quo vadis CT. Springer, Berlin Heidelberg New York London Paris Tokyo, S 194-211

Kalender W, Seissler W, Klotz E, Vock P (1990) Single breathhold spiral volumetric computed tomography (SVCT) by continuous patient translation and scanner rotation. Radiology 176: July 1990

Klöppel G (1986) Pathomorphology by pancreatic cancer. In: Malfertheimer P, Ditschuneit H (eds) Diagnostic procedures in pancreatic disease. Springer, Berlin Heidelberg New York, pp 277-284

Lammer J, Tölly E, Hörmann M, Zalaudek G (1984) Pankreaskarzinom: Staging mittels dynamischer CT. Digit Bilddiagn 4: 121-126

Rossi P, Bart A, Passariello R, Simonetti G, Pavone P, Tempesta P (1985) CT of functioning tumors of the pancreas. Amer J Roentgenol 144: 57-60

Zeman RK, Schiebler M, Clark LJ, Jaffe MH, Paushter DM, Grant EG, Choyke PL (1985) The clinical and imaging spectrum of pancreaticoduodenal lymph node enlargement. Amer J Roentgenol 144: 1223-1227

Discussion

R. Hupke, Erlangen: The Advantages of Fast and Continuously-Rotating CT Systems

v. Engelshoven, Maastricht:
What is the reason for Siemens' changing the KV values from the initial 120 KV to the present 137 KV?

Hupke:
The reason for this measure is to optimize the quantum output when using the 1 sec or subsecond scan times.

v. Engelshoven:
In addition, the focal spot was changed to a larger size which must result in a decrease of spatial resolution.

Hupke:
When using the 2 second high resolution mode a small focal spot size of 0,9 mm is always used. With a 1 second or subsecond scan a large focal spot size must be used in order to obtain sufficient quanta. The spatial resolution with 1 second scan and large focal spot size is about 0.5 mm, with the 2 second scans the resolution is about 0.35 mm. We consider that particularly in the lung the scan time is most important as the sharpening of the structures could be done by reconstruction kernels.

When scanning with an artefact reduction technique the same dose is applied as when scanning with a conventional 2 mm slice. When comparing the 8 mm slice to 4×2 mm slices, there is some increase due to the distribution of the dose profile. The dose is not much higher.

P. A. Gevenois, Brussels: Occupational Diseases of the Lung: Evaluation with High-Resolution CT

Bücheler, Hamburg:
More lesions were found with high resolution CT. But what is the clinical importance in the diagnosis of asbestosis or silicosis? The same question applies to the clinical importance of visualizing small lymph nodes.

Struyven, Brussels:
For silicosis, if a diagnostic score is to be made high resolution is not needed but for a full evaluation of the disease high resolution allows a more precise diagnosis. In asbestosis the diagnosis is not only made by subpleural plaques or calcification, but also by subpleural curvilinear lesions, which are visible with high resolution CT and may not be seen on conventional CT. Thus the diagnostic score for asbestosis was higher with HRCT.

M. Oudkerk, Rotterdam: Continuous Rotation CT of Hilar Adenopathy Using One-Second and Subsecond Scan Times

Struyven:
With reference to lymph node diagnosis it is correct that there were more small lymph nodes involved than large ones?

Oudkerk:
I refer to a study of Ekholm who did a study of lymph nodes in the hili during open biopsy. This author found that of all the lymph nodes checked, the small ones were malignant more often than the larger ones. This is completely the opposite to the situation in the mediastinum and in the abdomen.

Struyven:
It depends also what population you are screening. When screening mine workers there are many large nodes without malignant involvement, and even in a non selected population this may be seen.

Oudkerk:
The importance to diagnose small size lymph node pathology is the sensitivity. The higher the sensitivity is the more reliably lymph node pathology in the hili can be excluded, thus influencing the decision for surgical intervention.

Vock, Bern:
There seems to be no relevance of detecting small lymph nodes since surgeons will operate regardless of lymph node enlargement.

v. Engelshoven:
If no lymph nodes are visualized, the surgeon will operate immediately. If we identify lymph nodes of any size mediastinoscopy or -tomy will be performed.

Oudkerk:
I believe that hilar CT is useful in excluding hilar lymph nodes in patients who would otherwise, particularly with older CT equipment, be regarded as inoperable.

Vock:
But ipsilateral hilar lymph node involvement is of no surgical consequence.

Kramann, Homburg:
CT of the lung is very important in the full assessment of silicosis, particularly for insurance or compensation claims.

Struyven:
CT is mandatory in such an assessment of silicosis, as it is well known that CT demonstrates more nodules than conventional chest X-ray.

Adam, London:
You have shown that HRCT with thin slices misses nodules. Is it the slice thickness or the algorithm which is responsible? Would the high resolution algorithm and a 1 cm slice thickness be more sensitive?

Struyven:
The slice thickness is responsible, because in a larger volume nodules are more likely to be identified.
   But in the search for fine detail, e. g. septal lines, thin slices are needed.

Adam:
I accept that. I wonder, however, if a higher resolution algorithm should be used routinely for the lung.

v. Engelshoven:
Can the contrast injection be triggered by the SOMATOM PLUS?

Hupke:
Not at the moment.

v. Engelshoven:
What was the slice thickness in the assessment of hilar nodes?

Oudkerk:
5 mm.

W. Bautz, Tübingen: New Directions in the CT-Diagnosis of the Pancreas

Vock:
For visualizing 10 mm section slices, we prefer 5 mm slice thickness.

Bautz:
If we use 5 mm there is much noise which reduces the image quality. Therefore we do 10 mm, not 5 mm thick slices.

Fuchs:
Noise produces a granularity pattern in all images. Are there plans to reduce this granularity by applying special software?

Hupke:
One-second scans, particularly with thin slices in obese patients, can present problems. We would recommend the use of smoothening algorithms. The loss of reso-

lution is not very great, from 0.65 mm to 0.7 mm, and, especially in the abdomen, this is not significant. Most people work with the standard kernel, but when doing thin slices on an obese patient the soft detail kernel is helpful. There may be a possibility that additional image processing filters will become available, as for the DR 3, but in the meantime the soft kernels should be used.

Dixon, Cambridge:
Does this last statement also apply to the spine? There are some problems with noise on 5 mm slices in the spine in heavy patients.

Hupke:
Especially in the spine I would also recommend to use the smoother kernel.

Quantitative CT – Volume Scanning

Chairmen: J. Struyven, P. Gerhardt

Spiral CT Scanning for Fast and Continuous Volume Data Acquisition

W. A. KALENDER, P. VOCK, W. SEISSLER

Abstract

Continuous scanning of volumes during a single breathhold should provide decisive advantages in several clinical applications; continuously rotating CT scanners, in principle, offer the required technology. We modified the table feed mechanism of a SOMATOM PLUS to transport the patient at low, but accurately controlled speeds (0.1–11.0 mm/s) during continuous 1 s-scanning, resulting in a spiral scanning geometry. A special reconstruction software was developed to calculate artifact-free planar images from the volume data. As a particular advantage, it allows calculating images for arbitrary table positions. Physical performance characteristics are discussed; clinical examples are presented for lung nodule and contrast medium studies. Major advantages are the possibilities to scan extended volumes continuously and to retrospectively select arbitrary slice levels.

Introduction

The standard CT procedure in scanning a complete volume is a successive step-wise scanning of one slice after the other. Interscan delays are necessary for table feed and, possibly, for patient breathing. Thus, the total examination time is much longer than the actual scan time. This is of particular concern in contrast medium studies where imaging during the early vascular enhancement phase is desirable [1–3]. Also, the patient will not reproduce consistent levels of inspiration from scan to scan in whole-body CT. This problem becomes obvious in multiplanar reformatting and in 3D-displays when 'steplike' contours indicate the single slices being scanned in an unpleasant way. It can be a true diagnostic problem when certain levels are completely omitted; this has been reported in particular for the search and diagnosis of pulmonary nodules [4–7].

Continuous scanning of complete organs or volumes within a single breathhold would alleviate or even eliminate such problems. We have therefore developed and investigated a scanning mode for continuous volume data acquisition on the SOMATOM PLUS. It is based on transporting the patient continuously through the gantry during continuous multirotational scanning.

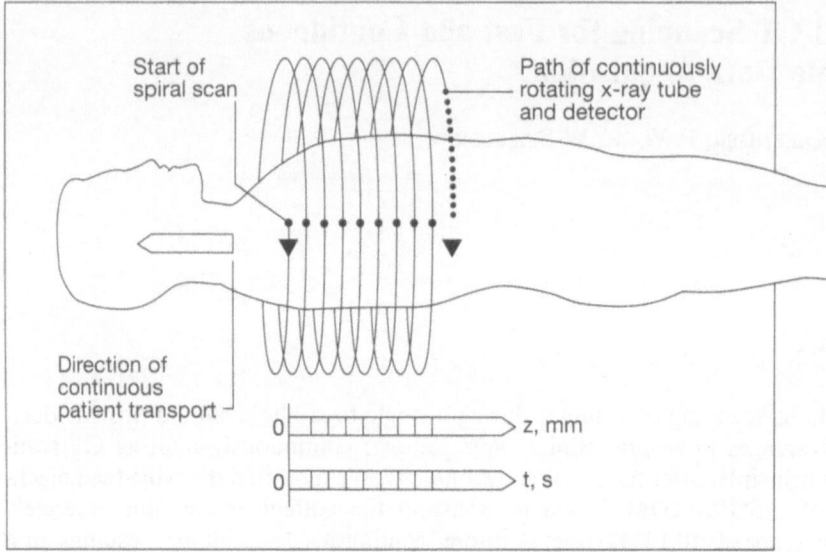

Fig. 1. Schematic presentation of spiral CT scanning geometry. The patient is transported continuously while X-ray tube and detector rotate continuously. The X-ray focus describes a spiral path on an imaginary cylinder surface (from [8])

Material and methods

Our work was carried out on a standard SOMATOM PLUS, a continuously rotating CT system which, at the present time, offers up to 12 consecutive 1 s-scans. It is equipped with a high-power X-ray tube rated at 3.5 million heat units storage capacity. Tube currents can be selected depending on the length of the scanning interval. They range from 250 mA for a 5 s-scan period to 170 mA for a 12 s-multiscan. We worked at 120 and 137 kV with slice thicknesses of 1, 2, 5, 8 and 10 mm. The scanner was operated in the DYNAMIC/MULTISCAN mode.

To allow for continuous patient transport during the multiscans, we developed an experimental setup which was attached to the scanner without changing or compromising any of its standard functions. A stepper motor was added to the table feed mechanism, allowing transport at 0.1 to 11.0 mm/s. A separate small microprocessor-based control unit, which can be placed next to the scanner console's keyboard, is used to select the table feed parameters and to start the multirotational scan in exact synchrony with patient transport.

The X-ray focus will follow a spiral path on a virtual cylinder surface with a constant radius equal to the distance of focus to center of rotation in this scanning mode (Fig. 1); we have therefore chosen the term **Spiral Volumetric CT (SVCT)**. The data obtained can be directly submitted to the regular image reconstruction process for immediate control purposes; however, artefacts have to be expected completely analogous to those resulting from patient motion. We therefore have

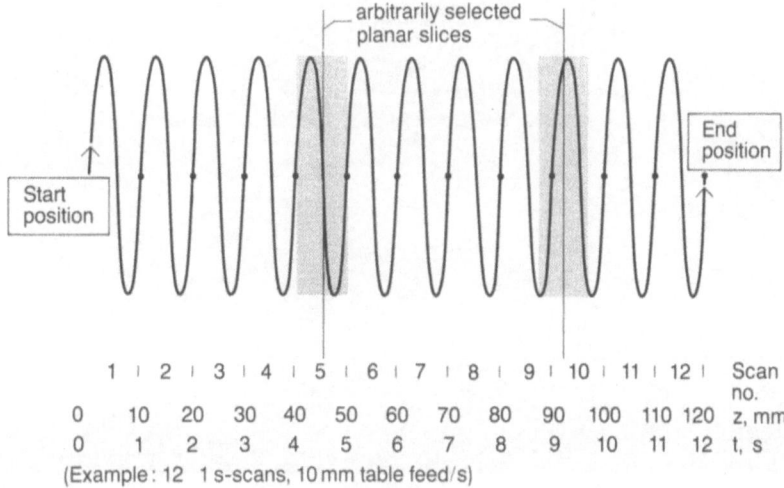

Fig. 2. Illustration of data processing in SVCT. Images can be reconstructed for arbitrary table positions within the scanned volume

developed a dedicated reconstruction algorithm which synthezises raw data representing a perfectly planar slice from the original spiral data by interpolation (Fig. 2) [8]. A particular advantage results from this procedure: planar data can be reconstructed for any table position within the scanned volume. In particular, this can be done repeatedly and in a retrospective fashion.

We have carried out a multitude of phantom experiments and clinical studies to establish the physical performance characteristics and the clinical value of SVCT.

Results

Image quality in SVCT is not significantly changed as compared to standard imaging [8]. The artefacts which had to be expected for direct reconstruction in spiral geometry can be demonstrated in phantom experiments (Fig. 3 a) and any clinical study (Fig. 4 a). However, they are completely eliminated when using the dedicated processing into planar data.

Slice sensitivity profiles are found to deteriorate to some degree; slice widths, measured as their full width at half maximum, are enlarged by about a factor of 1.3 [8]. This effective enlargement of slice thicknesses had to be expected due to the table feed during scanning. We have not observed significant image quality deteriorations in the type of studies conducted so far. Image noise is slightly reduced due to the interpolation process.

SVCT studies on patients with focal lung disease have demonstrated the advantage of continuous scanning in a consistent manner [3, 7]. In particular, solitary pulmonary nodules could be assessed in an optimal fashion in all cases, with the

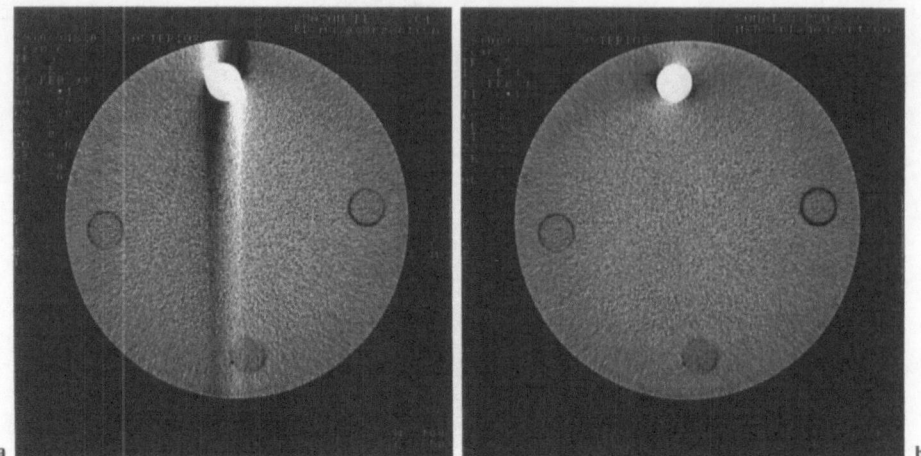

a   b

Fig. 3a, b. Image quality in spiral CT scans: Phantom study. **a** Direct reconstruction from the spiral data results in motion-like artifacts. **b** Reconstructions from synthesized planar data are free from such artifacts

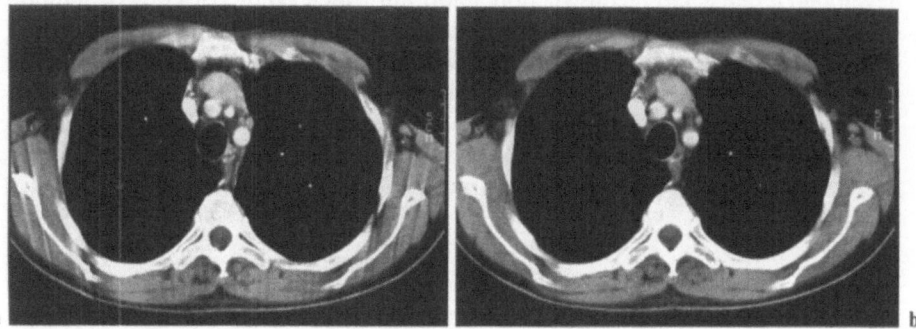

a   b

Fig. 4a, b. Image quality in spiral CT scans: Mediastinal study. **a** Direct reconstruction from the spiral data results in motion-like artifacts. **b** Reconstructions from synthesized planar data are free from such artifacts

center of the lesion determined retrospectively to assess size and density (Fig. 5). Liver contrast studies with SVCT were aimed at imaging as large a volume as possible in a single breathhold period of 12 s during the early enhancement phase. Examining a volume of 120 mm height using a bolus injection technique was always successful (Fig. 6).

Discussion

The demand for continuous and fast scanning of complete volumes is generally accepted; there have been no technical means until now, however. While the idea to use a helical or spiral geometry has been presented earlier in the patent literature [9], the technical basis for a respective scanner has not been available until the recent advent of continuously rotating CT systems. The SOMATOM PLUS with its high-power X-ray tube provided the necessary basis for investigations into this technique. The adaptation of the table feed mechanism to continuously transport the patient in synchrony with continuous data acquisition was only a minor but necessary step. Our efforts do not present a solution for all cases, but they demonstrate and prove that spiral scanning modes are a practical solution in a number of clinical studies without a loss in image quality.

In its present form as a work-in-progress project for experimental use, SVCT is limited to a 12 s scanning period. Data processing demands some extra efforts in the present experimental form. Data processing, however, does not constitute a principal problem; actually, the demonstration that an image quality equivalent to that of standard CT scanning can be achieved constitutes a major breakthrough. The principal limitation has to be seen in the X-ray power available for extended scan periods. The limitation of scanning to single breathhold periods constitutes a compromise between patient cooperation and X-ray tube limitations.

Our clinical investigations have focused on tasks where 170–250 mAs per scan appear sufficient. This is the case for lung nodule studies, since the high contrast of the nodule with respect to the surrounding lung tissue and the low attenuation of the thoracic region allow for low dose techniques. In contrast medium studies also, contrast is high enough during the early vascular enhancement phase so that the noise level due to the low-mAs technique does not constitute a limitation. Actually, the use of low mAs or low-dose techniques and the possibility to work with low amounts of contrast medium [3] can be considered a major advantage of SVCT.

SVCT is not limited to the applications demonstrated in this paper. Further contributions at this meeting give additional examples. SVCT potentially constitutes the CT scanning mode of the future.

Fig. 5. *(pp. 60, 61)* SVCT study on a pulmonary nodule (12 1 s-scans of a 24 mm subvolume, 2 mm nominal slice thickness, 2 mm/s table feed). 16 consecutive reconstructions spaced 1 mm apart are shown

Fig. 6. *(pp. 62, 63)* SVCT liver contrast study in multiple metastases from carcinoma of the colon (12 1 s-scans of a 120 mm subvolume, 10 mm nominal slice thickness, 10 mm/s table feed). 16 consecutive reconstructions spaced 5 mm apart are shown

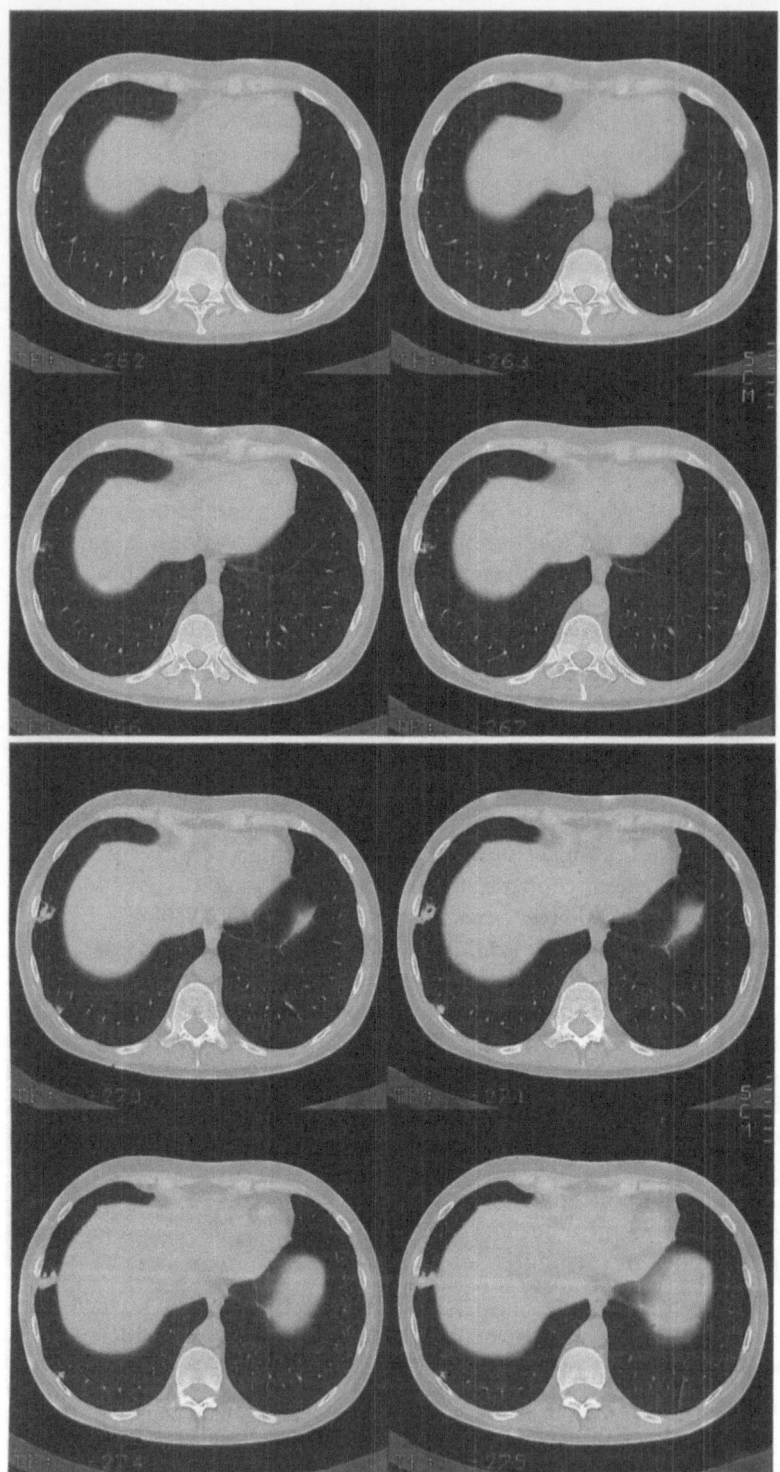

Fig. 5

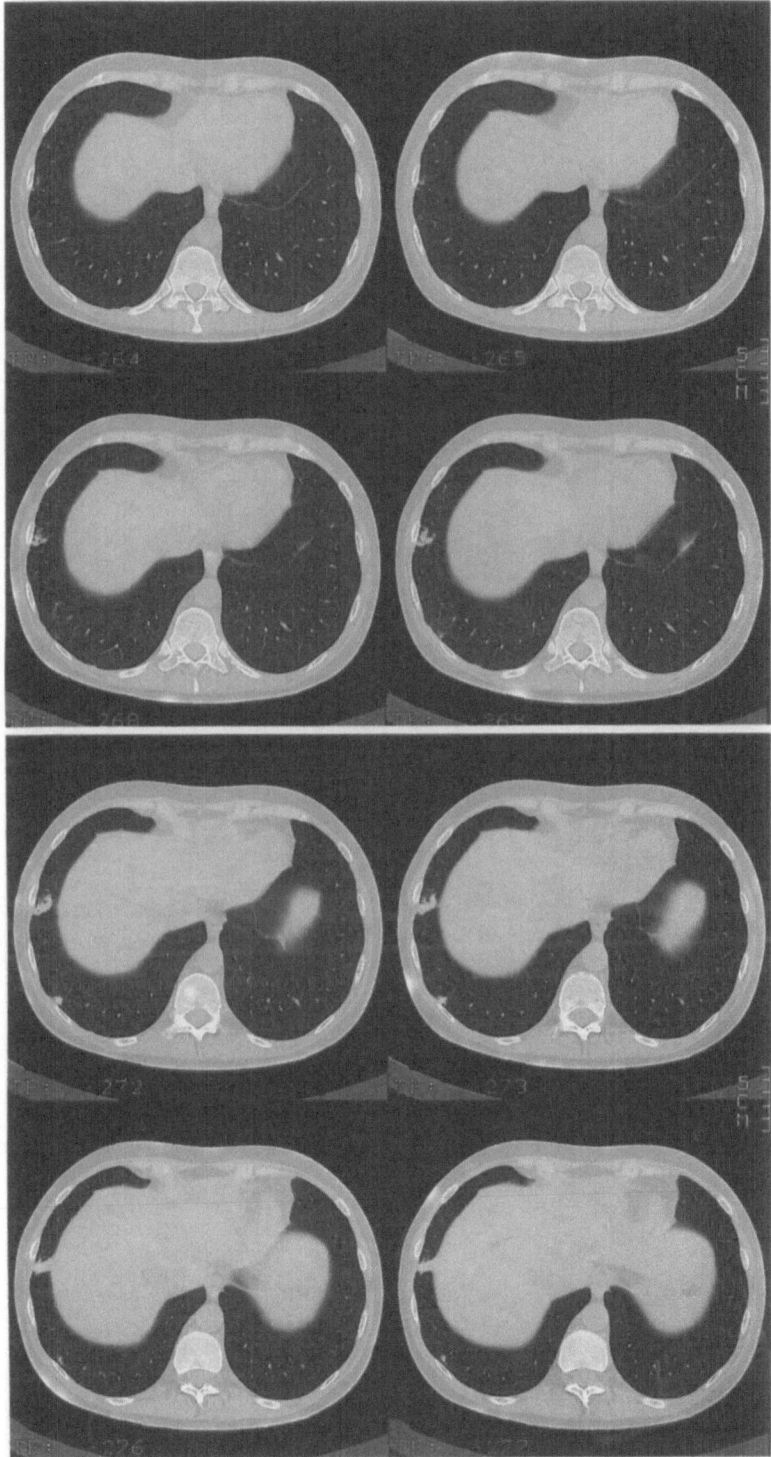

Fig. 5

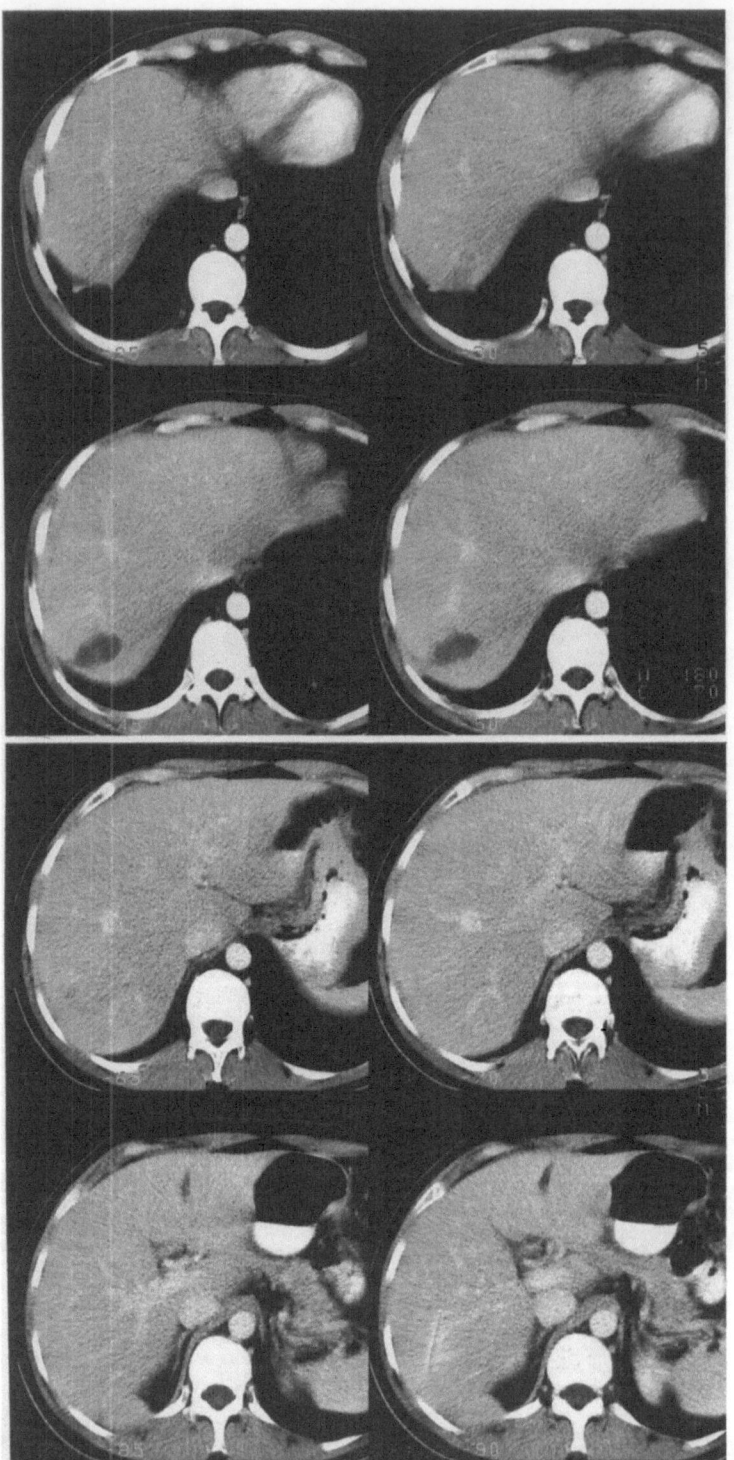

Fig. 6

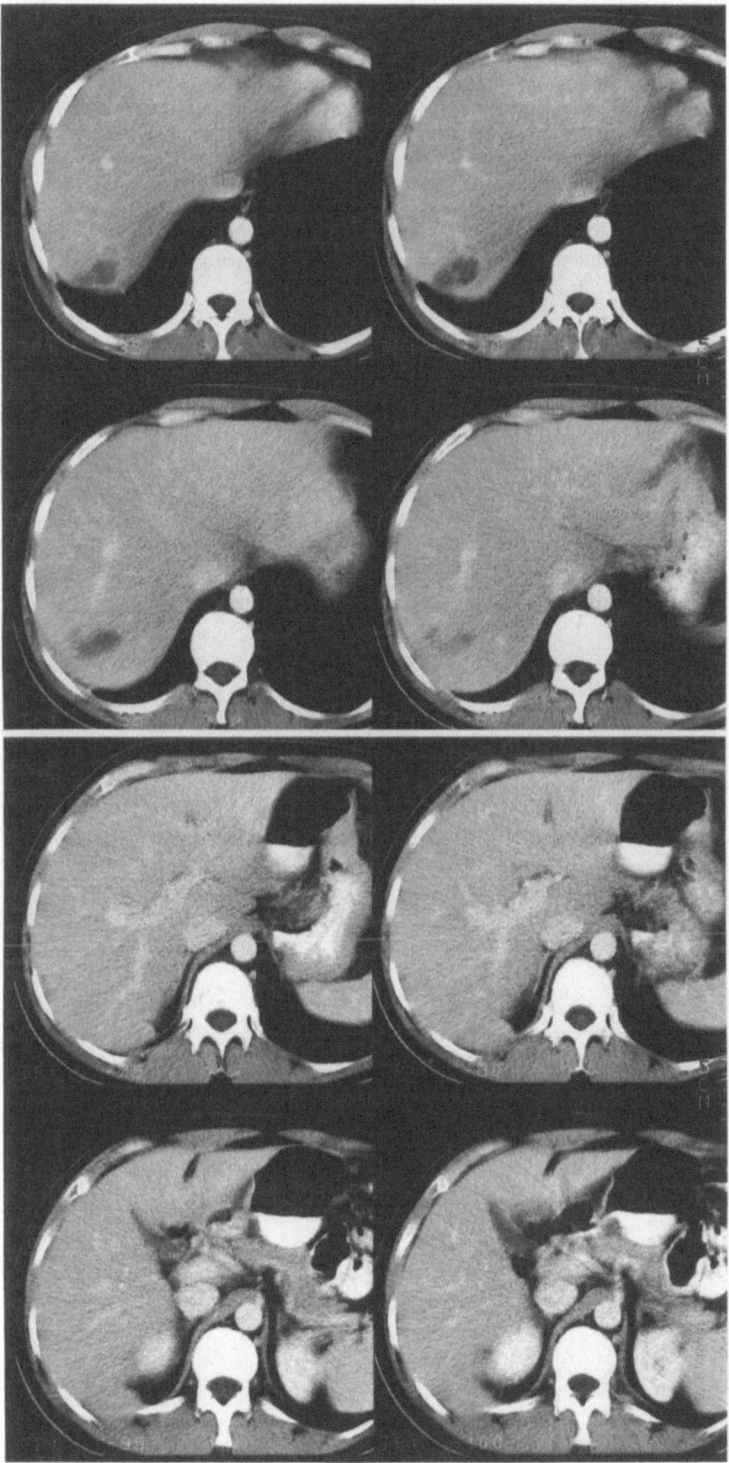

Fig. 6

References

1. Freeny PC (1988) Hepatic CT: State of the art. Radiology 168: 319–323
2. Zeman RK, Clements LA, Silverman PM, Paushter DM, Garra B, Jaffe MH, Clark LR (1988) CT of the liver: A survey of prevailing methods for administration of contrast material. Amer J Roentgen 150: 107–109
3. Vock P, Jung H, Kalender W (1989) Single-breathhold spiral volumetric CT of the hepatobiliary system. Radiology 173 (P): 377
4. Zerhouni EA, Spivey JF, Morgan RH, Leo FP, Stitik FP, Siegelman SS (1982) Factors influencing quantitative CT measurements of solitary pulmonary nodules. J Comput Assist Tomogr 6: 1075–1087
5. Siegelman SS, Khouri NF, Leo FP, Fishman EK, Braverman RM, Zerhouni EA (1986) Solitary pulmonary nodules: CT assessment. Radiology 160: 307–312
6. Shaffer K, Pugatsch RD (1989) Small pulmonary nodules: Dynamic CT with a single-breath technique. Radiology 173: 567–568
7. Vock P, Jung H, Kalender W (1989) Single-breathhold spiral volumetric CT of the lung. Radiology 173 (P): 400 (and Radiology 1990, in print)
8. Kalender W, Seißler W, Klotz E, Vock P (1990) Single-breathhold spiral volumetric computed tomography (SVCT) by continuous patient translation and scanner rotation. Radiology 176: July 1990
9. Slavin PE (1969) X-ray helical scanning means for displaying an image of an object within the body being scanned. United States Patent number 3432657.

Spiral Scanning: Phantom Studies and Patient Material

H. Rigauts, G. Marchal, A. L. Baert, R. Hupke

Abstract

A new method of computed tomography is proposed: "spiral scanning," obtained by continuous table incrementation during continuous scanning. This approach was successfully realised by implementing a continuous table incrementation on a commercially available third generation scanner with continuous measurement system and slip ring technology (SOMATOM PLUS).

Different phantoms were scanned with spiral scanning at different table incrementation speeds and with conventional scanning with regular sequential table incrementation. Image reconstruction of spiral scans was initially done with the commercially available software; later a special interpolation reconstruction algorithm was used.

Comparison of the results showed that in spiral scanning a table incrementation equal to the chosen slice thickness is the optimal compromise that allows covering a maximal acquisition volume at an acceptable level of artifacts. Experiments on geometrical distortion and contrast resolution revealed hardly any difference between volume scans and conventional scans.

Spiral scanning was used in 52 patients. Images were obtained in the thoracic, pelvic and upper abdomen. Image reconstructions of the spiral scans with the commercially available software are fast and easy to use. 30% of these reconstructed images showed to some extent streak artifacts, but in general the images were detailed and of good diagnostic value. Image reconstructions with the specially designed interpolation reconstruction algorithm showed images free of streak artifacts with a better signal to noise ratio. Drawbacks of the interpolation method are the occurrence of blurred images due to volume averaging and, at the present stage, the time consuming reconstruction.

Introduction

Most current CT scanners of the third generation apply the stop-and-go principle. In this type of scanner, which utilize a cable take-up assembly, minimal scan times are 2-3 seconds and cycle times up to 10 seconds. The interscan time is related to problems of rapidly accelerating and decelerating the large mass of the x-ray tube, collimator, data acquisition system and associated support structures [1].

Recently third and fourth generation scanners employing slip rings and continuously rotating x-ray tubes have been introduced. In this type of scanner the cycle times are reduced to 3-5 seconds, depending on the amount of table incrementation [2].

Reduction of cycle times (scan time and interscan interval) also improves the temporal resolution of fast sequential imaging or dynamic scanning [3].

In the past the diagnostic possibilities of dynamic scanning have been extensively explored. Dynamic CT can be used to study asymmetrical perfusion in the kidneys and brain [4, 5]. A significant arterial stenosis will decrease and delay the contrast uptake in the affected tissues. Dynamic scanning is also used to improve either lesion detection or characterization [6, 7, 8, 9, 10]. From liver studies it is well known that tumors display various patterns of perfusion and diffusion. To obtain a maximum detection rate, scan timing should be adapted accordingly. Particularly in hypervascular liver tumors, the period of optimal detectability can be limited to the early arterial phase after a bolus injection. Hence to optimize detection of this type of tumor the entire liver should at least theoretically be imaged during this optimal vascular phase.

This possibility is however not offered by present day scanners. Indeed, sequential table incrementation is a time consuming procedure, which limits the scan frequency to a maximum of 12 scans per minute, even in continuously rotating systems. Another drawback of sequential CT scanning is image acquisition during breath holding. As breath holding almost never corresponds to the same inspiration level, it is impossible to guarantee that a CT scan of the liver really explores the entire liver volume. This is a well known problem in clinical practice. Lesions smaller than 1 cm, well seen on ultrasound, can be very hard to confirm on CT.

It is to avoid these limitations of present day CT scanners that we explored the possibilities of spiral scanning, obtained by continuous table incrementation during continuous data acquisition. This possibility can easily be implemented on available continuously rotating systems with slip ring technology.

Materials and Methods

The volume scans were obtained with a commercially available SOMATOM PLUS scanner.

Initially, continuous table incrementation during continuous scanning was made possibly by a stabilized DC power supply with variable voltage implemented in parallel with the normal power supply of the table motor. For spiral scanning the table incrementation was experimentally calibrated by adjusting the power of the DC power supply. Table incrementation speed was obtained from the digital position indicator on the gantry.

Recently a dedicated software program was installed to control the table motion, together with a special interpolation program [11] to reconstruct the raw data obtained from spiral scans.

In the Dynamic Multiscan mode of the SOMATOM PLUS it is possible to accumulate the acquisition data of a 12 second scan period. The x-ray tube continuously radiates in this 12 second period, so that 1242 projections per second and 768 detection channels lead to more than 10 million data (ca. 22 Mbytes). This raw data set over a period of Tm seconds is available for reconstruction. (1 sec. < Tm < 12 sec.) (s. Fig. 1). In the commercially available software reconstructions with variable window R (0.7 sec. or 1 sec., corresponding respectively to a reconstruction angle of 240° and 360°) and variable time interval t (0.1 sec. to Tm sec.) can be made. The maximum number of available reconstructed images is (Tm · R)/t. The reconstructions are calculated with a standard back projection algorithm.

For experimental purposes a special linear interpolation algorithm was implemented in the system for reconstruction of the spiral scans [11].

At present the capacity of the central processor unit and not the x-ray tube is the limiting factor for the maximum duration of data acquisition (Tm). According to our experiments, it is possible to perform 5 volume scans, without image reconstruction, within a period of 3.5 minutes. After this series there is an x-ray tube cooling period of 3 minutes.

In order to evaluate the extent of artifacts due to continuous table incrementation during scanning, the method was first applied on an oval homogeneous plexiglas phantom using a central absorber with linearly decreasing attenuation in the z-axis (perpendicular to the image plane). This phantom was scanned during a period Tm = 8 seconds, with a table incrementation speed (Vt) of 1 cm/sec. and a slice thickness of 1 cm. Data were first reconstructed with reconstruction windows of 0.7 and 1 second and with different time intervals (1 and 0.5 seconds). Finally, two scans with R = 0.7 seconds and t = 0.5 seconds were averaged to evaluate the effect of image averaging on artifact reduction.

To determine the optimal compromise between table incrementation speed, slice thickness and artifact reduction, a body phantom was used. The body phantom consists of spinal and pelvic bones embedded in large body-shaped paraffin. Bowel structures are simulated by plastic tubing of two sizes, containing air and fluid. For a regular abdominal study, a slice thickness of 10 mm was chosen and volume scans were obtained at three different table incrementation speeds: 8 mm/sec, 10 mm/sec. and 12 mm/sec. Scan parameters were 1 sec, 120 kV, and 210 mA. These volume scans were subsequently compared with the regular 10 mm scans of the body phantom obtained with the same scan parameters and a sequential table incrementation of 10 mm. The pelvic region of the phantom was chosen as the critical test area, since in this area the pelvic bones cause important and rapidly changing local density differences, which make it particularly sensitive to artifacts.

To evaluate the influence of spiral scanning on spatial resolution, further experiments with an ATS high contrast phantom (minimal diameter of the holes in the absorber: 0.4 mm) were performed. This phantom was scanned within a conventional abdominal mode (120 kV, 210 mAs and 10 mm slices) and with spiral scanning. In addition, 1 mm slices of a skull phantom were obtained with regular scanning (sequential table feed of 1 mm) and with the volume scan method (Vt = 1 mm/sec). Parameters were identical in both methods.

The influence of the "spiral" scanning on geometric distortion was tested on a plexiglas cone phantom (maximum and minimum diameter 19 cm and 16 cm respectively, width: 3 cm). The geometry of the images of both conventional and volume scans were compared.

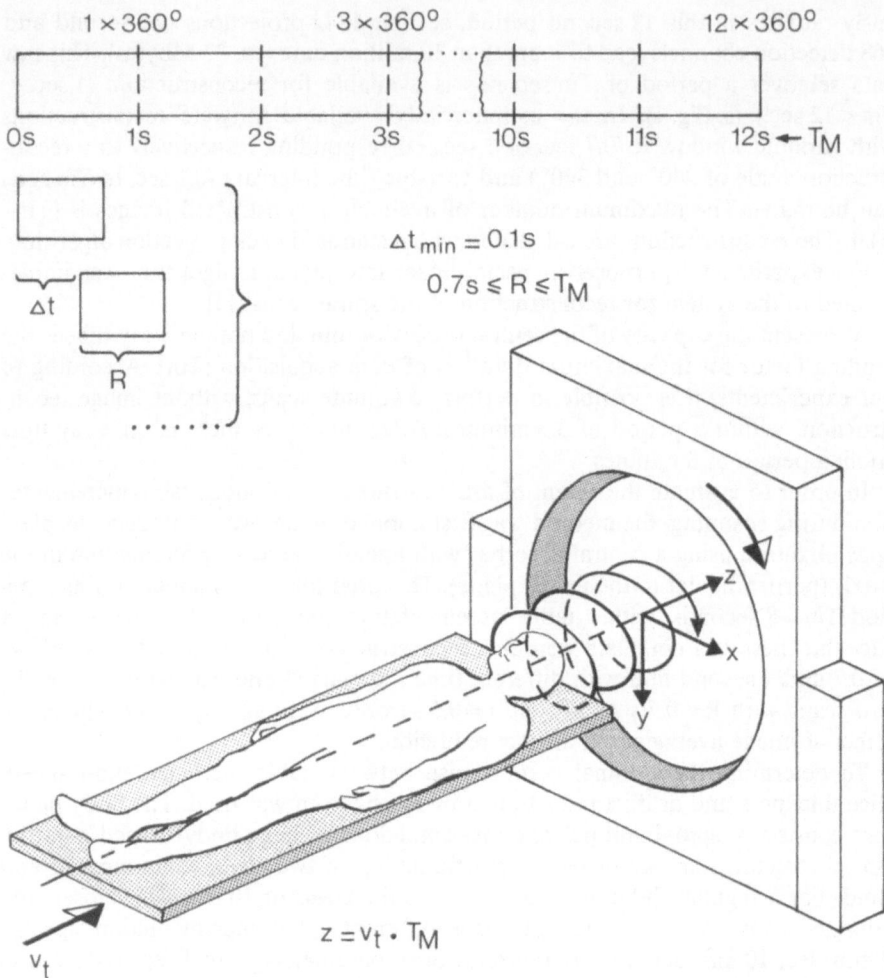

Fig. 1. Schematic representation of a raw data set for a scan period Tm. Reconstructions with variable time interval (t) and variable reconstruction window (R) are possible. Representation of spiral scanning during continuous table incrementation

Fig. 2a-e. Oval homogeneous plexiglas phantom using a central absorber with linearly decreasing attenuation parallel to the z-axis. **a** volume scan (slice thickness 10 mm; Vt = 10 mm/sec.) reconstructed with R = 1 sec. **b** volume scan reconstructed with R = 0.7 sec. **c** averaging of two volume scans reconstructed with R = 0.7 sec. interval. **d** volume scan (slice thickness: 10 mm; Vt: 10 mm/sec., t: 1 sec.) reconstructed with R = 1 sec. **e** averaging of two volume scans (slice thickness: 10 mm; Vt: 10 mm/sec., t: 0.5 sec). Compared with **a** the streak artifacts are already reduced with the 0.7 sec. reconstruction algorithm (**b**). Except for a better signal to noise ratio, the image quality is not significantly improved when two 0.7 sec. volume scans are averaged (**c**). Compared with **d, a** further reduction of streak artifacts is obtained when two volume scans are averaged

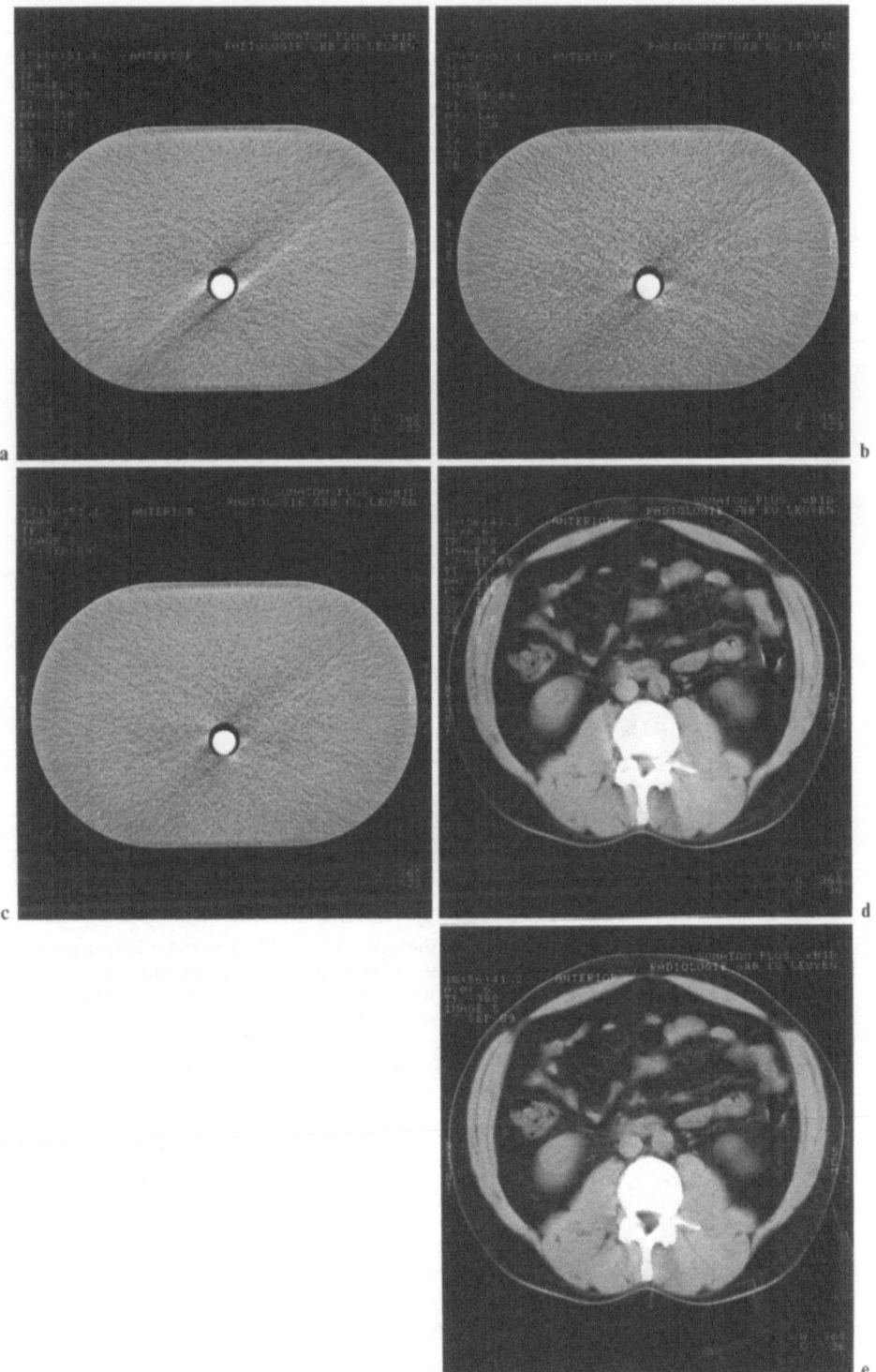

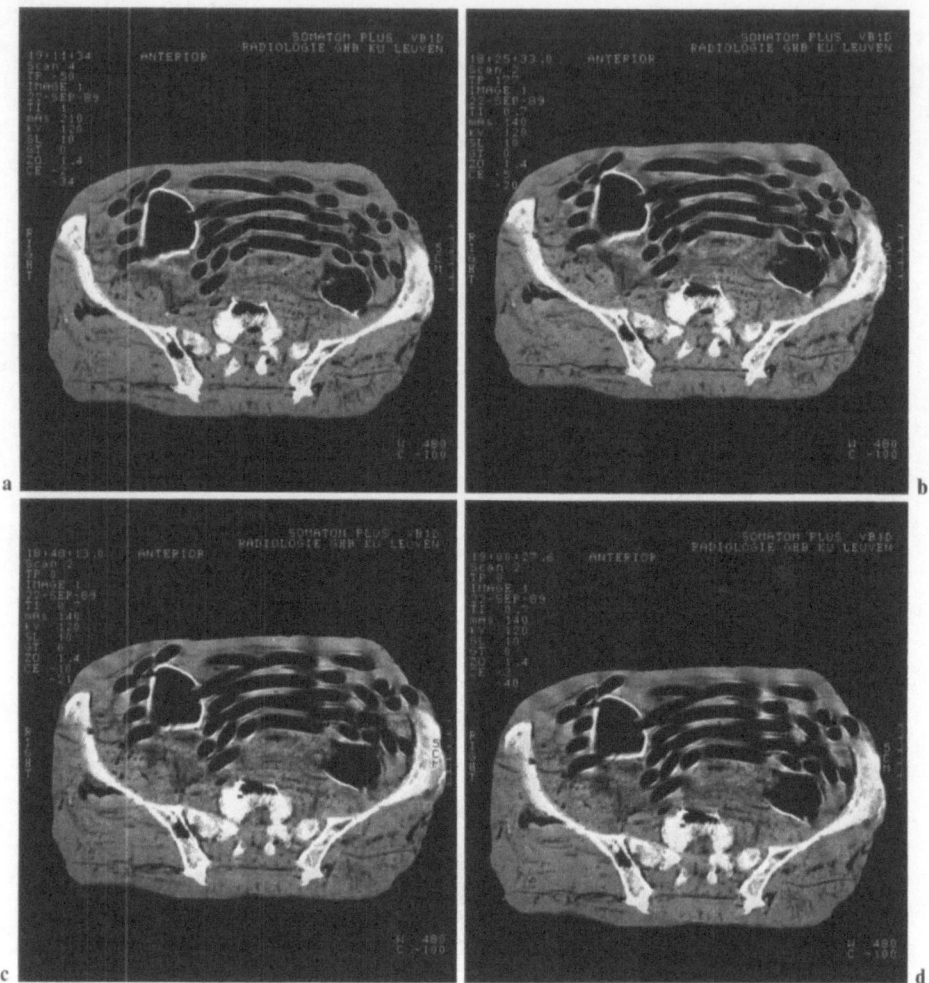

Fig. 3a–d. Body phantom. **a** Regular scan (slice thickness: 10 mm, kV: 120; mAs: 210; sequential table feed: 10 mm). **b** Volume scan (slice thickness: 10 mm, kV 120; mAs 210) with a table incrementation speed of 8 mm/sec. **c** Volume scan with table incrementation speed of 10 mm/sec. **d** Volume scan with table incrementation speed of 12 mm/sec. Compared with the conventional scan (**a**), the image quality progressively decreases in proportion to an increase in table incrementation speed. A table incrementation speed equal to the slice thickness was considered as the optimal compromise between maximal scan volume and an acceptable level of artifacts

Spiral scans were obtained in 52 patients. Initially, reconstructions were made with the commercially available software (R = 0.7 seconds and averaging of two R = 0.7 second images). Later on we compared the results of this software with the results of the specially designed interpolation reconstruction algorithm, both calculated from the same interpolation data.

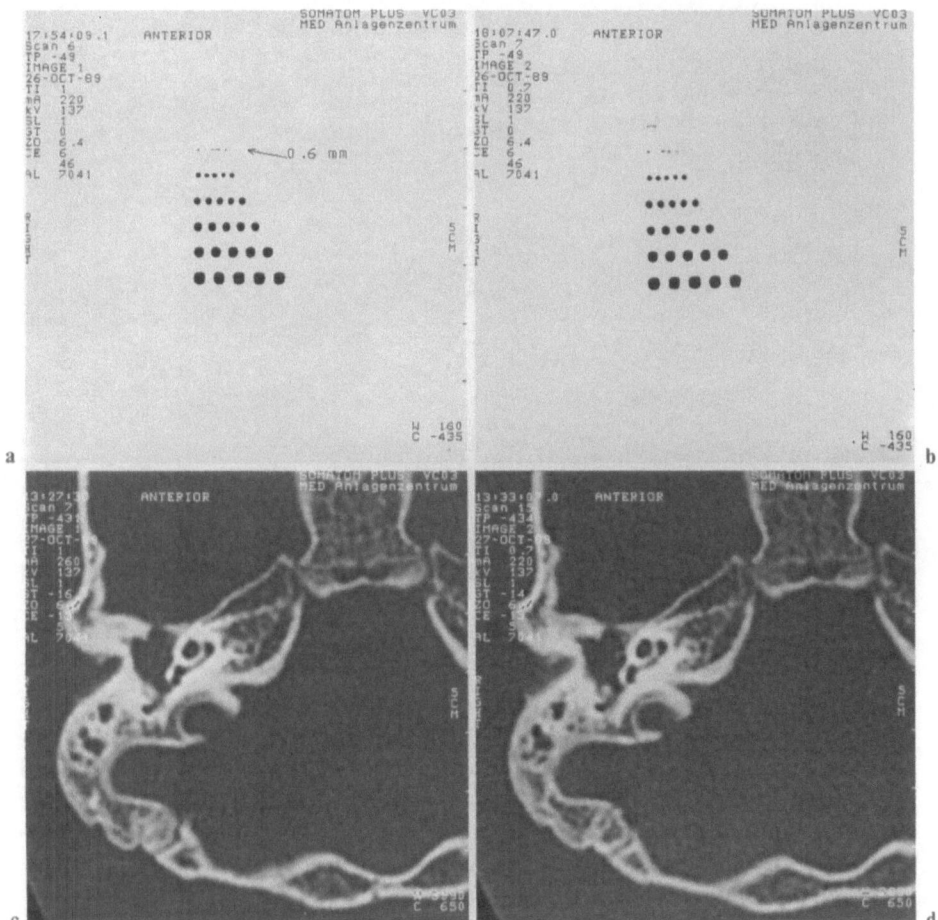

Fig. 4a-d. ATS high resolution phantom. **a** Regular scan, resolution of 0.6 mm, **b** volume scan, same resolution as **a**. Similar for planar resolution of both conventional and volume scan. Skull phantom, scanned in the region of the inner ear **c** conventional scan (slice thickness of 1 mm), **d** volume scan (slice thickness 1 mm, Vt = 1 mm/sec.). This test was used to evaluate the total spatial resolution (in the x, y and z axes). Here also there is no significant difference between both scan techniques

Results

Initial experiments with the oval, in the z-axis homogeneous, plexiglas phantom showed that reconstructions with R = 0.7 sec. produce less artifacts than reconstructions with R = 1 second (Fig. 2). Averaging two 0.7 second images improved the signal to noise ratio, but had no significant effect on artifact reduction. The 0.7 sec. reconstruction parameter was used in the further experiments.

Comparison of regular scans of the body phantom (Fig. 3) and volume scans showed that the best results were obtained at the lowest table incrementation

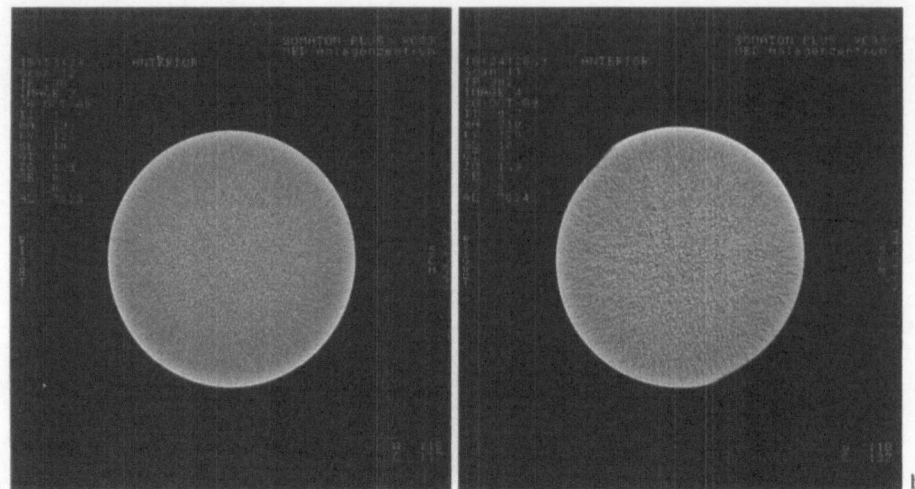

Fig. 5a, b. Cone plexiglas phantom. **a** Regular scan (slice thickness = 10 mm), **b** volume scan (SL = 10 mm, Vt = 10 mm/sec). An axial scan of the cone phantom is a regular circle (**a**). When the phantom is moved during the scan procedure (**b**), the resulting image shows a symmetrical spiral geometrical distortion

speed. Minimal volume averaging artifacts occurred at 8 mm/sec. table incrementation. At an incrementation speed of 12 mm/sec. the volume averaging artifacts began to blur anatomical details. 10 mm/sec. table incrementation speed offered good anatomical detail with an acceptable level of artifacts. In order to cover the largest possible scan volume with an acceptable level of artifacts, a table incrementation speed equal to the slice thickness was selected and used in further experiments.

The ATS high contrast phantom scanned in a conventional abdominal mode gives a spatial resolution of 0.6 mm. A volume scan performed with the same scan parameters and a table incrementation equal to the slice thickness offers a similar spatial resolution (Fig. 4). This phantom is, however, homogeneous in the z-axis. We therefore performed additional high resolution experiments on a skull phantom in the region of the inner ear. Conventional 1 mm scans with a sequential table incrementation of 1 mm were compared with 1 mm volume scans (1 mm slice thickness and table incrementation). As illustrated in Fig. 4, both series offer a similar spatial resolution (the difference in the signal to noise ratio is due to the difference between 210 mAs in the regular scans and 140 mAs in the 0.7 sec. reconstructed volume scans). Furthermore, hardly any artifacts can be recognized in the R = 0.7 sec reconstructed volume scan images.

As shown in Fig. 5, the conventional CT of the cone phantom is a normal circle. The image of the same region obtained with spiral scanning (10 mm slice thickness, Vt = 10 mm/sec) shows only a discrete localized distortion of the circle (local deviation of 1-2 mm).

The patient material reconstructed with R = 0.7 sec. in general displayed detailed images of the abdominal and thoracic regions. 30% of the images suffered to some extent from streak artifacts (Fig. 6). In obese patients, the low radiation dose at 0.7 sec was the main cause of image degradation.

Despite these disadvantages, reconstructions with the commercially available software are fast and easy to use. However these must be performed during or immediately after data acquisition.

The images reconstructed with the special interpolation reconstruction algorithm showed images free of streak artifacts, with a better signal to noise ratio than the 0.7 sec. reconstructed images.

However, the interpolation algorithm can induce volume averaging artifacts and image blurring. Particularly the volume artifacts can be very misleading. Typically, this can occur at an oblique interface between high and low density tissues. At the lower pole of the kidney it might simulate a subscapular effusion (Fig. 6). Image blurring mainly occurred in the chest because of the cardiac motion and vascular pulsation (Fig. 6).

A current disadvantage of the special reconstruction program is the time needed for calculation (about 1 min per image), so that this program cannot yet routinely be applied.

Discussion

As demonstrated by the phantom and patient studies, the diagnostic value of the images is not affected by spiral scanning. This is the result of an optimized combination of table incrementation speed, slice thickness, data acquisition and image reconstruction. The best compromise for image acquisition is a table incrementation speed equal to the slice thickness. This permits covering a maximum acquisition volume with an acceptable level of artifacts. Additional artifact reduction is obtained by reconstructing the images with a reconstruction window of $R = 0.7$ sec. or by using the special spiral scan reconstruction algorithm.

Our preliminary clinical results show hardly any difference between the results obtained by regular scanning and spiral scanning. There is no difference in spatial resolution between the conventional and the volume scans. This is because, in the scan plane, resolution is primarily defined by the detector spacing [12]. In the z-axis (or perpendicular to the image plane), however, changes in slice thickness can interfere with the volume resolution. Initial calculations [13] indicate that the effective slice thickness of a volume scan (where the physical slice thickness equals the table incrementation speed) is increased for 2 mm slices by about 30%, compared with the effective slice thickness of a regular scan. However, this can be reduced to about 20% when a reconstruction window of $R = 0.7$ sec. is used. For 10 mm slices the effective slice thickness for spiral scanning is only 10% greater than for regular scanning, with a reconstruction window of 1 sec. [13]. The dose to the patient per volume is the same for both techniques.

Although motion artifacts are apparently more prominent in the spiral scans (reconstructed with $R = 0.7$ sec.) than in conventional scans, these hardly affect the anatomical detail and do not interfere with image interpretation. The same applies to the minimum geometrical distortion, which is not even visible in the patient images.

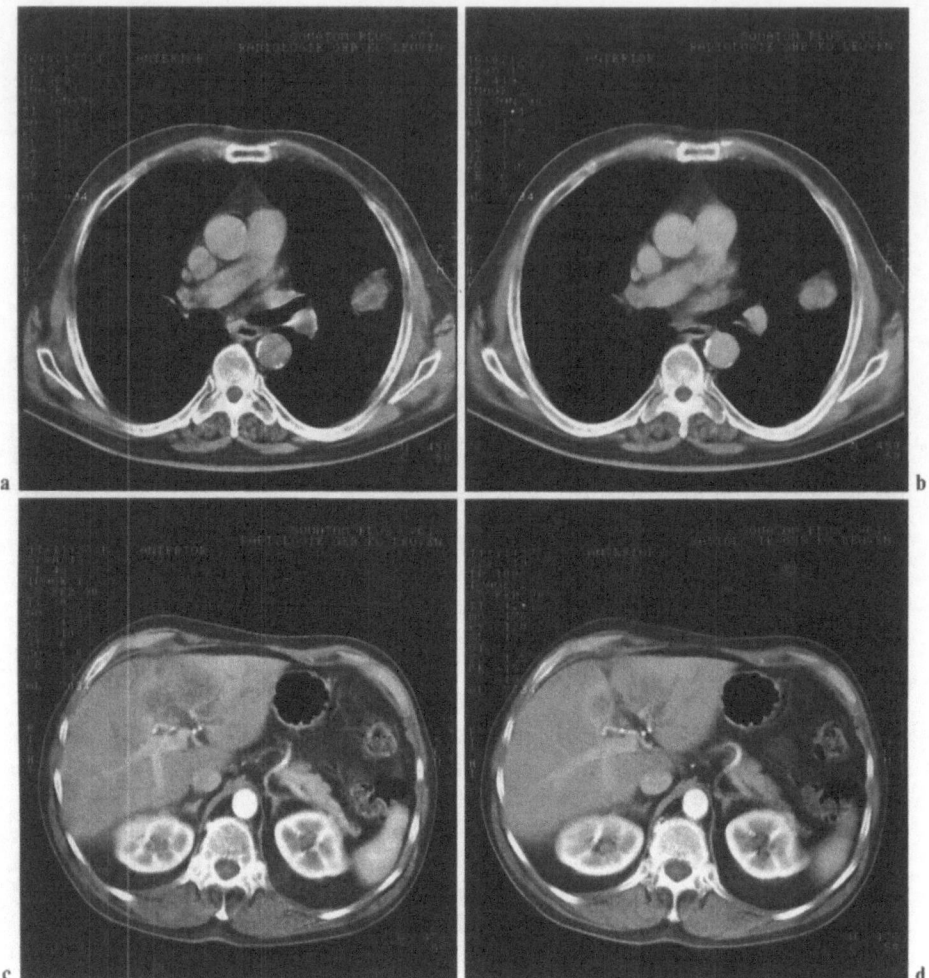

Fig. 6a-d. Patient material reconstructed with R = 0.7 sec., and with the special spiral scan interpolation program. **a** Reconstructed spiral scan (R = 0.7 sec.) of the thorax, **b** interpolated spiral scan of the same acquisition data as (**a**) (R = 1 sec.). Notice that in image **b** the bronchi are somewhat blurred. This is due to pulsatile motion of the heart, which becomes more prominent when the images are reconstructed over 1 second. **c** Reconstructed spiral scan (R = 0.7 sec.) of the abdomen, **d** interpolated spiral scan of the same acquisition data as (**c**). Notice the reduction in signal to noise in **d** compared with **c**

Both reconstruction methods – R = 0.7 sec. and the special interpolation reconstruction algorithm – have advantages and drawbacks. Reconstructions with R = 0.7 sec. are fast and produce very sharp images. Disadvantages are the streak artifacts seen in about 30% of the images and the poor signal to noise ratio in obese patients.

Advantages of the interpolation reconstruction algorithm are the excellent image quality, without any streak artifacts, and the better signal to noise ratio. Draw-

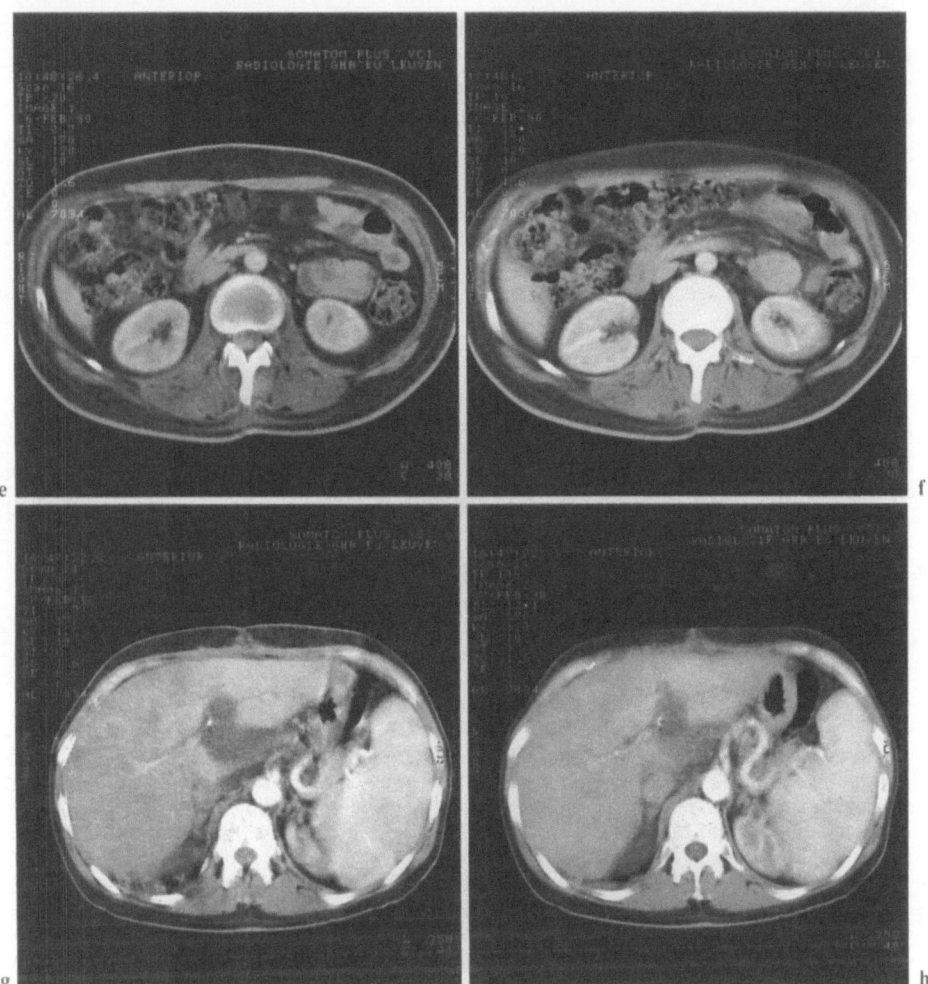

Fig. 6e-h. e Reconstructed spiral scan (R = 0.7 sec.) of the kidney, **f** interpolated spiral scan of the same acquisition data as (e) (R = 1 sec.). Notice the false double contour of the left kidney (f), suggesting a subscapular haematoma. This is not seen in (e) and is the result of volume averaging artifacts over normal renal paraenchyma and perirenal fat. **g** Reconstructed spiral scan (R = 0.7 sec.) of the abdomen, **h** interpolated spiral scan on the same acquisition data as (g) (R = 1 sec.)

backs of this method are the occurrence of blurred images due to volume averaging. Another disadvantage at present is the time consuming reconstruction.

The phantom tests have shown that the feasibility of spiral scanning and the image quality obtained with the first patients is encouraging.

The technique of spiral scanning offers many new approaches in scanning the body and has real advantages over regular scanning. These include the possibility of scanning an entire organ during a very short period after bolus injection of a contrast medium. This should at least theoretically improve the possibilities for using nonselective contrast agents.

Spiral scanning, particularly when images are calculated with an interval smaller than the reconstruction window, produces a series of overlapping images. This guarantees the complete exploration of the imaged organ. Overlapping images also allow visualizing the scan volume in a cine loop mode. An improved patient throughout is also a major advantage that can be expected.

References

1. Lee SK, Sagel SS, Stanley R (1989) Computed body tomography: Physical principles and image quality considerations. Raven Press, New York, second edition, pp 1-20
2. Rigauts H, Marchal G, Baert AL, Hupke R (1989) A six month clinical evaluation with the SOMATOM PLUS. Electromedica
3. Shepard JAO, Dedrick CG, Spizarny DL, Mc Loud TC (1986) Dynamic sequential computed tomography of the pulmonary hilus using a flowrate injector. J Comput Assist Tomogr 10: 369-371
4. Tiffany TF, Kou-Kou H (1988) Acute stroke: Detection of changes in cerebral perfusion with dynamic CT scanning. Radiology 169: 469-474
5. Drayer BP, Heinz ER, Dujovny M, Wolfson SK, Gur D (1979) Patterns of brain perfusion: Dynamic computed tomography using intravenous contrast medium. J Comput Assist Tomogr 3: 633-640
6. Foley WD (1989) Dynamic hepatic CT. Radiology 170: 617-622
7. Moss AA, Dean BP, Axel L, Goldberg HI, Glazer GM, Friedman MA (1982) Dynamic CT of hepatic masses with intravenous and intraarterial contrast material. AJR 138: 847-852
8. Matsui O, Kadoya M, Suzuki M et al. (1983) Dynamic sequential computed tomography during arterial portography in the detection of hepatic neoplasm. Radiology 146: 721-727
9. Foley WD, Berland LL, Lawson TL, Smith DF, Thorsen MK (1983) Contrast enhancement technique for dynamic hepatic computed tomography scanning. Radiology 147: 797-803
10. Young SW, Moon MA, Nassi M, Castellino RA (1980) Dynamic computed tomography body scanning. J Comput Assist Tomogr 4: 168-173
11. Kalender WA, Seißler W, Klotz E, Vock P (1989) Single-breathhold spiral volumetric computed tomography (SVCT) by continuous patient translation and scanner rotation. Radiology 1990 (in print)
12. Glover GH, Eisner RL (1979) Theoretical resolution of computed tomography systems. J Comput Assist Tomogr 3: 85-91
13. Vestner effective slice thickness calculations in spiral scanning (1989) Private communications. Siemens AG Erlangen, W Germany

Single-Breathhold Spiral Volumetric CT (SVCT) of the Lung and the Hepato-Biliary System

P. VOCK, M. SOUCEK, M. DAEPP, W. A. KALENDER

Abstract

We adapted the table feed mechanism for patient transport during continuous rotation scanning with the intention to examine complete subvolumes of the lung and the hepato-biliary system during a single breathhold. 21 adult patients for each of the two areas were scanned during up to 12 continuous 1-second rotations; data acquisition was synchronized with longitudinal patient motion at 1 slice thickness per second. Interpolated planar raw data were obtained retrospectively for any level within the volume. Image quality was comparable to standard images. Due to the continuous scanning process, pulmonary nodules and focal hepatic lesions were never omitted, their center could always be depicted, and secondary reformations as well as 3D-reconstructions were easily obtained. We conclude that SVCT, by completely surveying a subvolume of the lung or the hepato-biliary system, is an attractive new application of CT.

Introduction

Interscan respiration in ordinary CT prolongs contrast enhancement studies beyond the early vascular phase and, due to irreproducible lung volumes, makes anatomically continuous scanning difficult (Vock et al. 1989). Pulmonary nodules or focal upper abdominal lesions may be missed and other levels scanned twice, secondary reformations are often of poor quality.

Our hypothesis was that a spiral scanning geometry based on longitudinal table motion with simultaneous tube rotation might investigate complete subvolumes within the lung or hepato-biliary system during a single breathhold. This approach which we term "single-breathhold spiral volumetric computed tomography (SVCT)" would allow us to achieve anatomically continuous scanning and to optimally use the early phase of intravenous contrast enhancement.

Methods

42 patients of age 19 to 90 years were studied. Among the 21 patients with pulmonary disease, 3 had lung cancer, 9 lung metastases, 3 benign mass lesions and 6 localized benign lung disease without any mass effect. Among the 21 patients with

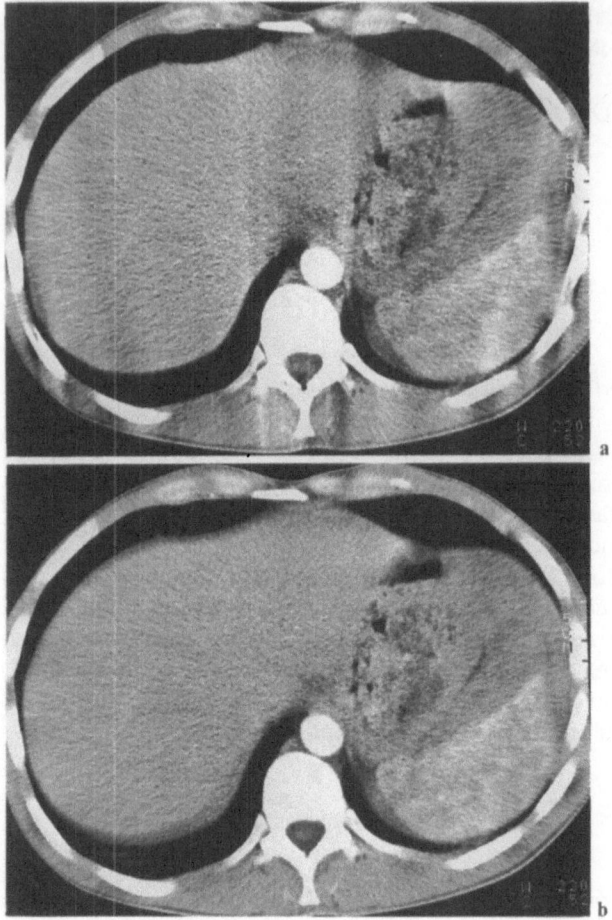

Fig. 1a, b. Non-corrected (upper) and corrected (lower) image of abdominal SVCT study. The disturbing streak artifacts on the upper image are no longer present on the lower corrected image

hepato-biliary disease, 4 had a hepatocellular carcinoma, 4 liver metastases, 6 non neoplastic focal liver disease and 7 biliary disease.

Ordinary single-slice CT examination consisted of 10 mm thick slices spaced at 10 to 15 mm, using 120 kVp in the abdomen and 137 kVp in the chest, 200 to 250 mA and 1 second scan time. Some patients also had scans at 2 to 8 mm collimation.

Our SOMATOM PLUS allows up to 12 continuous 1-second rotations at 170 mA or up to 5 rotations at 250 mA. To realize SVCT, we used an experimental setup with a modified integrated table feed mechanism and a dedicated reconstruction algorithm. Scanning was synchronized with longitudinal table motion, as used for scout views, at a speed of one slice thickness per second (Kalender et al. 1989). Depending on the clinical problem, a slice thickness of 2 mm, 5 mm, 8 mm or 10 mm was selected. The table speed was 2 to 10 mm per second accordingly,

Table 1. SVCT versus CT of the lung (N=21)

Nominal slice thickness		2 mm (N=7)		5-8-10 mm (N=14)	
Quality		SVCT=CT	SVCT>CT	SVCT=CT	SVCT>CT
Lung cancer	3			3	
Lung metastases	9	4	1	1	3
Benign mass	3	1	1	1	
Benign, no mass	6			5	1
Total	21	5	2	10	4

Table 2. SVCT versus CT of the hepatobiliary system (N=21)[a]

Quality		SVCT<CT	SVCT=CT
Hepatocellular Ca	4	0	4
Liver metastases	4	2	2
Benign liver dis.	6	0	6
Biliary disease	7	2	5
Total	21	4	17

[a] Nominal slice thickness of SVCT always 8 mm (n=4) or 10 mm (n=17)

mostly for a 10- to 12-second scanning time. In the current experimental configuration, data transfer and processing had to be carried out immediately after the spiral scan; the scanner was blocked for up to ten minutes. Therefore SVCT scans were always the final scans of the total study. After transfer from the image processor to the harddisk, adjacent helical raw data were interpolated in order to retrospectively synthesize non-distorted planar raw data for arbitrary table positions (down to 1 mm-intervals) within the volume (Kalender et al. 1989); according to the clinical problem, subsequent calculation of images was performed for any field of view, any slice center, using standard and/or bone algorithms.

Scan quality was assessed by two radiologists comparing the detectability and distinctness of normal vessels, bronchi and of morphologic details of pathology. SVCT was called inferior, equal or superior to single scans of the same area.

Results

Non-corrected spiral volumetric scans exhibited significant streak artifacts on soft tissue windows and minor ones on lung windows, whereas these artifacts were no longer present on interpolated images (Fig. 1). Corrected scans compared well with single scans both of the lung (Fig. 2) and the upper abdomen (Fig. 3) and demonstrated the lesions in a continuous sequence, allowing morphologic analysis and differentiation of pathology. As the images could be reconstructed for arbi-

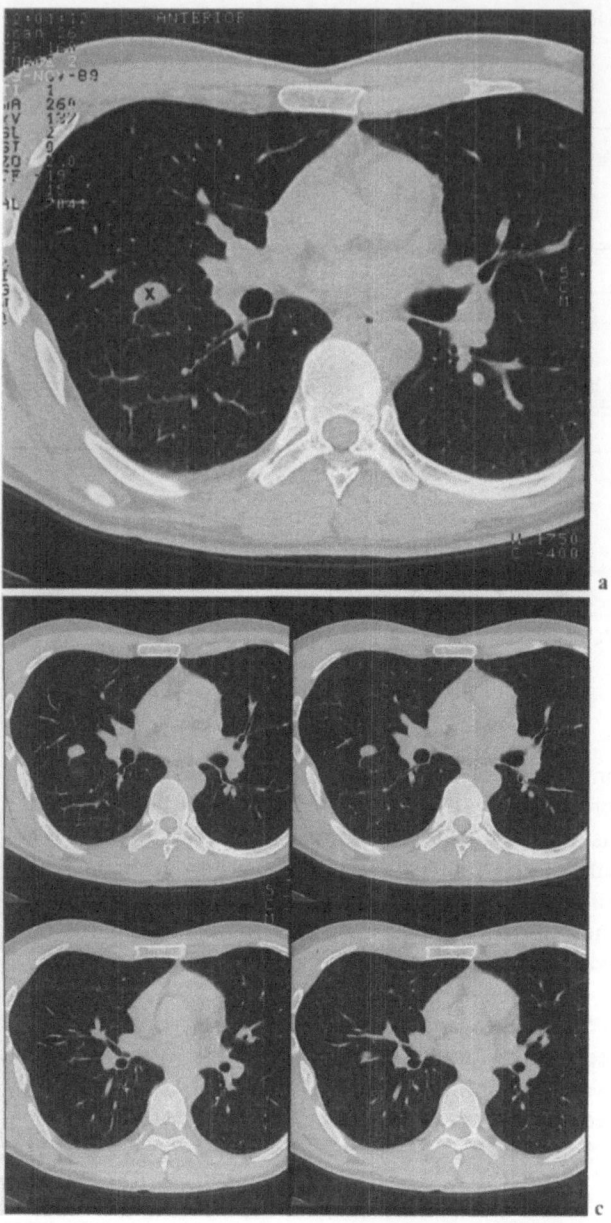

Fig. 2a–d. Small posttraumatic subpleural pulmonary hematoma (x) in front and contiguous to the right oblique fissure. Similarly detailed normal anatomy and pathology are demonstrated on the conventional 2 mm-thick section (260 mAs, **a**) and on the corresponding SVCT image

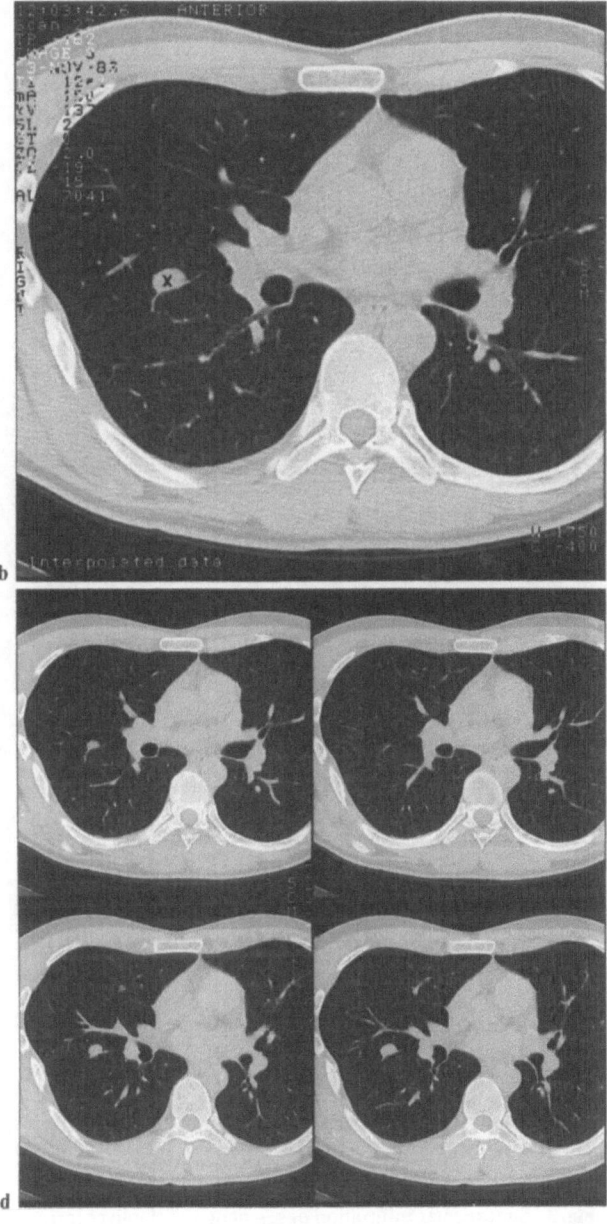

Fig. 2. (Continued) (150 mAs, **b**) using the same nominal thickness. **c, d** The lower eight images represent contiguous slices through the hematoma reconstructed from the same SVCT scan

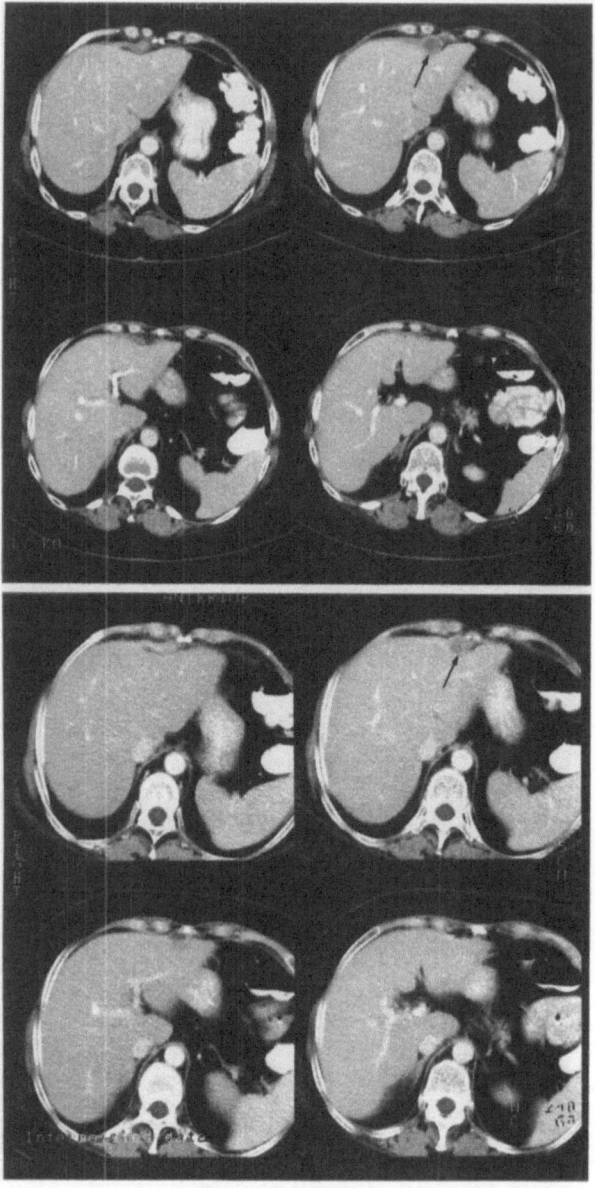

Fig. 3. Subcapsular infiltration of segment 3 of the liver (arrow) in peritoneal metastases from carcinoma of the uterus. The upper four scans were taken during a dynamic contrast-enhanced sequence whereas the lower four corresponding images were selected from the subsequent SVCT study

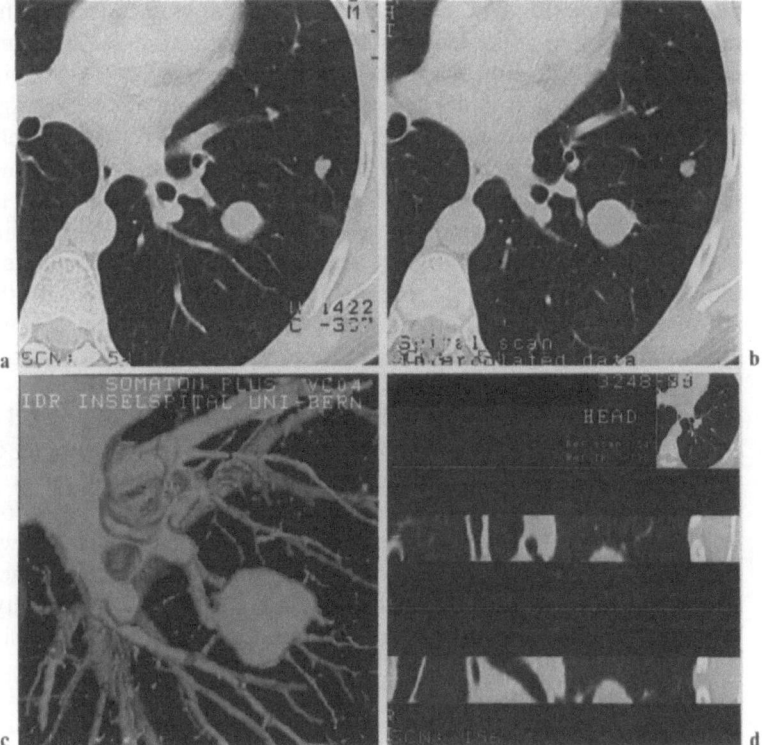

Fig. 4a–d. 29 years old female patient with Carney's triad. SVCT study of two pulmonary hamartomas of the left lower lobe (**a, b**). **c** Shows a three-dimensional view from above of the larger lesion, **d** an oblique coronal reformation with the relation of the upper pole of the hamartoma to the left main and lower lobe bronchus

trary table positions within the scanning volume, the center of a pulmonary nodule or a focal hepato-biliary lesion could always be selected. Secondary reformations were superior to those from a series of single scans (Fig. 4). In the lung, the quality of SVCT was judged as good as or better than that of conventional scans (Table 1). In the enhanced studies of the upper abdomen, SVCT was as good as or slightly inferior to the dynamic sequence obtained earlier (Table 2).

Discussion

Our early results demonstrate the practicality of SVCT of the lung and the hepato-biliary system for a subvolume of up to 12 cm with a scan quality comparable to single scans. The artifacts resulting from the spiral scanning geometry are adequately removed by linear interpolation into planar data.

   The technique is currently limited by tube heating and the storage capacity of the image processor. The time needed for data transfer to the harddisk was the reason for our using SVCT at the end of patient studies. With contrast enhancement of the upper abdomen, this allowed either a pure SVCT technique or a second look by SVCT after the initial bolus injected during a dynamic sequence. In most of these cases, in order to keep the total amount of contrast agent injected at a normal level, the second bolus for SVCT was reduced (40 to 60 ml). This and the reduced contrast between normal parenchyma and lesions due to interstitial diffusion of the contrast agent injected earlier were probably the main reasons for the inferiority of SVCT in some abdominal studies. Although the nominal slice thickness is increased by 30 to 40% by the helical interpolation procedure, partial volume effects did not turn out to become a significant problem. In the lung, SVCT allowed reconstruction of more levels within a given volume, as compared to normal contiguous scans. We think that this was the reason for a sometimes better behavior of SVCT in detecting small anatomical structures.

Already now, single-breathhold spiral volumetric CT can be used during routine clinical studies and affords anatomically continuous scanning of organ subvolumes. Therefore, focal lesions are not missed, and their center can retrospectively be selected both for densitometry and for optimal morphologic analysis. Radiation dose is lower than for a comparable conventional study with contiguous slices. Finally, the timing of vascular and parenchymal enhancement studies can be optimized, sometimes even the contrast dose reduced. Continuity of slices also offers better quality of secondary reformations and three-dimensional presentations.

References

Vock P, Jung H, Kalender W (1989) Single-breath-hold Spiral Volumetric CT of the lung. Radiology 173 (P): 400 (and Radiology 1990, in print)
Kalender W, Seissler W, Vock P (1990) Single-breath-hold Spiral Volumetric CT by continuous patient translation and scanner rotation. Radiology 176: July 1990
Vock P, Jung H, Kalender W (1989) Single-Breathhold Spiral Volumetric CT of the hepatobiliary system. Radiology 173 (P): 377

Quantitative CT of the Lung with Spirometrically Controlled Respiratory Status and Automated Evaluation Procedures

W. A. KALENDER, R. RIENMÜLLER, J. BEHR, W. SEISSLER, H. FICHTE, M. WELKE

Abstract

Quantitative determination of lung density and structure by CT can be of high clinical value, but suitable procedures are needed to ensure reproducibility and objectivity. We present a newly developed, complete protocol for this task which addresses CT measurement as well as image evaluation.

A microcomputer-controlled pocket spirometer is employed to measure vital capacity, to control the level of inspiration during the CT examination and to trigger the scan at a user-selected respiratory level. Evaluation is based on semi-automated algorithms which isolate lung parenchyma by fast contour tracing and define subregions by shrinking and radial and anteroposterior subdividing of the left and the right lung. Global and regional mean density values and histogram parameters are extracted.

Lung density changes by more than a factor of 2 were found in clinical studies as a function of inspirational status. This is a clear indication that tight control of respiratory status is absolutely necessary for reproducible lung density measurements. The evaluation software also improves reproducibility, but above all supports the investigator in his work and provides the possibilities for an extended analysis.

Introduction

High-resolution CT imaging of the lung parenchyma constitutes a wide-spread clinical CT application [e. g. 1-4]. Diagnosis is usually based on a subjective, qualitative assessment of changes in morphology and density by an experienced radiologist. Quantitative evaluation of CT images with respect to density, on the other hand, has also been investigated in numerous studies. Applications focussed on assessing pulmonary emphysema [5-10], sarcoidosis [11], panbronchiolitis [12], and silicosis [13], on determining post-irradiation lung density changes [14], bleomycin-related lung damage [15-17] and the relation of pulmonary density to pulmonary mechanics [18]. However, it cannot be postulated at this time that quantitative applications are well-established and generally accepted. Quantification appears to pose more difficult problems than imaging.

The respective methodological aspects of quantitative assessment of lung density by CT have also been addressed in numerous studies [19-27]. Some of these indicated a principal problem of lung density measurements: the respiratory status, ranging from full expiration to full inspiration, will drastically affect density measurements [5, 19, 20, 22, 26, 28, 29]; this will also be demonstrated below. An exact control of the degree of inspiration appears mandatory. We therefore have developed and here present a means for the definition and control of the respiratory status and for respiratory gating.

Evaluation of CT images may also pose significant problems, both with respect to user efforts and to reproducibility. Manual insertion of regions of interest (ROIs) is a time-consuming and responsible task, above all if regional or segmental analysis is required [12, 16–20, 22, 26–28]. We therefore propose and present semi-automated algorithms for ROI definition. These include definition of regional or segmental ROIs, an extended histogram analysis and determination of a.-p. gradients.

Methods

Apparatus for Respiratory Gating

We developed an experimental set-up which has been described in an earlier report [30]. Its purpose is to trigger scans at a user-selected level of respiration and to interrupt air flow during the scan. The definition of the level of inspiration is achieved by a spirometric measurement. We employ a small-size hand-held transducer (Micro Medical Instruments, Rochester, UK) through which the patient is asked to breathe (Fig. 1). In this open spirometer system, rotational air flow is created by a set of turbines and is directed onto a vane. Two light barriers are incorporated to detect the frequency and direction of rotation of the vane. Flow and volume measurements are achieved by counting the rotations of the vane. Accuracy is specified to be 2%; BTPS (Body Temperature Pressure Saturated) corrections are applied.

A microcomputer was connected to the transducer to determine vital capacity (VC) and to generate trigger signals at a user-selected level of inspiration. These levels can be chosen either in percent of vital capacity or as an absolute volume in liters above residual lung volume. A typical breathing curve is sketched in Fig. 1. Simultaneous to generating and sending a trigger signal to the CT scanner, air flow is inhibited by closing a valve attached to the transducer, i. e. the momentary respiratory status is kept constant for the duration of the CT scan. By practicing the breathing maneuver before the CT examination, the patient is prepared for this. Since he can remove the spirometer at any time, there is no risk involved.

CT Scanning Technique

CT scans were obtained on a SOMATOM PLUS; the preferred scan parameters were 1 s scan time, 250 mA tube current, 1 or 2 mm slice thickness and 120 kVp voltage. Scans were triggered from the respiratory gating device (dynamic modes)

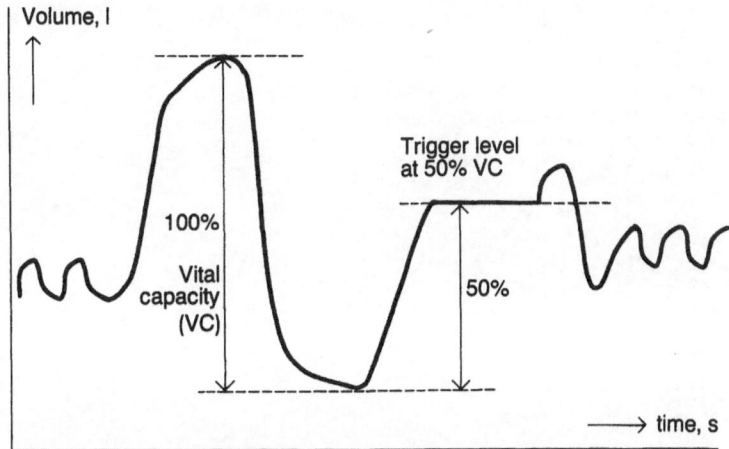

Fig. 1. Typical breathing curve for obtaining CT scans at a defined inspiratory volume. After a vital capacity measurement, the CT scan is triggered at a user-selected level, defined in percent of the VC

or started manually, observing the spirometer signals. Three slices per patient were selected via a localizer radiograph, one through the carina and one each at 5 cm above and below that cut. Before taking the CT scans, a spirometric measurement of the vital capacity was obtained. Thereafter, the trigger level was chosen; we typically measured at 50% of vital capacity. In several studies, scans were obtained at 20%, 50% and 80% for the same position.

Image Evaluation

Our aim was to automate the evaluation of the total study to as high a degree as possible; speed and the extraction of parameters beyond mean density values were of further importance [31]. A detailed description of the algorithm and a performance evaluation are given in a separate report [32]. The primary objective is to isolate the left and the right lung in each CT scan in a semi-automated fashion. The algorithm first determines an approximate center of mass of each lung field by determining the coordinates of all pixels in the image with values between two threshold values, typically -800 and -500 Hounsfield Units (HU), and calculating the center of mass of these determined pixels, separately for the left and the right half of the image matrix. Using these starting points for both lung fields initial points on the lung contour are determined by searching towards the lateral border; i. e., line profiles are read and a threshold value for the soft tissue-to-lung interface is used, typically -200 HU. To prevent intermediate intra-lung structures from being erroneously accepted as lung contour points, several profiles are read out above and below the approximate center of mass. The outermost point is accepted as the starting point for contour tracing. To trace the lung contour, which

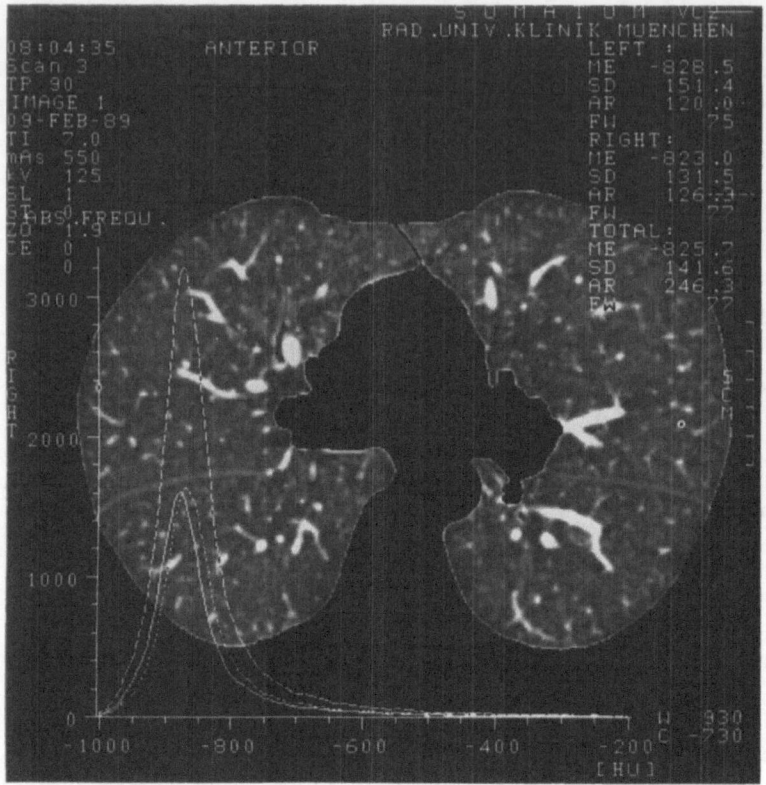

Fig. 2. Isolated lung parenchyma and corresponding histograms for the left (——), for the right (. . . .), and for the total lung (---)

represents a transition of several hundred HU in most cases, a standard algorithm [32] has been adapted. The possibility for user interaction is provided for every step of the algorithm.

When the contour is accepted, the image background, i. e. everything but the lung parenchyma, is erased. Histograms are determined for the left, the right and the total lung. In their analysis, mean values, standard deviations, most frequent values, full widths at half maximum (FWHM) and arbitrary percentiles of the histograms are calculated (Fig. 2). Images may be segmented in several ways. An arbitrary number n of subregions in the anterior-posterior direction is generated by calculating those lines which divide the left and right lung, respectively, into equal areas (one n-th of the total area each). Anteroposterior differences are thus calculated directly; an estimate of the a.-.p. gradient can be calculated as the linear fit line to the subregion mean values (Fig. 3). Alternatively, peripheral lung ROIs can be generated by calculating a second contour in parallel to the lung contour at a fixed distance in millimeters (Fig. 4).

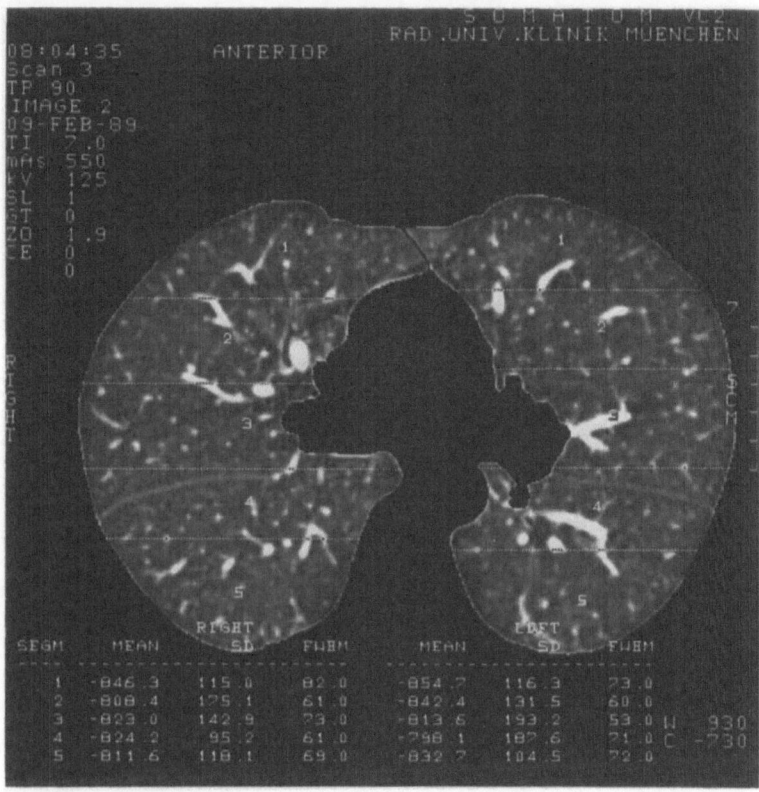

Fig. 3. Definition of lung segments in anteroposterior direction. The left and right lung are divided into an arbitrarily selected number of subsegments of equal area. The a.-p. gradient can be estimated as the fit to the mean CT values of the subsegments

Results

The use of the spirometer system did not pose any problems with respect to patient compliance. The inhibition of respiration for about 5–10 s was tolerated well; the patients were instructed and were aware that they could remove the spirometer mouthpiece at any time. We tested how well patients reproduced the triggering point at 50% VC in three consecutive spirometry trials. Healthy volunteers ($N = 10$) exhibited a mean deviation of 1.0% ($\sigma = 4.2\%$); in patients with obstructive and restrictive ventilation disturbances, a mean deviation of 5.7% ($\sigma = 7.3\%$) was found. Particular problems for repeatedly performing expiratory VC maneuvers are given in patients with obstructive disease. Compared to a standard closed spirometer (Jäger, Würzburg, FRG), no significant differences with respect to accuracy were found [33]. Although calibrated according to BTPS conditions, the spirometer system exhibited some drift. For a three-minute breathing period, the baseline may fluctuate by up to 0.2 liters typically, depending on the

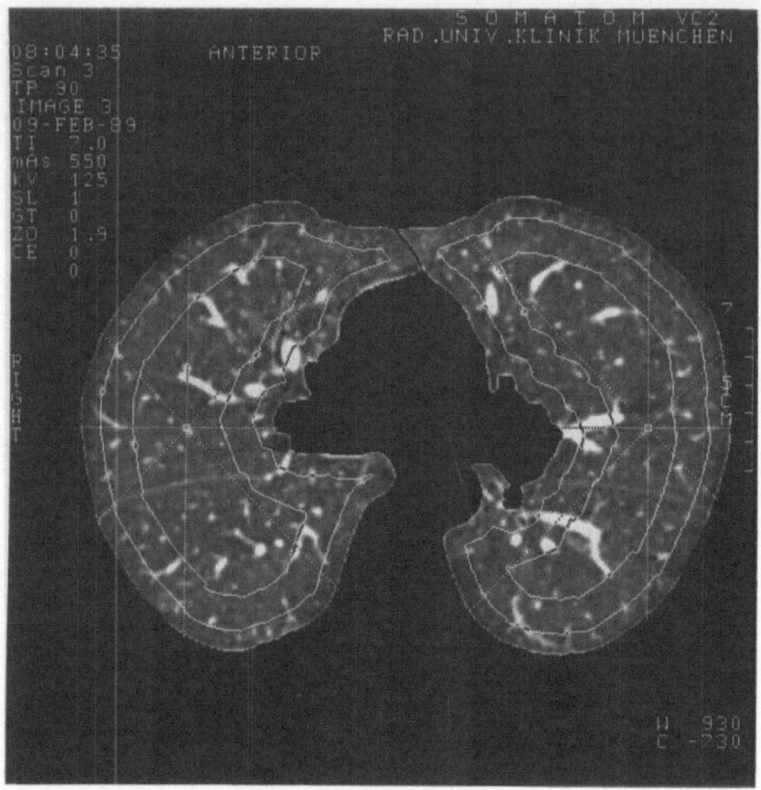

Fig. 4. Definition of peripheral lung ROIs by shrinking. Peripheral lung segments can be defined in an arbitrary, but reproducible manner by contour shrinking and radial divisions. Here, contours with a distance of 8 mm and 20 mm, respectively, measured normal to the lung boundary are shown

individual breathing behavior. To exclude drift influences with certainty, we decided to repeat the VC maneuver before each of the three scans.

Contour tracing for both lungs takes about 2 s per image without interaction; possible interaction, background deletion, segmentation and histogram analysis take additional time depending on the interaction, the number of segments, etc. The frequency of user interactions depended on the degree of anatomical variations and pathology. Studies on normals and the more cranial slices appear less critical; central and basal scans of the lung and pathological findings may demand interaction rather frequently. In the first 50 clinical studies, interaction was necessary in about half of the images.

The precision of the whole procedure was tested in one volunteer study. The complete study was repeated three times with the subject being repositioned every time. A standard deviation of 2.1 HU (1.2%) resulted; reproducibility for single slices was 3.1 HU, 6.7 HU and 3.6 HU, respectively [30]. The influence of respiratory status was also measured in this volunteer study at 20%, 50% and 80% of vital capacity for the central slice. When going from 20% to 80% inspiration, mean CT values dropped from -763 HU to -862 HU, corresponding to lung densities of approximately 237 and 138 mg/ml, respectively [30]. A 10% change in inspirational status resulted on average in a change of about 16 mg/ml in density. Using linear extrapolation to estimate lung density at 0% and 100% vital capacity, 105 and 270 mg/ml would result, corresponding to a density change by about a factor of 2.6.

Discussion

Quantitative computed tomography presents a measure of the attenuation of an x-ray beam by a volume element of tissue. Since attenuation in the lung is very closely related to density, CT may provide absolute, rather than relative density estimations. This is a unique advantage as compared with other radiographic techniques. Both accuracy and reproducibility of CT density measurements of the lung have been discussed previously [23, 25, 26]. In our study, we above all addressed the question of reproducibility. We accordingly present and discuss methodological aspects of CT measurements of lung density in this paper.

It is obvious that lung density depends on the status of inspiration; this dependence has been measured both by CT [5, 19, 20, 22, 26, 28] and by Compton densitometry [29]. These studies did not present a practical solution to the problem, however. We have developed a respiratory gating device based on spirometric measurements which may alleviate this problem. Any level of inspiration can be reproduced, according to objective criteria. Previously used subjective descriptions of respiratory status like "in arrested inspiration" [5], "at a lung volume slightly above functional residual capacity" [6], "during suspended mid-inspiration" [15], "scanned during breathholding midway between normal volume inspiration and expiration" [28] or similar statements can be replaced by more precise and objective statements.

Compared to a standard closed spirometer the open system showed no significant disadvantages with respect to accuracy and compared favorably with respect to handling, patient reactions and the fact that it intrinsically offers electronic output. Drift of the system is the only limitation which we see at this time. For our present work this does not constitute a principal problem, since we repeat the VC measurement before any scan to reset the system. However, it would be clearly advantageous and easier for the patient if a single VC measurement were sufficient for a complete study. Such a system would lend itself to a number of other applications.

A general limitation of any spirometric technique for longitudinal measurements may result if the patient fails to reproduce the levels of full expiration and inspiration required for the measurements of vital capacity in successive examinations. In particular, this may be the case in patients with obstructive respiratory disease. If so, careful patient monitoring and instruction can improve the situation. It has been pointed out, for example, that "the degree of inflation achieved on the 'deep inspiration' instruction varied greatly among subjects" [20]. Apparently, trust is not sufficient to minimize patient-related errors. It therefore appears to be an improvement that the spirometer provides an objective and reliable control if the patient cooperates successfully.

Reproducibility errors due to the operator's intervention in the evaluation process may be considered smaller than the patient-related effects discussed above. Still, such errors have to be expected, for example when manually entering ROIs. Such effects become more pronounced in more detailed evaluations, e.g. for regional density values or for quantitative descriptors of morphology. Automated evaluation algorithms ensure reproducibility and objectivity. A practically much more important and relevant aspect is, however, that such automated procedures will facilitate the operator's work and relieve him of a tedious, time-consuming and responsible task.

The control of both the measurement conditions and of the evaluation procedures should lead to improved reproducibility. Our first and only volunteer study yielded better results than we had expected and than we will generally claim at this stage. We will await further evaluations, possibly by independent groups. A reproducibility in lung density measurements of better than 10 mg/ml or 10 HU, i. e. typically an error $\leq 5\%$ (assuming an average density of about 200 mg/ml), appears to be a high, but realistic aim, however. Ignoring all other error sources, this implies that the respiratory level has to be known within about $\pm 6\%$, measured in percent of VC. This can only be ensured by spirometric control and respiratory gating. We conclude that objective and reproducible measurements of lung density by CT can be achieved by using respiratory gating at defined levels of inspiration, short scan times and automated procedures for ROI definition and evaluation.

References

1. Zerhouni EA, Naidich DP, Stitik FP, Khouri NF, Siegelman SS (1985) Computed tomography of the pulmonary parenchyma. II. Interstitial disease. J Thorac Imaging 1: 54–64
2. Mayo JR, Webb WR, Gould R et al. (1987) High-resolution CT of the lungs: An optimal approach. Radiology 163: 507–510
3. Munk PL, Müller NL, Miller RR, Ostrow DN (1988) Pulmonary lymphangitis carcinomatosis: CT and pathologic findings. Radiology 166: 705–709
4. Mathieson JR, Mayo JR, Staples CA, Mueller NL (1989) Chronic diffuse infiltrative lung disease: Comparison of diagnostic accuracy of CT and chest radiography. Radiology 171: 111–116
5. Goddard PR, Nicholson EM, Laszlo G, Watt I (1982) Computed tomography in pulmonary emphysema. Clinical Radiology 33: 379–387
6. Hayhurst MD, MacNee W, Flenley DC et al. (1984) Diagnosis of pulmonary emphysema by computerised tomography. Lancet 8: 320–322
7. Bergin C, Müller N, Nichols DM et al. (1986) The diagnosis of emphysema. A computed tomographic-pathologic correlation. Am Rev Respir Dis 133: 541–546
8. Sanders C, Nath PH, Bailey WC (1988) Detection of emphysema with computed tomography. Correlation with pulmonary function tests and chest radiography. Invest Radiology 23: 262–266
9. Mueller NL, Staples CA, Miller RR, Abboud RT (1988) An objective method to quantitate emphysema using computed tomography. Chest 94: 782–787

10. Gould GA, MacNee W, McLean A et al. (1988) CT measurements of lung density in life can quantitate distal airspace enlargement – an essential defining feature of human emphysema. Am Rev Respir Dis 137: 380–392
11. Gilman MJ, Laurens RG, Somogyi JW, Honig EG (1983) CT attenuation values of lung density in sarcoidosis. J Comp Ass Tomogr 7: 407–410
12. Murata K, Itoh H, Senda M et al. (1989) Stratified impairment of pulmonary ventilation in 'diffuse panbronchiolitis': PET and CT studies. J Comp Ass Tomogr 13: 48–53
13. Rienmüller R, Schätzl M, Kalender W, Krombach F, Fiehl E (1988) Quantitative CT-Untersuchungen der Lunge am tierexperimentellen Modell der Silikose. Fortschr Röntgenstr 148: 347–486
14. Van Dyk J, Hill RP (1983) Post irradiation lung density changes as measured by computerised tomography. Int J Radiation Oncology Biol Phys 9: 847–852
15. Bellamy EA, Husband JE, Blaquiere RU, Law MR (1985) Bleomycin-related lung damage: CT evidence. Radiology 156: 155–158
16. Rimmer MJ, Dixon AK, Flower CDR, Sikora K (1985) Bleomycin lung: computed tomographic observations. British J Radiology 58: 1041–1045
17. Bellamy EA, Nocholas D, Husband JE (1987) Quantitative assessment of lung damage due to bleomycin using computed tomography. British J Radiology 60: 1205–1209
18. Wollmer P, Albrechtsson U, Brauer K et al. (1986) Measurement of pulmonary density by means of X-ray computerized tomography. Relation to pulmonary mechanics in normal subjects. Chest 90: 387–391
19. Wegener OH, Koeppe P, Oeser H (1978) Measurement of lung density by computed tomography. J Comp Ass Tomogr 2: 263
20. Robinson PJ, Kreel L (1979) Pulmonary tissue attenuation with computed tomography: Comparison of inspiration and expiration scans. J Comp Ass Tomogr 3: 740
21. Doehring W, Linke G (1979) Die Grundlagen der quantitativen pulmonalen Computertomographie. Fortschr Roentgenstr 130: 133–143
22. Rosenblum LJ, Mauceri RA, Wellenstein DE et al. (1980) Density patterns in the normal lung as determined by computed tomography. Radiology 137: 409–416
23. Rhodes CG, Wollmer P, Fazio F, Jones T (1981) Quantitative measurement of regional extravascular lung density using positron emission and transmission tomography. J Comp Ass Tomogr 5: 783–791
24. Keller JM, Edwards FM, Rundle R (1981) Automatic outlining of regions on CT scans. J Comp Ass Tomogr 5: 240–245
25. Hedlund LW, Anderson RF, Goulding PL, Beck JW, Effmann EL, Putman CE (1982) Two methods for isolating the lung area of a CT scan for density information. Radiology 144: 353–357
26. Hedlund LW, Vock P, Effmann EL (1983) Evaluating lung density by computed tomography. Seminars in Respiratory Medicine 5: 76–87
27. Wandtke JC, Hyde RW, Fahey JP et al. (1986) Measurement of lung gas volume and regional density by computed tomography in dogs. Invest Radiol 21: 108–117
28. Vock P, Malanowski D, Tschaeppeler H, Kirks DR, Hedlund LW, Effmann EL (1987) Computed tomographic lung density in children. Invest Radiol 22: 627–631
29. Reiss KH, Schuster W (1972) Quantitative measurements of lung function in children by means of compton backscatter. Radiology 102: 613–617
30. Kalender W, Rienmüller R, Seissler W, Behr J, Welke M, Fichte H (1990) Spirometric gating for measuring pulmonary parenchymal density by quantitative computed tomography. Radiology 175: 265–268
31. Kalender W, Rienmüller R, Welke M (1988) Algorithm for automated evaluation of high-resolution CT images of the lung. Radiology 169 (P): 116
32. Kalender W, Fichte H, Bautz W (1990) Semi-automatic evaluation procedures for quantitative CT of the lung. Submitted to J Comp Ass Tomogr
33. Behr J, Merin M, Rienmüller R, Kalender W, Fruhmann G (1989) Quantitative analysis of interstitial lung disease with spirometrically standardized high resolution tomography. Europ Respiratory J 2 (8): 672

CT Examinations of Lung Ventilation with Stable Xenon

W. Bautz, R. Klier, H. Bongers, W. A. Kalender

Abstract

CT diagnosis of lung morphology often correlates poorly with clinical findings and lung function test results. Stable xenon constitutes an inhalation contrast medium for CT which allows assessing lung ventilation both in a quantitative and a qualitative manner. We describe the method and report on our first clinical results.

Introduction

In spite of the great success of high-resolution CT in the diagnosis of lung morphology, CT results often do not show satisfactory correlation with clinical findings and the results of lung function tests. Earlier efforts to achieve clinically meaningful results focussed on densitometry [5, 14]. These methods were prone to error [7], however, and have not been accepted for routine diagnosis due to methodological problems. For successful quantitative computed tomography (QCT) studies of the lung, images of high quality and free of artifacts are required as well as high reproducibility of all measurement parameters, including the inspiratory level of the patient.

The new continuously rotating scanners offer significantly improved image quality due to higher spatial resolution and shorter scan times, as compared to standard CT scanners which work with conventional start-stop technique. Partly, the gain in spatial resolution can be attributed to minimizing motion blurring by subsecond sanning. In addition, Kalender et al. have presented means for triggering CT scans at freely selectable inspiratory or expiratory breathing volumes [10]. Also, automated evaluation programs for the lung have been developed on the basis of fast contour tracing algorithms; with a minimum of operator interaction, they allow isolating the lung parenchyma and defining regions for density measurement and further analysis [9]. Thus, new methods are available which, in combination with the improved image quality, might lead to a breakthrough in QCT of the lung. There remain doubts, however, if densitometry and structure analysis of the lung will allow statements on lung function in all cases.

The use of stable xenon as an inhalation contrast medium opens new perspectives for examinations of the lung. Earlier efforts in conventional radiography [13] and digital radiography [3] did not yield satisfactory results for clinical use or, similar to digital dual energy radiography [2], are not available for routine diagnosis.

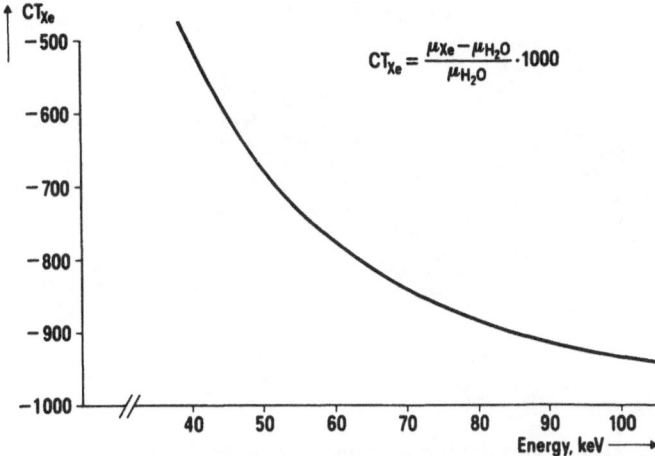

$$CT_{Xe} = \frac{\mu_{Xe} - \mu_{H_2O}}{\mu_{H_2O}} \cdot 1000$$

Fig. 1. CT numbers of pure xenon as a function of energy

The new high-resolution CT scanners with continuously rotating measuring system and the methodological advances described above provide an adequate basis for CT ventilation studies with xenon for the first time. We want to demonstrate the potential of the method by means of volunteer studies and our first clinical results.

Material and Methods

CT values of xenon exhibit the strong dependence on photon energy which is typical for contrast media (Fig. 1). This is due to the high atomic number of this element ($Z = 54$), very close to that of iodine ($Z = 53$), which gives rise to strong absorption of X-rays mostly due to the photoelectric effect. For a 120 kVp spectrum (corresponding to an effective energy of about 70 keV) stable xenon yielded CT values of about -860 Hounsfield units (HU), i.e. 140 HU above air. To avoid side effects of xenon in patient examinations, we used xenon/oxygen gas mixtures containing 40–60% xenon, resulting in an enhancement of 50–80 HU in the lung.

Our examinations were done on a continuously rotating scanner (SOMATOM PLUS, Siemens AG, Erlangen). Following a standard CT examination of the lung, the ventilation studies were carried out in dynamic CT mode for selected slices (dynamic sequence at 120 kVp, 170 mAs, 10 mm slice thickness, 2s cycle time, 9 scans, standard reconstruction). All scans were taken at maximal inspiration. The reference scan of the dynamic CT series served as plain scan for the qualitative and quantitative evaluations after xenon inhalation (contrast scans). Immediately before starting the dynamic CT series, the patient exhales maximally and then inhales the Xe/O_2 mixture through a mouthpiece from the gas bag until maximal inspiration is reached.

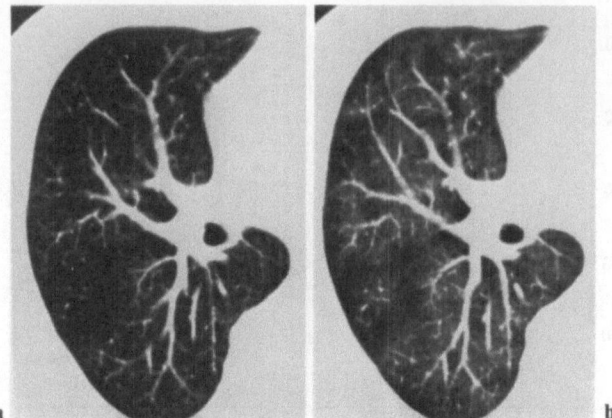

Fig. 2a, b. Xenon distribution in the lung. **a** Plain scan, **b** Xenon inhalation. Immediately after xenon inhalation, strong enhancement is seen in the central zones of the lung lobuli

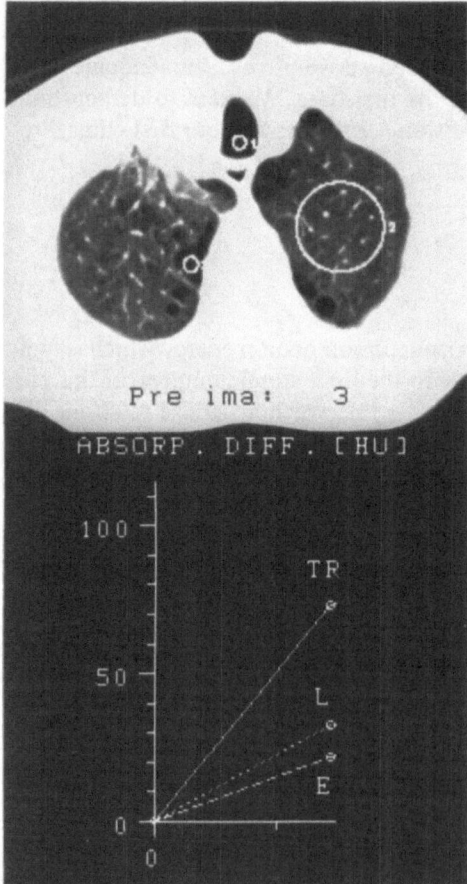

Fig. 3. Subpleural emphysema bullae. After inhalation of stable xenon, only a small enhancement is seen in the emphysema (E) as compared to the trachea (TR) and the left upper lung field (L). The emphysematous regions enhanced to different degrees indicating differences in their ventilation

To evaluate the studies, we determined the time density curves for both the total lung and the left and right lung separately with the integrated semi-automated program for lung isolation and evaluation (as described in a separate chapter by Kalender et al.). The program provides mean CT values and areas of the lung and an extended histogram analysis. In addition, the enhancement due to xenon was measured in pathologically altered lung regions by selecting circular and irregular ROIs as part of the standard evaluation functions. Xenon enhancement in the lung was also assessed qualitatively by use of subtraction images (temporal subtraction of contrast and plain scans). We examined 10 normal healthy volunteers and 15 patients with pathological changes of lung parenchyma.

Results

For testing purposes, the 10 volunteers inhaled pure xenon. In one case, slight dysasthesia in the fingers and euphoria for a period of about 2 minutes were experienced. We did not notice any anesthetic effects of xenon for this single-breath technique.

In patients with normal lung ventilation, the increase of xenon density in the alveoli (Fig. 2) could be seen for the first scans of the dynamic CT series. After a few seconds, a homogeneous enhancement of the total lung with a CT value increase of about 40–60 HU was reached. Histogram analysis of the dynamic CT scans showed double-peak curves shortly after xenon inhalation representing the higher xenon concentration in the bronchi and bronchioli. The histogram curves changed to normal in all cases towards the end of the series; we found single-peak curves, very similar to those for plain scans, but shifted to higher attenuation values due to xenon.

Our efforts to calculate perfusion parameters from time-density measurements have not been successful up to now. The time density curves showed an increasing tendency for the duration of the 12s dynamic CT series. Analysis of the measured lung cross-section areas as a function of time showed that the patients and volunteers pressed during the phase of inhibited respiration. They thereby unvoluntarily performed a Valsalva manoeuvre resulting in a reduction of lung volume and an increase in lung density. Further clarification, including physiological aspects, is needed.

Fig. 3–5 give examples of our results in patient examinations. Hpyoventilated lung regions could be recognized after xenon inhalation with high sensitivity; the degree of hypoventilation can be quantitated. For qualitative assessment of ventilation disturbances, temporal subtractions of scans proved to be a useful tool, although with limited image quality due to changes in respiratory volumes (Fig. 5).

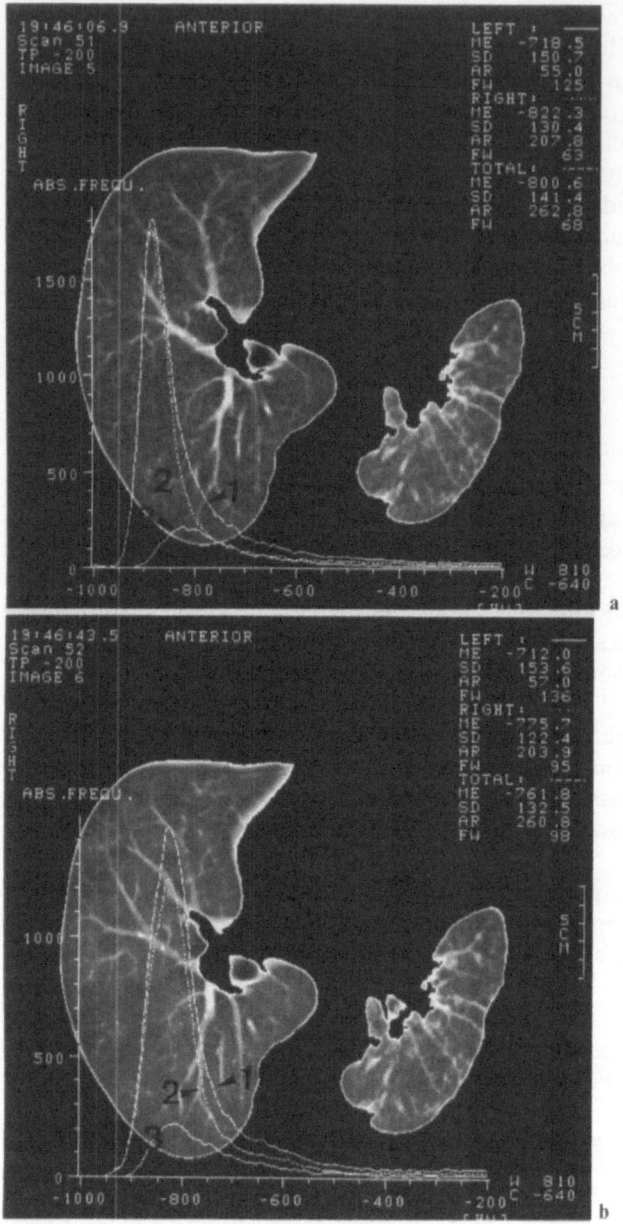

Fig. 4a, b. Ventilation disturbance of the left lower lung lobe in a patient with central bronchus carcinoma. Evaluation with a semiautomated program for lung isolation and densitometry. Histogram analysis: curve 1 = both lungs, curve 2 = right lung, curve 3 = left lung. Numerical results are presented in the upper right corner. **a** Plain scan, **b** Xenon inhalation. In the right lower lung lobe an enhancement due to xenon of 53.7 HU is found, in the left it only amounted to 6 HU

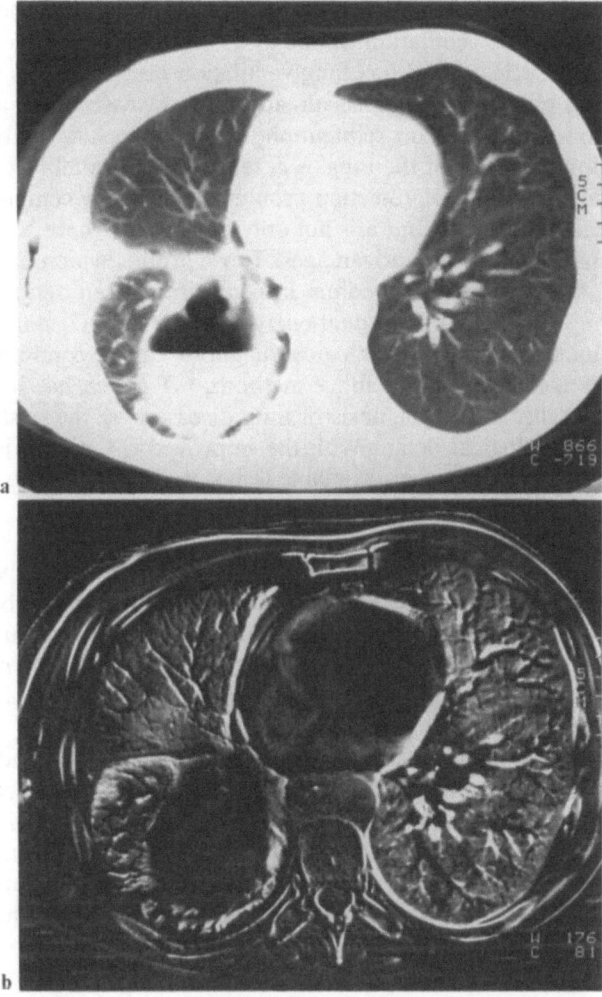

Fig. 5 a, b. Cavity formation in the right lung after surgical resection of oesophagus diverticula. The question if there is a connection to the cavity in the airpaths can be negated on the basis of the xenon inhalation studies. The subtraction image (b) does not show enhancement in the cave

Discussion

In many pneumological problems, measurements of lung density alone have only limited predictive power. In fibrotic lungs, for example, an integral measurement of lung density will combine emphysematic and fibrotic zones. Even in the case of massive parenchymal alterations, possibly a 'normal' mean density value can result. The use of morphometric methods, e.g. an extended histogram evaluation, will improve the situation; however, there remain doubts with respect to the validity of density or structure measurements for describing changes in lung function.

With stable xenon, we have an inhalation contrast medium available to us with which lung ventilation can be assessed both qualitatively and quantitatively.

In nuclear medicine, lung ventilation measurements with radioactive xenon are part of routine diagnosis already. In most cases, they are performed in combination with perfusion scintigraphy to deliniate lung emboli from secondary perfusion disorders of the lung, e. g. related to a bronchus carcinoma [1, 11]. However, due to radiation protection problems only a few centers are equipped for such inhalation studies. But it is not only this aspect where X-ray studies of the lung with stable xenon offer advantages. Those groups which have used stable xenon as an inhalation contrast medium in conventional radiography [13], in digital radiography [3] and in digital dual-energy radiography [2] pointed out the advantage that functional and morphological diagnosis can be combined in a single examination. As compared to the above methods, CT which has become the leading imaging modality in the diagnosis of lung disease over the past years provides even more morphological detail. With the improved CT measuring equipment and the extended analysis tools available today, we continued the work of Winkler et al. [15], Foley et al. [6] and Gur et al. [8] who tried previously to use stable xenon in CT examinations of lung ventilation.

Our preliminary clinical results indicate that even ventilation disturbances of small extent can be demonstrated with CT using stable xenon as an inhalation contrast medium (Fig. 3). The enhancement of up to 80 HU associated with inhaling gas mixtures of 40–60% xenon is very high. This, in combination with the improved spatial resolution, should provide a higher sensitivity for ventilation disturbances than any other imaging modality (Fig. 4, 5).

So far, we have carried out all xenon ventilation studies at maximal inspiration without using respiratory gating [10]. In the future we will use the spirometric technique and scan at 80% or 90% of vital capacity to provide better results in the temporal subtraction of successive scans. Up to now, subtraction images have been of unsatisfactory quality (Fig. 5). Anesthesizing effects of xenon do not have to be considered for the single-breath technique described here. The cost of xenon per examination can be considered acceptable.

References

1. Alderson PO, Biella DR, Gottschalk A, Hoffer PB, Kroop SA, Lee ME, Ramanna L, Siegel BA, Waxman AD (1984) To-99m-DTPA serosol and radioactive gases compared as adjuncts to perfusion scintigraphy in patients with suspected pulmonary embolism. Radiology 153: 516–521
2. Bautz W (1988) Digitale Zwei-Spektren-Radiographie. Habilitationsschrift, Universität Tübingen
3. Bjork L, Bjorkholm PJ (1982) Xenon as contrast agent for imaging of the airways and lungs using digital radiography. Radiology 144: 476–478
4. Cullan SC, Gross EG (1951) The anaesthetic properties of xenon in animals and human beings, with additional observations on krypton. Science 113: 580–582
5. Doehring W, Linke G (1979) Die Grundlagen der quantitativen pulmonalen Computertomographie. Fortschr Roentgenstr 130: 133–143

6. Foley WD, Haughton VM, Schmidt J, Wilson CR (1978) Xenon contrast enhancement in computed body tomography. Radiology 129: 219–220
7. Gilman MJ, Laurens RG, Somogyi JW, Honig EG (1983) CT attenuation values of lung density in sarcoidosis. J Comput Assist Tomogr 7: 407–410
8. Gur D, Drayer BP, Borovetz HS, Griffith BP, Hardesty RL, Wolfson SK (1979) Dynamic computed tomography of the lung: Regional ventilation measurements. J Comput Assist Tomogr 3: 749–753
9. Kalender W, Rienmüller R, Welke M (1988) Algorithm for automated evaluation of high-resolution CT images of the lung. Radiology 169(P): 116
10. Kalender W, Rienmüller R, Seißler W, Behr J, Welke M, Fichte H (1990) Spirometric gating for measuring pulmonary parenchymal density by quantitative computed tomography. Radiology 175: 265–268
11. Katz RD (1981) Ventilation-perfusion lung scanning in patients detected by a screening program of early lung carcinoma. Radiology 141: 903–907
12. Pittinger GB, Moyers J, Cohen SC, Featherstone RM, Gross EG (1953) Clinicopathologic studies associated with xenon anaesthesia. Anaesthesiology 14: 10–17
13. Rockoff SD, Mendelsohn ML (1962) Evaluation of xenon as gaseous roentgenographic contrast material. A preliminary report. Am Rev Resp Dis 86: 434–438
14. Wegener OH, Koeppe P, Oeser H (1978) Measurement of lung density by computed tomography. J Comput Assist Tomogr 2: 263–273
15. Winkler SS, Holden JE, Sackett JF, Fleming DC, Alexander SC (1977) Xenon and Krypton as radiographic inhalation contrast media with computerized tomography: Preliminary note. Invest Radiol 12: 19–22

Spirometrically Standardized Quantitative High Resolution CT of Interstitial Lung Diseases

R. Rienmüller, I. Altmann, J. Behr, F. Krombach, W. A. Kalender

The following is based on an experimental animal study of Javanese macaques examined by high resolution CT at the end of 27 months exposure to defined amount of quartz and/or high atmospheric pressure [1].

The intention of this study was to evaluate possible sequels of occupational exposure to high levels of quartz-dust and/or atmospheric pressure on the lungs of the tunnel workers which may cause morphological and functional changes of the lung parenchyma. Over a period of 27 months, 8 hours/day, five times per week, four groups of monkeys were exposed to the following conditions as shown in Table 1.

Table 1. Classification of animal groups

group A (control)	$1.0\,bar_a$
group B (quartz)	$1.0\,bar_a + DQ\ 12$
group C (quartz-pressure)	$2.5\,bar_a + DQ\ 12$
group D (pressure)	$2.5\,bar_a$

DQ 12: "Dörentruper Quartz", $<5\ \mu m$, $5\ mg/m^3$

Bronchoalveolar lavage and the analysis of its samples, lung biopsies and its patho-histological work up and functional studies of the lungs were performed at constant time intervals.

Material and Methods

2–5 days before the end of this experimental study high resolution CT of the lungs were obtained in all animals. The CT scans were performed in supine position at the level of carina as well as 5 cm above and below. The animals were anesthetized, intubated and exposed at an intratracheal pressure of 15 cm of water. The CT exposure time was 7 seconds and the slice thickness was 1 mm.

The isolation of the right and left lung parenchyma succeeded automatically using a fast contour tracing algorithm. The quantitative analysis of CT images included:

- the determination of regional and global CT density values of both lungs separatively
- the assessment of dorso-ventral CT density gradients
- a quantitative histogram analysis and
- a correlation with histological and functional data.

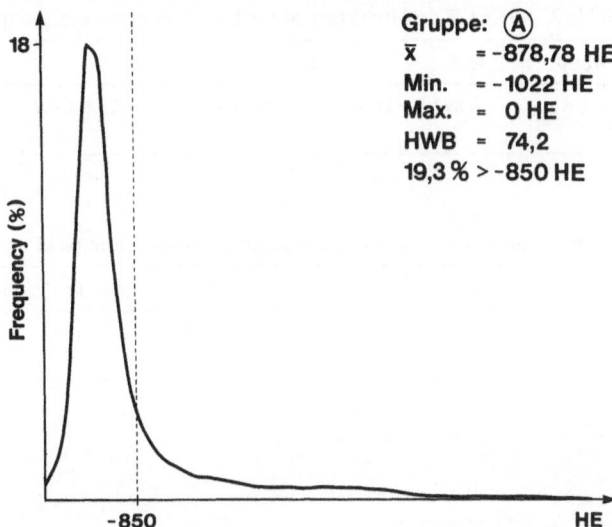

Fig. 1. Frequency histograms of CT density values of the right lung at the level of the carina of an animal of the group A ($\bar{x}$ = mean CT density value, *HE* = Hounsfield units, *Min.*, *Max.* = minimal and maximal CT density value, *HWB* = full widths of half maximum, *Häufigkeit* = frequency (Rienmüller R., Fortschr. Röntgenstr. 148, 4 (1988)

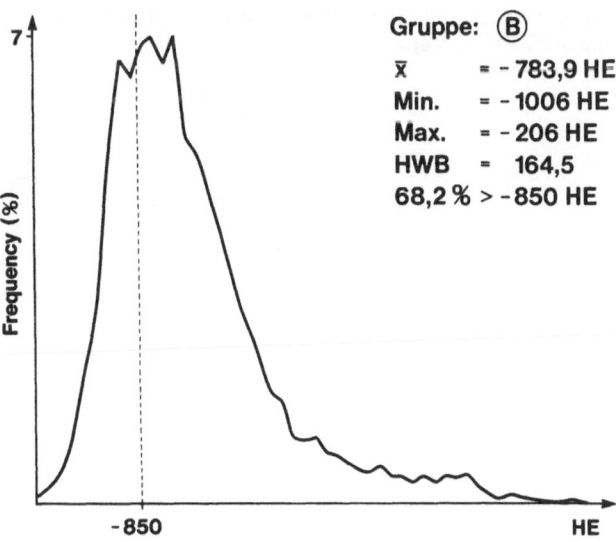

Fig. 2. Frequency histogram of CT density values of the right lung at the level of carina of an animal of the group B (Rienmüller R., Fortschr. Röntgenstr. 148, 4 (1988)

Table 2. Mean CT density values of the lungs in the studied groups of animals

Group:	A	B	C	D
$\bar{x} \pm SD$	-892.3 ± 19.1	-734.6 ± 72.8	$-799,8 \pm 4.9$	$-908,6 \pm 17.5$
n	5	7	4	5

Table 3. Lung area (%) of reduced air in the studied groups of animals

Group:	A	B	C	D
$\bar{x}$ (%)	16.9	76.7	62.0	15.6
n	5	7	4	5

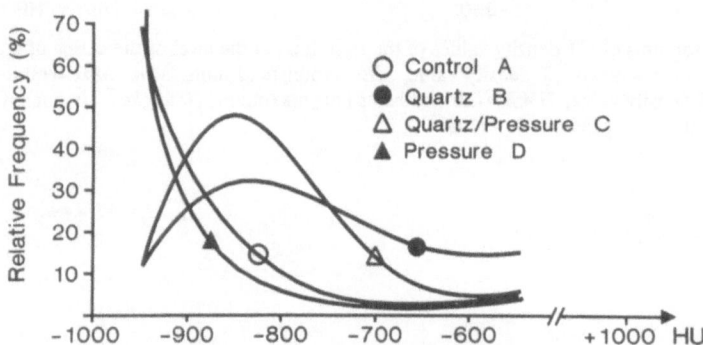

Fig. 3. Frequency histogram of accumulated CT density values of both three levels of the lungs of the four animal groups

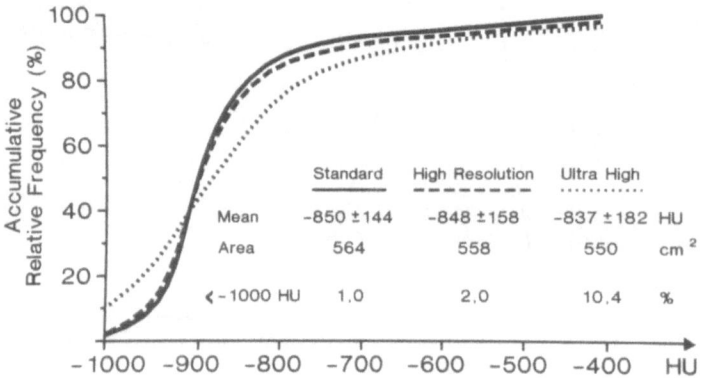

Fig. 4. Frequency histogram of accumulated CT density values of a CT scan of the lungs reconstructed by standard, high resolution and ultra high resolution mode

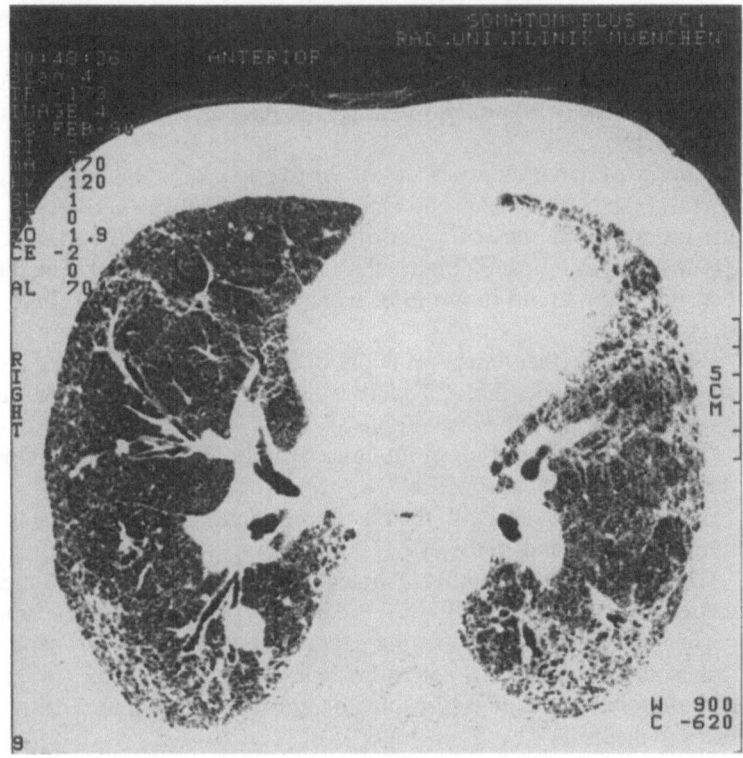

Fig. 5. High resolution CT scan five cm below the carina of a 74 years old patient with idiopathic pulmonary fibrosis performed in inspiration at 50% of actual vital capacity

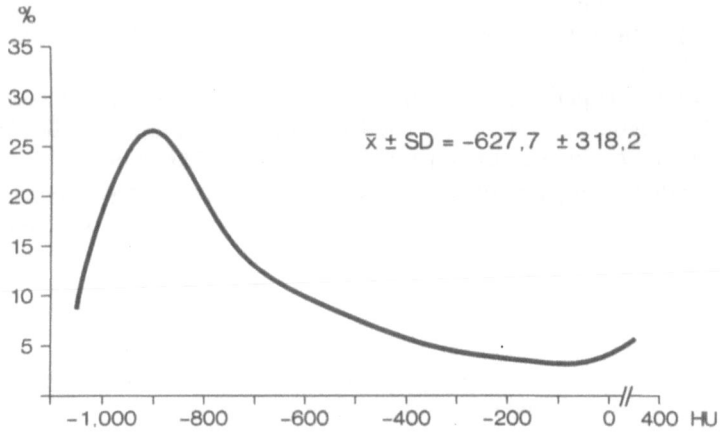

Fig. 6. Frequency histogram of accumulated CT density values of the patient of Fig. 5 with increased frequency of CT density below −1000 HU (suggesting increase amount of an emphysema) and above −800 HU as a result of pulmonary fibrosis. The frequency of CT density values between −1000 and −800 HU is also reduced if compared with results of Fig. 8

Figures 1 and 2 are typical histogram curves of the right lung of a monkey from the control group A and of a monkey from the quartz group B, demonstrating not only a difference of the mean CT density values (x) but also of the full widths at half maximum (FW) and of the ranges of lung areas with CT density values above -850 HU.

The quantitative analysis of the histograms of both lungs at all three levels reveals (Table 2) for the group D somehow lower mean CT density values than for the group A. The mean CT density values of group C (quartz and high pressure group) were significantly higher than in the group A and D. The highest mean CT densities were found in group B, which was exposed just to high level of quartz dust.

Based on the theoretical principle of the meaning of CT densities it seems reasonable to assume that CT density values above -850 HU suggest reduced amount of air per CT voxel (Table 3).

The area of reduced air in the lung is similar between the groups A and D and the groups B and C respectively.

These data correlate with the histomorphometric determined gas volumes of the lungs in this animal study [2].

There was found significant linear correlation between the mean CT density values and the vital capacity ($r = 0.84$; $p < 0.001$). The close linear, significant correlation between the diffusing capacity ($r = 0.75$; $p < 0.001$) and the percentage of histomorphometrically determined gas space ($r = 0.91$; $p < 0.001$) with the corresponding mean CT density values demonstrates the high sensitivity of these CT measurements [3].

These excellent results come to perform a more subtle analysis of CT density values in the quantitative evaluation of the lungs. Accordingly, a new software package was developed in close cooperation with the co-workers at Siemens Company and fitted in the new CT machine SOMATOM PLUS, giving the possibility to show that the analysis of relative frequencies of accumulated CT density values enables additional quantitative data in our animal study (Fig. 3).

For the CT studies of our patients' lungs we developed a standardized method [4]. Spirometric measurements of the vital capacity are performed before the CT study. The patients are instructed how to use the pocket spirometer by means of a few preliminary exercises. The following topogram is already done in inspiration at 50% of the measured actual vital capacity. Thereafter three scanning levels are defined at the level of carina and 5 cm below and above. At these three levels high resolution CT scans are obtained again at the same controlled inspiration. The scanning parameters are: 1 s scan time; 250 mA tube current, 120 kVp and 1 mm slice thickness.

If no motion artefacts are visible on the CT scans of the lungs, an isolation of the lung parenchyma succeeds by using a fast contour algorithm. In case of artefacts the CT procedure must be repeated. Out of various threshold values those of -1024 and -200 HU revealed to be most suitable. From the different reconstruction algorithms (standard, high resolution, ultra high) we selected the high resolution one, allowing a quantitative and morphological analysis of the lung parenchyma as well (Fig. 4). Then a quantitative analysis of CT density values follows for the left and right lungs respectively, as well as for the total lung. The anal-

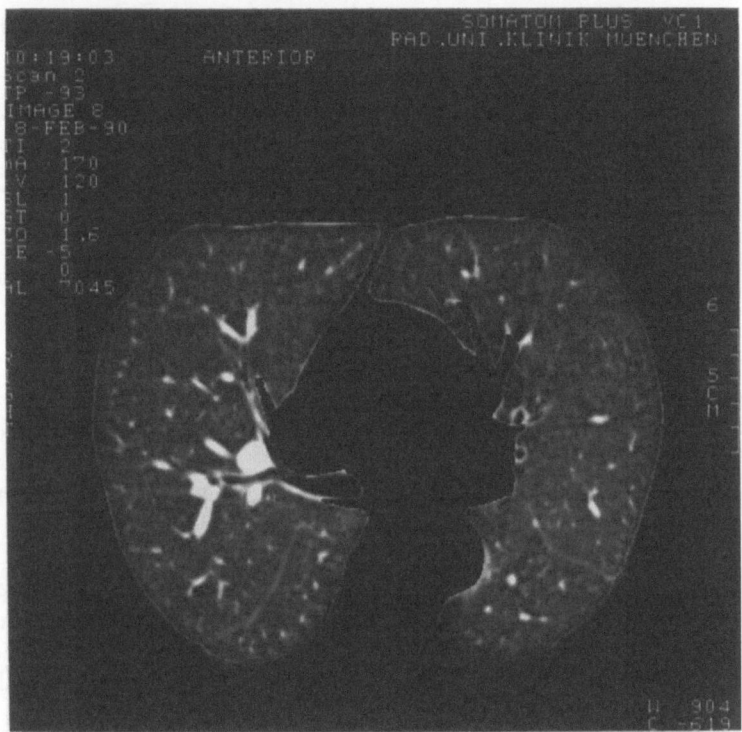

Fig. 7. Isolated parenchyma of the lungs of a high resolution CT five cm below the carina of a 60 years old patient with mild extent of systemic sclerosis treated with cortisone performed in inspiration at 50% of actual vital capacity

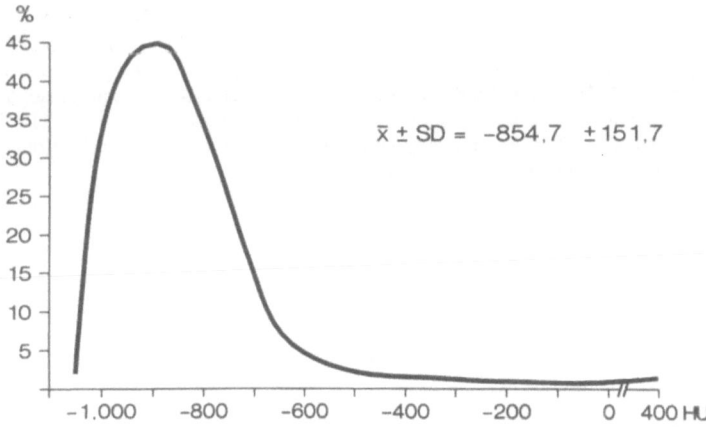

Fig. 8. Frequency histogram of accumulated CT density values of the patient of Fig. 7 with normal distribution of CT density values in all parts of the histogram and normal functional data of the lungs

ysis includes: the mean CT density values, the full widths at half maximum (FWHM), standard deviations, histogram evaluation in steps of 25 or 100 HU, as well as the quantification of the area of the lungs.

Two patients, one with severe idiopatic pulmonary fibrosis, the other with mild extent of systemic sclerosis will be presented instead of more than 50 patients with various pulmonary diseases studied by SOMATOM PLUS (Figs. 5, 6, 7, 8).

The essential advantages of SOMATOM PLUS are:

I. Shorter exposure time, reducing the extent of motion artefacts in patients with respiratory insufficiency, making this study not only easier, but in some cases, even possible at all.
II. More simple handling of the new pocket spirometer not only for the patient but also for the physician.
III. Automatic isolation of the lung parenchyma with reproducible contour tracing.
IV. Improved software for a more extended evaluation of global and regional frequencies of CT density values.

Our preliminary results of comparative studies of different frequencies of CT density values with pulmonary functional data show, that standardized quantitative high resolution CT will play a clinically important role in the diagnosis, staging and follow up of patients with various pulmonary diseases, especially of the interstitial and occupational type.

References

1. Rienmüller R, Schätzl M, Kalender W, Krombach F, Fiehl E (1988) Quantitative CT-Untersuchungen der Lungen am tierexperimentellen Modell der Silikose. Fortschr Röntgenstr 148 (4): 367–373
2. Rosenbruch M: Med Inst für Umwelthygiene, Düsseldorf (unpublished data)
3. Krombach F, Ronge R, Hildemann S, Fiehl E, Wanders A, Burkhardt D, Aimelling A, Hammer C (1987) A model of experimental silicosis in a compressed invironment. In: Baethmann A, Messmer K (eds) Surgical research: Recent concepts and results. Springer, pp 59–68
4. Kalender W, Rienmüller R, Seissler W, Behr J, Welke M, Fichte H (1990) Quantitative CT of the lung with spirometrically controlled respiratory status and automated evaluation procedures. Radiology 175 (1): 265–268

Discussion

W. A. Kalender, Erlangen: Spiral CT Scanning for Fast and Continuous Volume Data Acquisition

zur Nedden, Innsbruck:
What additional equipment is necessary to operate the SOMATOM PLUS for spiral CT?

Kalender, Erlangen:
There will be a product available for clinical application in the near future.

P. Vock, Bern: Single-Breath Hold Spiral Volumetric CT of the Lung and the Hepatobiliary System

Schmitt, Würzburg:
At what level do you set the window level in imaging to demonstrate a particular lesion?

Vock:
It is difficult to define the adequate window level. One has to move the window level according to the given problem.

v. Engelshoven, Maastricht:
Spiral scanning induces a lower radiation dose compared to normal scanning. This must be because the mA values are lower. Are there additional factors?

Vock:
This is the main explanation. The other reason is that by performing slices at many levels within a volume, one has to repeat overlapping single slices. For this reason more radiation dose is applied than with volume scanning and secondary reconstruction of slices from raw data.

W. A. Kalender, Erlangen: Quantitative CT of the Lung with Spirometrically Controlled Respiratory Status and Automated Evaluation Procedures

v. Engelshoven:
Is there a reference phantom necessary in quantitative CT of the lung, as for osteo-densitometry?

Kalender:
The reference phantom for bone mineral measurements is above all used to check the X-ray quality, that is the effective energy, because one has to convert from CT numbers to bone mineral density in grams per cubic centimeter. In lung there is hardly any dependence on the effective energy, because one is concerned about soft tissue only, the range of Hounsfield numbers from minus 1000 to 0. So, if your scanner is stable and the CT values – which you can check with a water phantom – are set to 0 and minus 1000, you would not need it, definitely not to the same extent as in bone mineral. However, we are currently exploring the necessity of the reference values.

Fuchs, Zürich:
May CT densitometry measure lung water and identify e. g. early transsudation in left ventricular heart failure?

Vock:
This method does not differentiate between various causes leading to an increased density. If there is fibrosis, there are means to differentiate it from water, either by spiral scans or densitometry.

Kalender:
We can only determine differences in density. It is not possible to make a differentiation through the density measurements.

Rienmüller, Munich:
Very subtle histogram analysis may contribute to the evaluation of fluid in the lung, because the CT density measurements are very sensitive. We have already studied a few patients with left heart failure, measuring the CT density values before and after treatment. This might be of importance for patients in intensive care units.

Vock:
We did some animal studies in a model of left ventricular failure and in overhydrated dialysis patients. An increase in lung density can be measured, but I doubt whether one really can specifically differentiate such conditions from other pathology, such as fibrosis or another interstitial disease.

Bautz, Tübingen:
In cases with increased lung fluid, there must be an increase of lung density over time.

Rienmüller:
We also measured the dorsoventral gradient in healthy persons and found substantial differences between the upper and the lower part of the lung. In left heart

failure the patient stays mainly in a supine position. For this reason higher CT density values in the depending parts of the lungs are encountered. By moving the patient into a different position density values will change accordingly.

W. Bautz, Tübingen: New Means of the CT Examination of Lung Ventilation with Xenon

Schmitt, Würzburg:
To demonstrate hypoventilation as with Xenon may CT scans performed in expiration and inspiration also demonstrate pathology by measuring density values within the diseased areas?

Bautz:
Such a method would most likely be hampered by the limited reproduceability of density measurements.

Oudkerk, Rotterdam:
Did you perform CT Xenon ventilation studies in cases with pulmonary embolism?

Bautz:
No such investigations were attempted because of methodological problems.

R. Rienmüller, Munich: Spirometrically Standardized Quantitative High-Resolution CT of Interstitial Lung Diseases

Deininger, Darmstadt:
Clinical spirometry is a rather global method to evaluate lung diseases. Can spirometrically standardized quanitative CT give more precise information?

Rienmüller:
In my opinion with quantitative evaluation of CT images of the lungs more precise information may be achieved. CT quantitation seems to be a more sensitive method by which better quantification is obtained.

Struyven, Brussels:
Did you notice any relationship between the length of the exposure to quartz and density measurements in patients with silicosis?

Rienmüller:
There was only one single CT examination performed, no follow-up studies are available.

v. Engelshoven:
What topographical subdivision of the lung, anterior-posterior, segmental, cortex-medulla should be applied?

Rienmüller:

This depends on the pathological condition investigated. It is reasonable to perform at least three or four slices through the chest, one at the level of the carina 5 cm cranially and twice 5 cm caudally.

Regional quantitative analysis is mandatory since the pathological changes may be localized in particular areas of the lung for a given disease.

3 D Reconstruction

Chairmen: H. Riemann, W. Fuchs

Three-Dimensional Imaging: Technical Aspects

J. HODLER, W. KUONI, M. RODRIGUEZ

Abstract

Three-dimensional (3 D) imaging was performed in 60 cases, most often in dysplasia and osteochondritis dissecans of the knee and in trauma of the shoulder and
lumbar spine. Identical imaging parameters were used as for axial imaging. Slice
thickness and table increments were normally both 2 mm. Software manipulation
with its few interactive commands was easily done. Segmentation was performed
by thresholding and was the most time consuming part of the examination.
Manipulation of the 3 D data was achieved simply by using a light pen. Rotation
and secondary cuts were accomplished. A simulated, freely movable light source
was very important to improve image quality. 3 D images were documented by
laser printed images with a good quality. In the future quantitative measurements
and interactive capabilities such as the extraction of an irregular region of interest
and preoperative simulation will be important.

Three-dimensional imaging (3 D imaging) is rapidly gaining importance as a
diagnostic tool. Several publications have discussed principles and clinical use of
3 D imaging [1-4].

Case Material and Data Acquisition

We have performed 3 D imaging in the musculoskeletal system in 60 cases. The
knee, the shoulder and the lumbar spine were most often examined. The most
important indications were dysplasia and osteochondritis dissecans of the knee,
while trauma predominated in the examinations of the shoulder and spine.
Patients were instructed to take a convenient position and were told that inad-
vertant movements could ruin the whole study. For knee studies the feet were
taped together, for shoulder studies the hand was taped to the thigh. Slice thickness and table increments were important for the quality of the 3 D reconstructions. In most cases we used 2 mm slice thickness and 2 mm table increments.
Even with this protocol steps were visible in structures cut almost tangentially,
such as the femoral condyles or the upper pole of the humeral head. If the femoral
condyle was the main region of examination the table increment was reduced to
one millimeter. Depending on the examined region and the pathology 14 to
92 slices were acquired, the smallest number only being large enough for a small
structure like a hand or a single vertebral body. To reduce examination times in
trauma patients with the examination of more than four spinal segments we

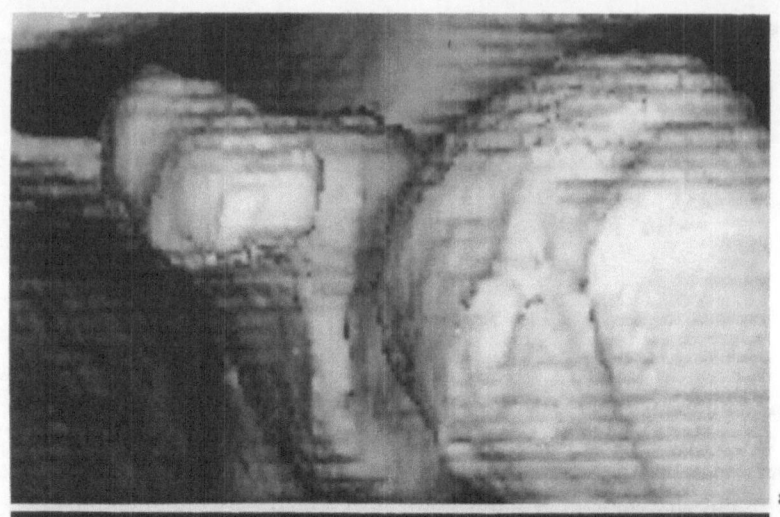

a

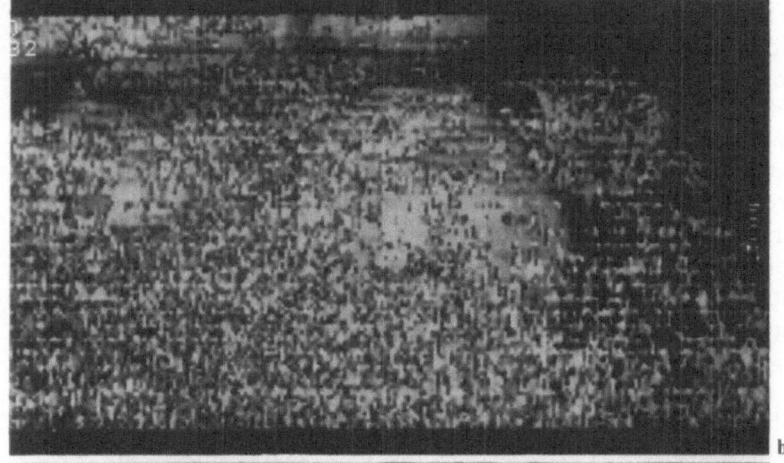

b

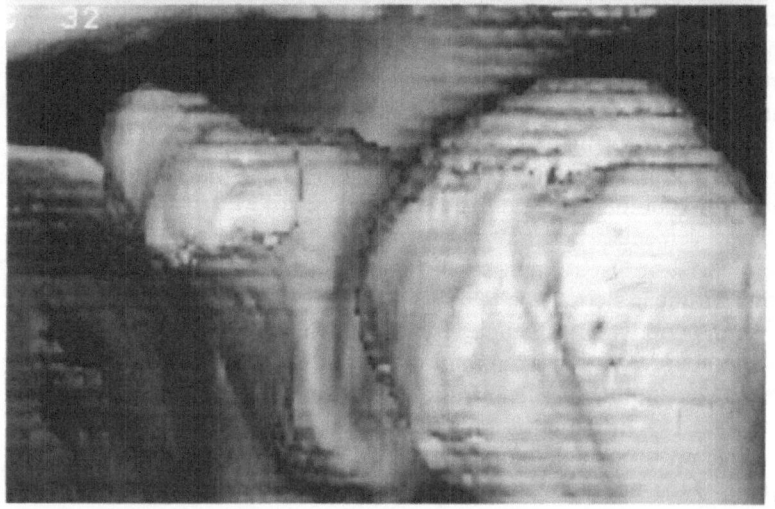

c

Table 1. Knee

Positioning	Feet first, feet taped together
Program	Extremity
mAs	330
kV	120
Algorithm	high resolution
Slice thickness	2 mm
Table increments	2 mm
Region of interest	cranial pole of patella to fibular head
Threshold	Window center 150
	Window width 2
Reconstruction matrix	256

Table 2. Shoulder

Positioning	Head first, hand taped to the thigh
Program	Shoulder
mAs	870
kV	137
Algorithm	high resolution
Slice thickness	2 mm
Table increments	2 mm
Region of interest	cranial end of acromion to axillary recess
Threshold	Window center 150
	Window width 2
Reconstruction matrix	256

Table 3. Lumbar spine

Positioning	Head first, slight flexion of the hip (pillow under knee)
Program	Spine
mAs	870
kV	137
Algorithm	high resolution
Slice thickness	2 mm
Table increments	2 mm
Gantry tilt	adjusted to most important vertebral end plate, no change during examination
Region of interest	from upper end plate of last normal vertebral body to lower end plate of first normal vertebral body inferior to pathologic process
Threshold	Window center 150
	Window width 2
Reconstruction matrix	256

Fig. 1a-c. 3D reconstruction of the left shoulder: thresholding. **a** Correct threshold (window center 150, window width 2). **b** Window center too low (window center 80, window width 2), with overlying skin and soft tissue. **c** Window center too high (window center 300, window width 2), with artifactual hole within scapular bone

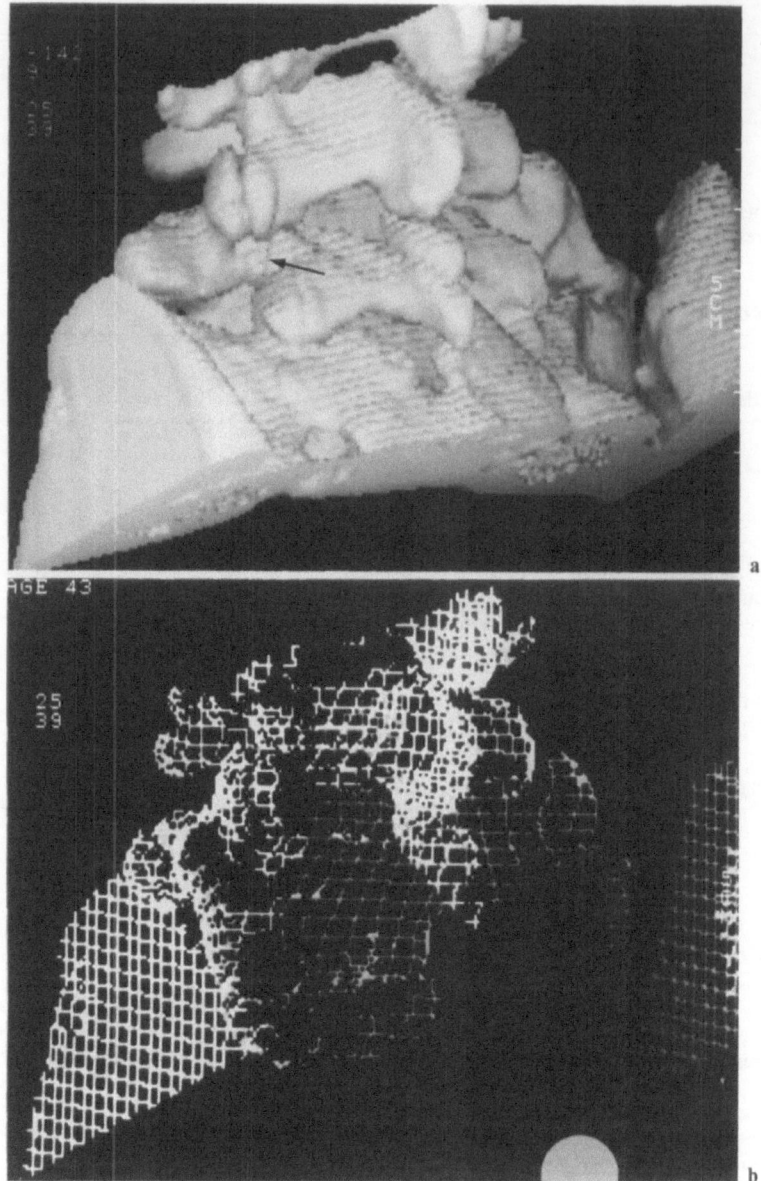

Fig. 2a, b. 3 D reconstruction of the lumbosacral region, spondylolysis: rotation. **a** View from behind and left. Spondylolysis L5 left (arrow). **b** Lattice image used to rotate image. Spondylolysis not visible

adapted the protocol in so far as we performed imaging with a slice thickness of 5 mm and table increments of 5 mm. The most important region was then re-scanned with the usual 2/2 protocol and an adapted gantry tilt. In five knee and two shoulder joints arthrogram CT was performed for a pathology of the retropat-ellar cartilage or the glenoid labrum. While the contrast medium was very impor-tant for the diagnosis in axial images it was disturbing in 3 D imaging.

High quality axial images were the main diagnostic tool in our cases. So we did not reduce mAs when performing 3 D imaging, and there was no decrease in radia-tion dose, contrary to other groups [5].

3 D Reconstruction

3 D reconstructions can be performed on the fast SMI image computer, or during image acquisition by its REP subunit [6]. We did not perform 3 D reconstructions on the separate DSC console during the examination of the subsequent patient, because the second console was then used to look at bone windows and for dis-tance and density measurements. 3 D reconstructions were performed outside rou-tine imaging time.

With the prereleased VC04 software the reconstruction time was between 7 and 34 minutes (mean 19 minutes) in our first 20 consecutive patients depending on the slice number and the number of reconstructions. The number of slices varied between 14 and 49, the number of 3 D reconstructions used for documentation between 4 and 23.

Segmentation took about 4 times longer with the use of the 512 reconstruction matrix instead of the 256 matrix. Although images were sharper with the larger matrix, we usually used the 256 matrix to reduce calculation time [6].

The SOMATOM PLUS software was easy to handle with few interactive com-mands. 3 D-reconstruction was based on a segmentation by thresholding as in most currently available systems. We found the default value (window width of 2 HU, window center of 150 HU) useful in most cases of bone imaging. A low window center obscured smaller gaps in non-displaced fractures and extracted skin and soft tissue, which overlaid bone. With a too high window center thin bony structures got lost, such as parts of the scapular body. When the threshold had been incorrectly chosen, the segmentation had to be started from the begin-ning to get different image information. This meant a significant time loss. Because with thresholding, voxels are within the chosen limits or not, there remained only binary image information after the segmentation. Only surfaces were shown and the internal structure was lost.

Rotation of the image was simple, but rather time consuming. In a first step the image was reduced to a lattice image which allowed real time control of the rota-tion by moving a light pen. Details were not visible on the lattice image and thus it could be difficult to project freely minor pathologic changes or anatomic details. The next step was calculation of a complete surface image which was done within a few seconds. In most cases a series of rotations about a vertical axis by steps of 30 to 45 degrees was useful. It had to be performed image by image by manipulat-

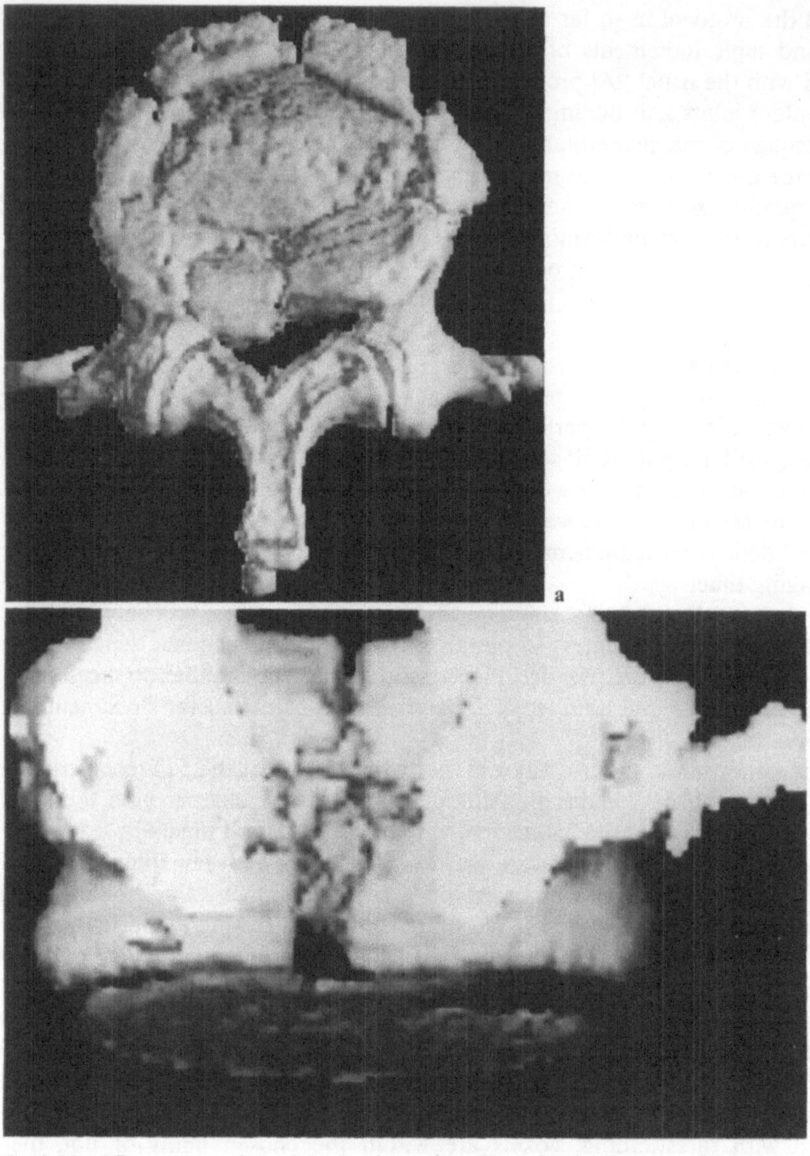

Fig. 3a, b. 3D reconstruction of the lumbar spine. Comminuted fracture of L2: secondary cut. **a, b** View from above and behind after removal of the dorsal parts of L2

ing the lattice images. No automatic rotation was available, nor was there a cine-loop mode.

Secondary cuts could be performed, but their quality was limited due to the binary character of the data set available. We used this feature for instance to cut disturbing structures such as calcified abdominal vessels in examinations of the lumbar spine. By a combination of two cutting planes removal of convex structures could be performed. We removed the distal femur to show the articular surface of the patella for instance. More complex operations like the simulated exarticulation of the femoral head from the acetabular groove was not possible.

The position of a simulated *light source* could quickly be changed and was very important in improving the quality and legibility of reconstructed images. Certain pathologies like an irregularity of the retropatellar surface could be visible or hidden depending on the position of the light source. In addition, steps in the reconstructed image were hidden or enhanced depending on its position.

Documentation

The reconstructed images were printed with an AGFA Scopix Compact L Laser-printer and demonstrated in the clinical conference like any other CT examination on the day of the examination or the following day. This was important to increase acceptance of 3 D imaging by clinicians and to improve indications for 3 D imaging. In addition to these hard copies the 3 D image data were stored on the optical disc.

Comparison with the Siemens MIP System

3 D reconstructions were also performed with the MIP system provided by Siemens working on a VAX 11/780 system in the Federal Institute of Technology in Zurich. Although the MIP software was not up-to-date this system provided several advantages, because of the greater computer capacity and additional software features.

The complete imaging data were available for image manipulation and not only the binary data provided after thresholding. Changing the threshold or any other type of reconstruction like rotation or secondary cuts for instance was possible within 10 seconds. Another important feature was the possibility of producing movies with rotating images or a so called clipping. This means a series of consecutive secondary cuts. On the other hand the system was not adequate for routine use: The patient data had to be copied onto a magnetic tape because the computer was located outside the hospital. The assistance of a computer specialist was necessary.

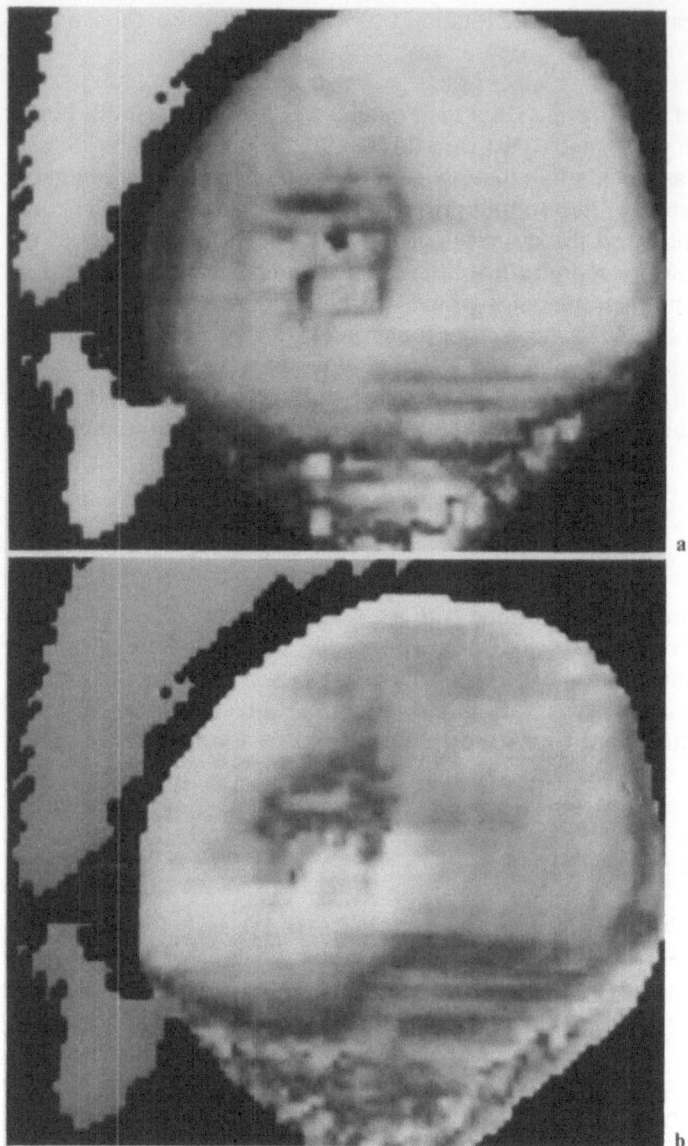

Fig. 4a, b. 3 D reconstruction of the knee. Osteochondrosis dissecans: simulated light source. **a, b** Different spatial impression due to different position of the simulated light source

Future Developments

Scanner based 3 D imaging is cost effective because no additional hardware is needed, software commands are known and manipulation is not time consuming [3]. Additional development of the Siemens SOMATOM PLUS system with its easy handling are still necessary to achieve an ideal working instrument. Interactive capabilities like extraction with an irregular ROI, angle, distance and volume measurements and preoperative simulation of osteotomies and arthroplasties would be helpful for orthopedic surgeons. The direct transfer of the 3 D data to a computer-controlled milling machine to produce solid polyethylene models is feasible [2]. Software for the production of video movies is of importance. Data transfer to other systems like the MIP system for scientific work should be less complicated. The large magnetic tapes should eventually be replaced by normal Video-8-cassettes with a capacity of 1 Gigabyte.

The production of 3 D images by thresholding is relatively simple and needs limited storage capacity. Small structures like the thin scapular body or non-displaced fractures may be lost. Methods have been described to overcome these problems: In volume rendering each voxel represents the percentage of material present within it. The thinner an object becomes, the more translucent it appears. So the integrity of very thin objects is preserved. Objects of the same material separated by even a small gap will be shown as separated. Fracture gaps smaller than one voxel have been demonstrated in this manner [7]. The main disadvantage of volume rendering is its need for a great storage capacity. Even more sophisticated systems using artificial intelligence to extract important structures based on topographical and density information after a learning process have been investigated [8].

Conclusion

Direct 3 D imaging on the SOMATOM PLUS CT has several advantages compared to stand-alone workstations concerning cost, handling and time. The 3 D software provided for the SOMATOM PLUS allows 3 D imaging of good quality within a reasonable time. More interactive capabilities such as the extraction of an irregular region of interest, preoperative simulation and quantitative measurements will be required in the future to improve clinical relevance of 3 D imaging.

References

1. Totty WG, Vannier MW (1984) Complex musculoskeletal anatomy: analysis using three dimensional surface reconstruction. Radiology 150: 173–177
2. Pate D, Resnick D, Andre M, Sartoris DJ, Kursunoglu S, Bielecki D, Dev P, Vassiliadis A (1986) Perspective: Three-dimensional imaging of the musculoskeletal system. AJR 147: 545–551

3. Herman GT (1988) Three-dimensional imaging on a CT or MR scanner. Journal of Computer Assisted Tomography 12: 450-458
4. Fishman EK, Magid D, Ney DR, Kuhlman JE (1989) Three-dimensional imaging: orthopedic applications. In: Udupa JK, Herman GT (eds) Computer aspects of 3 D imaging in medicine: a tutorial. Lewis Publishers, Inc, Chelsea, MI
5. Scott WW, Fishman EK, Magid D (1987) Acetabular fractures: optimal imaging. Radiology 165: 537-539
6. Imhof K (1989) Die dreidimensionale Darstellung von CT-Bildern: Methode und Möglichkeiten. Electromedica 57: 154-159
7. Fishman EK, Drebin B, Magid D, Scott WW, Ney DR, Brooker AF, Riley LH, Ville JA, Zerhouni EA, Siegelman SS (1987) Volumetric rendering techniques: applications for three-dimensional imaging of the hip. Radiology 163: 737-738
8. König HA, Laub G (1988) Verarbeitung und Darstellung dreidimensionaler Datensätze in der Kernspintomographie. Electromedica 56: 42-49

Evaluation of Three-Dimensional CT in Orofacial Surgery

C. Zwicker, F. Astinet, M. Langer, B. Erdtmann, R. Felix

Summary

Fifty-two patients with tumors and fractures of the visceral cranium were tested to demonstrate what additional information could be obtained with three-dimensional CT reconstructions as compared to conventional transaxial CT slices. 3D CT was seen to reproduce the spatial relationships in complex bony destructions more cleary and thereby contribute towards an improved therapeutical plan and postoperative follow-up controls. Transaxial CT, however, remains the basis for diagnostic information.

Introduction

The complex, anatomical structures of the visceral cranium can be displayed morphologically exact and free of superposition. High resolution CT with thin slices has proved to be the investigative method of choice for diagnosing tumorous or traumatic changes in the bones of the face. Multiplanar, two-dimensional image reconstructions have made further improvements in CT diagnostics possible. However, 2D CT has at times provided only insufficient spatial information for the surgeon, especially in operations on complex anatomical structures. The 3D CT introduced in recent years has gained increased popularity, because of its improved display of spatial relationships following alterations in the craniofacial region and the axial skeleton. The goal of this study was to evaluate the information provided by 3D CT in orosurgical illnesses, as compared to that of transaxial CT examinations.

Patients and Methods

Three-dimensional image reconstructions from the data files of fifty-two patients (36 males, 16 females, mean age 54 ± 9 years) were collected. Forty patients presented with tumor destruction and twelve with craniofacial fractures.

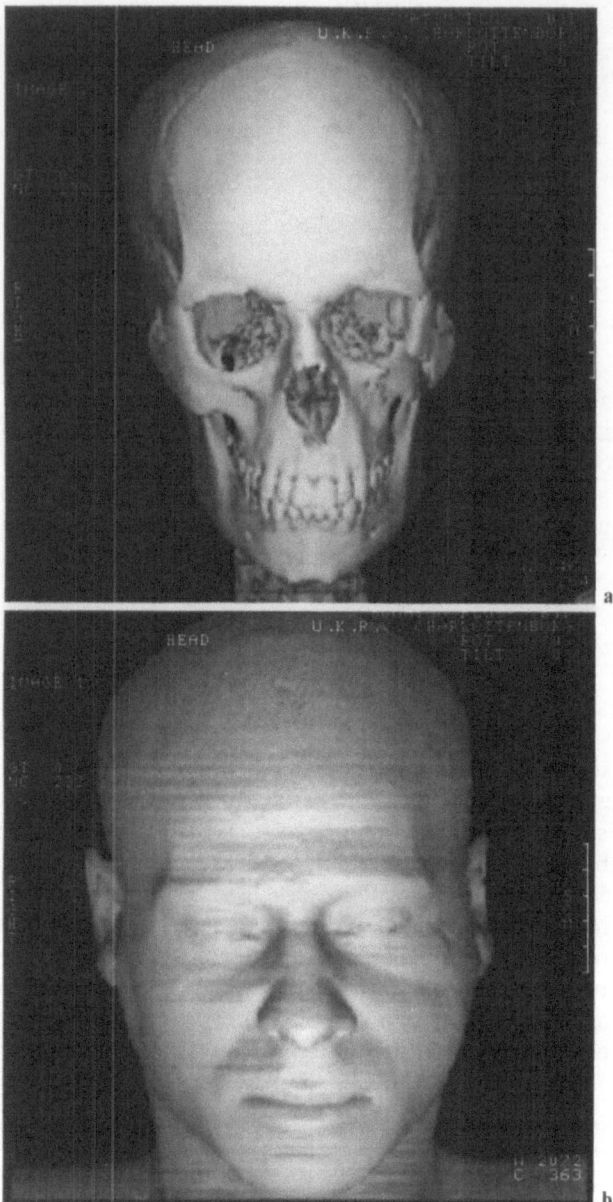

Fig. 1a, b. Fracture of the lateral orbital wall, orbital floor and zygomatic bone, left **a** bone reconstruction, **b** soft-tissue reconstruction

Table 1. 3D CT image quality in the area of the visceral cranium

very good image quality: n = 24
diagnostically sufficient image quality: n = 25
diagnostically insufficient image quality: n = 3

Each study was performed with a SOMATOM PLUS CT (1024 × 1024 pixel image matrix). The scans were made using overlapping slice technique (2 mm slice thickness and 1 mm table feed), the shortest scan time (0.7 sec) and minimal radiation intensity (60 or 170 mAs). The examination time lasted from 15–30 minutes, depending on the extent of the findings.

The standard 3D program implemented by the unit's software can generate surface images of bony structures and of the skin. This program permits the recording of only those pixels whose density lies above that of a freely selectable threshold. The reconstructed area can be localized by defining a square ROI. The threshold values for three-dimensional displays of the skull range from 150–180 HU, whereas values as high as −200 HU were required for reconstructing contours of the skin. These pixels were read slice-by-slice and their coordinates stored (contour extraction as per Vannier and Marsh, [11]). The 3D surface display offers a spatial presentation through the shaded reproduction of the object. The reflection of a light source with a frontal angle of incidence is simulated: Pixels nearer the viewer are imaged brighter, while structures further away are imaged darker. The spatial presentation can be varied by changing the light's angle of incidence. Furthermore, the object can be displayed in six standard projections or rotated as a wireframe model into any desired position for the evaluation of surface reconstructions. Freely selectable cutlines permit the projection of any internal view by eliminating the superimposed structures. The computation of a 3D data record from 100 individual scans takes approx. 10–15 minutes. Image reconstruction of any desired projection requires a matter of seconds. Furthermore, a square section of the image generated can be enlarged and displaced as desired.

Results

The evaluation of the information provided by the reconstructed three-dimensional CT images was limited to the spatial relationships and the clear demonstration of the findings. The 3D-CT images offer no additional information to that found in the underlying transaxial CT slices. Comparing the diagnostic information gained by this method to that of transaxial CT does not seem useful.

Twenty-four patients demonstrated a very good 3D-CT image quality (Fig. 1). Here, the complex bony destructions or fractures and the extension of defects after surgery were clearer and easier for the oral surgeon to understand than with transaxial CT slices (Table 1). Artifacts resulting from metal fragments were demonstrated in the three-dimensional display of twenty-five patients who received

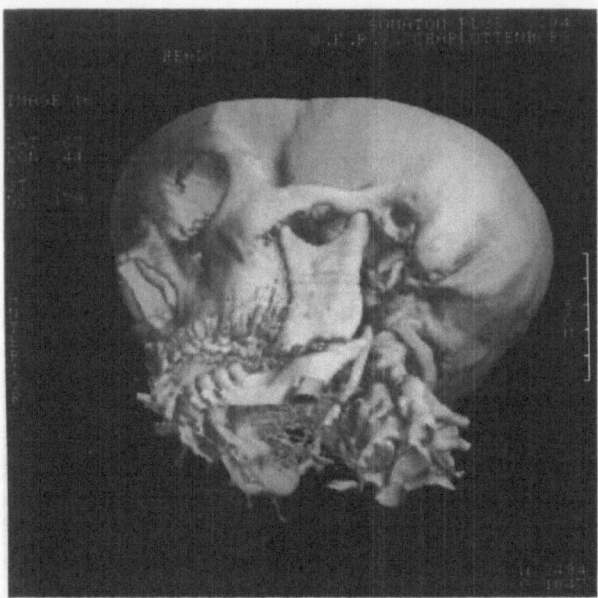

Fig. 2. Mandibular fracture, left. Considerable band-shaped metal artifacts do not interfere with evaluation

dental prostheses or prosthetic material (Table 1, Fig. 2). No relevant interference of image quality was found which compromised the diagnostic information obtained. Sufficient three-dimensional images could not be generated for three hyperkinetic patients (Table 1).

Discussion

Complex bony destructions present with tumors and fractures of the visceral cranium are often difficult to demonstrate to the operating surgeon with transaxial CT slices [11, 12]. The large number of scans necessary, especially for high-resolution CT examinations (HR-CT), can hinder the clarity of findings considerably. In concordance with Vannier, Grodd and Totty [5, 9, 11, 12], our experience has shown that three-dimensional imaging leads to significant improvement. A more vivid, three-dimensional view of the entire anatomical situation makes the findings easier to comprehend and to explain. From a diagnostic viewpoint, good three-dimensional reconstructions were performed in forty-nine cases and additional spatial information and clarity of the findings were obtained. We believe that better diagnostic information of the visceral cranium cannot be obtained with the 3D CT, since the image information of transaxial CT images provide the basis for this reconstruction. Discrete bony changes can be "subtracted" by contour smoothing of the three-dimensional images with the aid of the reconstruction algorithm. Therefore, these changes can only be demonstrated with certainty in transaxial HR-CT scans [5].

It has proved useful to choose as short a scan time as possible, along with a small mAs product (0.7 sec, 60 mAs) for examinations whose primary goal is the 3D reconstruction of thin, overlapping slices (2 mm, 1 mm table feed). In this way, the scan time and radiation exposure of the numerous resulting images can be limited [2, 5]. The network configuration available to us permitted calculations on a separate evaluation console with an average calculation and processing time of 30–45 minutes, independent of the ongoing examination.

Problems exist with the 3D surface reconstructions as a result of partial volume effects and anisotropic voxels due to high threshold values, leading to so-called "pseudo foramina". These are found on such fine lamellae as the anterior wall of the maxillary sinus or the medial wall of the orbit. One should not confuse these with destructions or fractures [5]. A sufficient three-dimensional display of the pituitary region is therefore presently impossible. "Pseudo foramina" can be avoided in image reconstructions by setting low threshold values. However, this leads to the inclusion of more structures demonstrating less absorption and which often represent disturbances in the reconstruction. The threshold value must therefore be chosen individually to suit the particular clinical problem. Further problems caused by metal artifacts were seen to appear in the form of typical striped bands extending beyond the skull contours of the 3D images generated. Nevertheless, as a rule rotating the reconstructed object in the proper direction generally makes a clear view of interesting regions of the jaw possible so that the loss of information can be limited. Three-dimensional CT permits, as a further advantage, the possibility of interactions with the observer, for example with computer-simulated surgery on a model or the production of three-dimensional models and individual prostheses based on the CT data file [1, 3, 4, 8, 10].

Conclusions

1. The three-dimensional reconstruction of CT images with its clear, spatial display provides an optimum demonstration of the findings from tumors and fractures of the visceral cranium.
2. Transaxial 2D CT slices continue to provide the basis for diagnostic information.
3. Thin, overlapping slices, a short scan time and reduced mAs products provide 3D-CT images of optimum quality.

References

1. Becker H (1988) Dreidimensionale kraniale und spinale Computertomographie. Radiologe 28: 239–242
2. Ernsting M (1989) 3-D-imaging: a program for the future? In: Lemke HU, Rhodes ML,

Jaffe CC, Felix R (eds) Computer Assisted Radiology '89. Springer, Berlin Heidelberg New York, pp 74-79

3. Fujioka M, Nakajima H, Yokoi S, Yasuda T, Toriwaki J (1986) Computer graphic simulation of craniofacial surgery in children. Radiology 161: 406-411

4. Fujioka M, Yokoi S, Yasuda T, Hashimoto Y, Toriwaki J, Nakajima H (1988) Computer-aided interactive simulation for craniofacial anomaly based on 3-D surface reconstruction CT images. Radiation Medicine 6: 204-212

5. Grodd W, Dannenmeier B, Petersen D, Gehrke G (1987) Drei-dimensionale (3-D) Bildrekonstruktionen von Gesichtsschädel und Schädelbasis in der Computertomographie. Radiologie 27: 3-11

6. Lang P, Genant HK, Steiger P, Stoller DW, Heuck AF (1989) 3-D reformatting asserts clinical potential in MRI. Diagnostic Imaging, May: 80-84

7. Lang P, Hedtmann A, Genant HK (1988) Three-dimensional computerized tomography in osteochondritis dissecans of the trochlea tali. Orthop Praxis 24: 779-782

8. Schmitz H-J, Tolxdorff T, Honsbrok J, Fritz T, Gross U (1989) 3-D-based computer assisted manufacturing of individual alloplastic implants for cranial and maxillofacial osteoplasties. In: Lemke HU, Rhodes ML, Jaffe CC, Felix R (eds) Computer Assisted Radiology '89. Springer, Berlin Heidelberg New York, pp 390-395

9. Totty WG, Vannier MW (1984) Complex musculosketal anatomy: analysis using three dimensional surface reconstruction. Radiology 150: 173-177

10. Tronnier U, Wolff KD, Trittmacher S (1989) A 3-D surgical planning system and its clinical application. In: Lemke HU, Rhodes ML, Jaffe CC, Felix R (eds) Computer Assisted Radiology '89. Springer, Berlin Heidelberg New York, pp 401-408

11. Vannier MW, Marsh JL, Warren JO (1984) Three dimensional CT reconstruction images for craniofacial surgical planning and evaluation. Radiology 150: 179-184

12. Vannier MW, Gronemeyer S, Gutierrez FR (1988) Three dimensional MRI of congenital heart disease. Radiographics 8: 857-871

High Resolution CT of the Petrosa with Two- and Three-Dimensional Reconstructions

F. ASTINET, M. LANGER, C. ZWICKER, U. KESKE, P. UHRMEISTER, R. FELIX

Abstract

HR-CTs were produced with a unit having a 1024×1024 pixel display matrix on 100 patients with illnesses of the petrosa. It was seen that high spatial resolution with the resultant possibility of differentiating even fine anatomical structures offers extended diagnostic possibilities for clarifying illnesses of the auditory and vestibular apparatus. The evaluation of the 2D secondary reconstruction showed that the use of the thinnest possible, continuous slices (1 mm) usually resulted in an image quality sufficient for diagnosis in 2D-CT. This is additionally combined with a substantial reduction in patient stress (no problems with positioning, no further radiation exposure) and a considerable saving in time. A three-dimensional display of the base of the skull was performed in cases with extensive bony destruction to permit a clear display of more complex bony structures. Disadvantages of these methods include the deficient display of soft-tissue structures and inferior spatial resolution. Furthermore, there is no possibility of producing detailed internal views, e. g. of the ossicular chain, or contour smoothing by means of a filtering algorithm. Differentiation of a soft-tissue tumor or finer bone arrosions is still impossible three-dimensionally. The primary or secondary reconstructed 2D-CT slice remains the basis for diagnostics.

Introduction

High resolution computed tomography of the petrosa is an undisputed method of examination which displays a superiority over other imaging techniques. Goal of the prospective study presented here is to demonstrate the extensive diagnostics made possible by using a display matrix of 1024×1024 pixels. This leads to further possibilities of multidimensional image reconstruction as well as to an improved spatial resolution.

Aside from the improved imaging qualities, the present paper goes into specific details in regard to extending the potential of secondary image reconstructions, both two- and three-dimensional. These possibilities result from shortened examination times and increased computer capacity. Various scan parameters are also compared and their use discussed in relation to the particular problem in question.

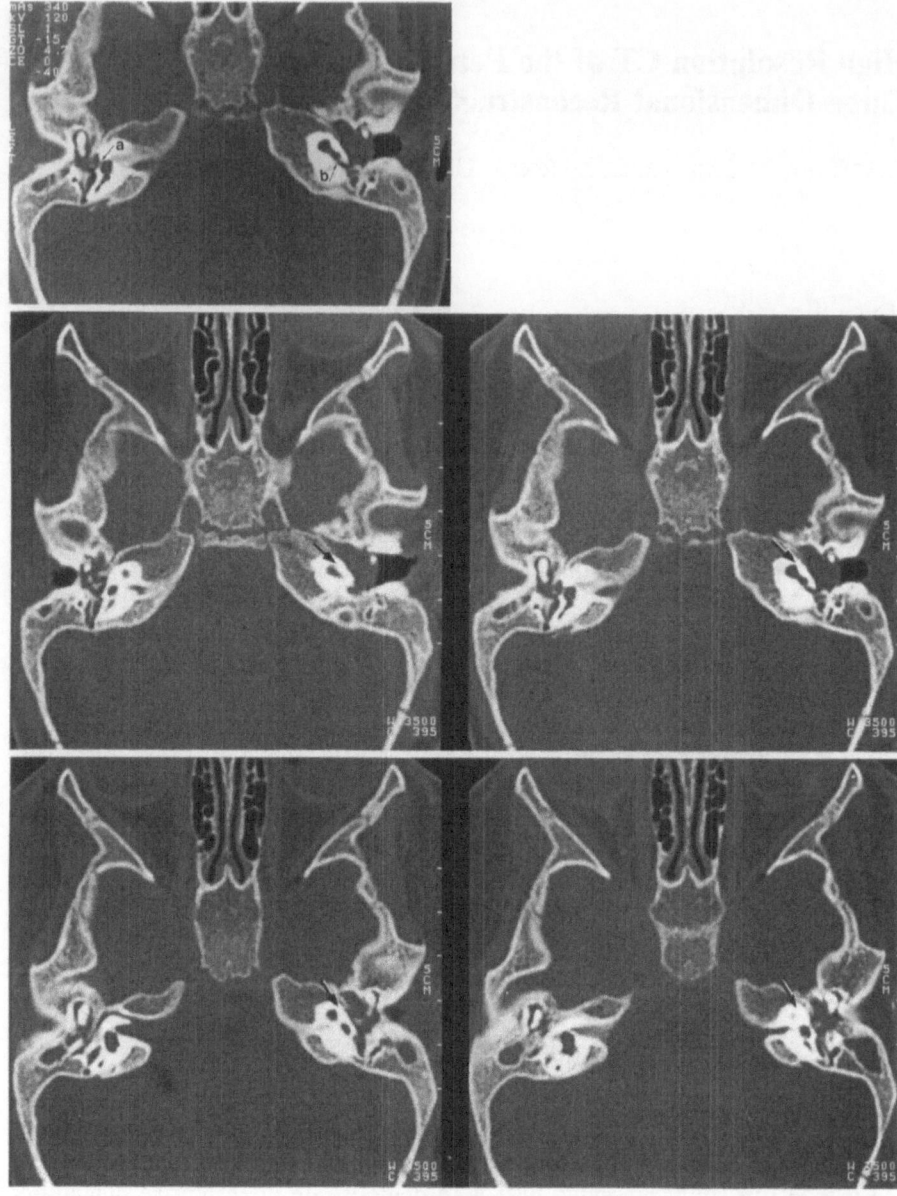

Fig. 1a, b. a 2 year-old female patient with congenital deformities of the middle/inner ear: aplasia of the cochlea's apical spiral canals and soft tissue consolidation of the tympanic cavity. In the
left petrosa, good differentiation of the oval window bordering on the vestibulum (<‑‑a) with the
posterior semicircular canal. The dense soft tissue shadow of the left tympanic cavity extends into
the considerably narrowed epitympanic recess and surrounds the incudomalleolar joint entirely
from caudal. Right: basal section of the cochlea's spiral canal with the round window (<‑‑b) bordering laterally on the tympanic cavity. An uninterrupted, dense soft tissue shadow of the meso-
tympanum is also seen here with displacement of the manubrium ventrolaterally. **b** The scan sequence documents the total aplasia of the cochlea's apical canal (<‑‑). The girl's chromosome
analysis revealed a "de-novo" translocation of the long arm of chromosome 8 to the short arm of
chromosome 9. Objective audiometry showed no evaluable brain stem reflexes

Patients and Methods

High resolution transaxial images of the petrosa were performed on 100 patients with illnesses of the middle or inner ear in a prospective study. SOMATOM PLUS, with a display matrix of 1024 × 1024 pixels and a reconstruction matrix of 512 × 512 pixels, was used for the examinations. The tube voltage was 120 kV in each case, and the cathode current was 340 mAs with a scan time of 2 seconds or 510 mAs at a scan time of 4 seconds. Examinations were performed with the assistance of a special inner ear algorithm with an edge-enhancing algorithm. Computed tomograms were produced in axial projection with the examination slice tipped 10–20 degrees cranially from the orbitomeatal plane. This avoids radiation exposure to the crystalline lenses and improves the conditions for imaging the middle and inner ear. Here, the tympanic part of the facial nerve as well as the entire course of the lateral semicircular canal can be displayed. Enlarged image cutouts were produced additionally by the renewed reconstruction of raw data. An additional examination in the coronal plane (offset 105 degrees to the orbitomeatal line) followed in 60 cases. Axial slices were reconstructed secondarily in the coronal plane and results were compared to the coronal scan produced primarily.

Findings could only be displayed in a second plane with the coronary secondary reconstruction in cases entailing problems with problem positioning (n = 40). Such cases resulted, for example, due to advanced age, a poor state of health and limited mobility of the cervical spine.

Continuous slices of 1 mm thickness were produced in 72 cases and in the remaining 28 cases with 2 mm slices. A comparison of imaging conditions was also made here between slices of 1 and 2 mm thickness.

In the presence of extensive bony destruction (n = 38), three-dimensional reconstructions of the base of the skull were obtained from data files of the axial examination. Three-dimensional images were produced according to the principle of surface reconstruction with contour extraction as described by Vannier and Marsh [28]. This method only reads out those pixels for which the density lies above that of a freely selectable threshold. A threshold between 150 and 200 Hounsfield Units (HU) is generally used. A "pseudo" light source provided the spatial presentation, whereby pixels nearer the viewer are displayed brighter and structures further away are displayed darker. Enlarged cutouts via a zoom offer a further possibility for image processing. Furthermore, the object can be viewed in six standard projections or rotated in real-time with one degree graduation as a wire-frame model for the evaluation of surface reconstructions. A cutout function (CUT) provides a detailed internal view.

In individual cases (n = 10), an i.v. contrast medium administration was performed for improved soft tissue contrast.

Results

Display matrix of 1024 × 1024 pixels

The high resolution of the 1024 × 1024 pixel display matrix proved to be advantageous for displaying the ossicular chain and especially the stapes and the crura of the incus. Imaging the stapial head and base within the recess of the oval window was possible in axial and coronal planes in 100% of the cases. At least one limb of the stapes could be identified 77% of the time in the axial or 81% in the coronal slice. Even minute otosclerotic plaque or active, otospongiotic foci can be identified in the region of the cochlea and semicircular canals as well as in the oval and round windows (Figs. 2b + c). Bony juxtapositions or synostoses of the ossicular chain with one another or with the tympatic attic could also be displayed in the course of otosclerosis or malformations. Fixation of the stapedial footplate in the oval window alone is not possible with computed tomography. These structures are therefore not amenable to quantitative evaluations, even with the maximum available image resolution. Bony destruction of the ossicular chain could be demonstrated more accurately, whereby even arrosions on the long crus of the incus and the stapedial footplate could be displayed. The intrapyramidal part of the facial nerve could be displayed completely in 100% of the examinations. The axial projection proved to be especially suitable for evaluating the labyrinthine and tympanic parts. On the other hand, the mastoid part can be evaluated better in the coronal plane. Even the lamellae, which usually only surround the proximal tympanic part of the facial nerve, could be displayed in 80% of all cases. Nonpathologic changes of the tympanic membranes (physiological thickness from 0.08–0.1 mm [1] as well as the tensor tympani muscle could be displayed in both planes for each examination performed. The tendon of the tensor tympani muscle

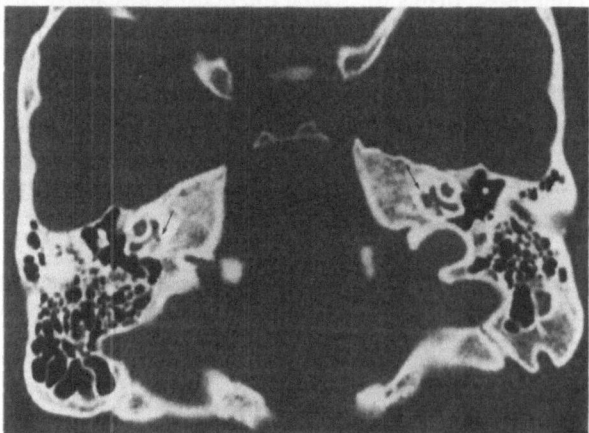

Fig. 2a. 38 year-old male patient with extensive pericochlear otospongiosis (< --) in the course of an otosclerosis. Axial 1 mm slice at the level of the cochlea's spiral canal. Clinically, the patient demonstrated a severe combined conductive and neural hearing loss, right worse than left

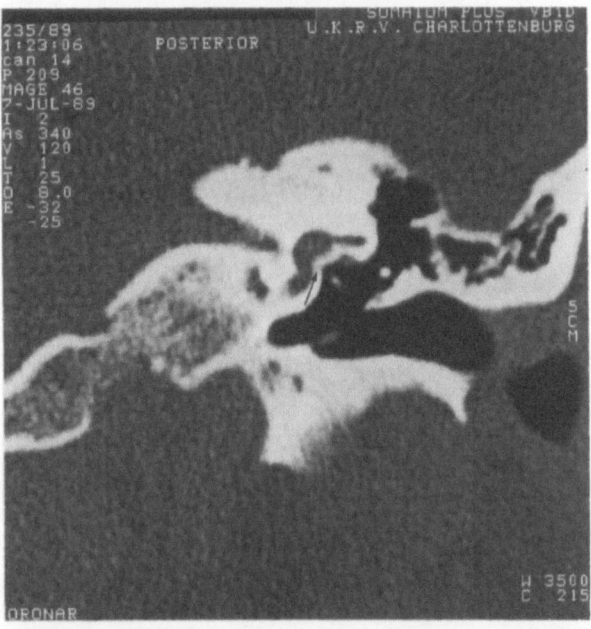

Fig. 2b. Enlarged cutout of a 1 mm coronal slice of the right petrosa in the same otosclerosic patient. Good differentiation of the consolidation on the stapedial base, whereby the inactive sclerotic foci lead to an uninterrupted bony deposition of the oval window adjacent to the vestibulum (<--)

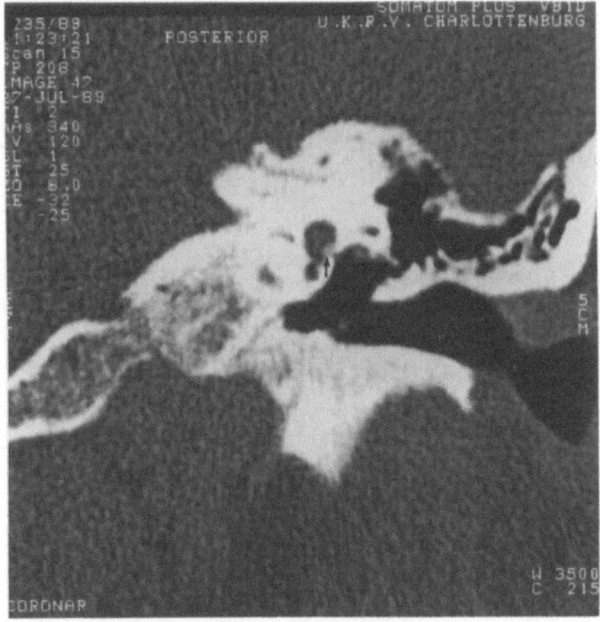

Fig. 2c. 1 mm slice directly dorsal to 2b showing an active otospongiotic focus (<--) projecting into the vestibulum

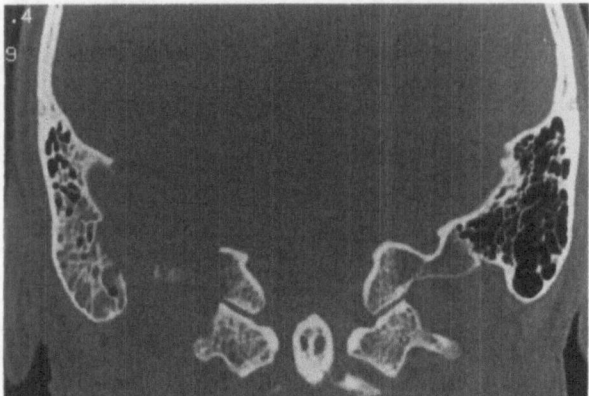

Fig. 3a. 42 year-old male patient with a histologically established squamous cell carcinoma of the external auditory canal. Coronal 1 mm primary slice through the dorsal part of the petrosa. Along with the mastoidal destruction, a nearly complete obliteration of the condylar part of the occipital bone can be seen where the tumor extends beyond the base of the skull inframastoidally. Additionally, arrosions of the occipital condyle and the left arch of the atlas can be seen

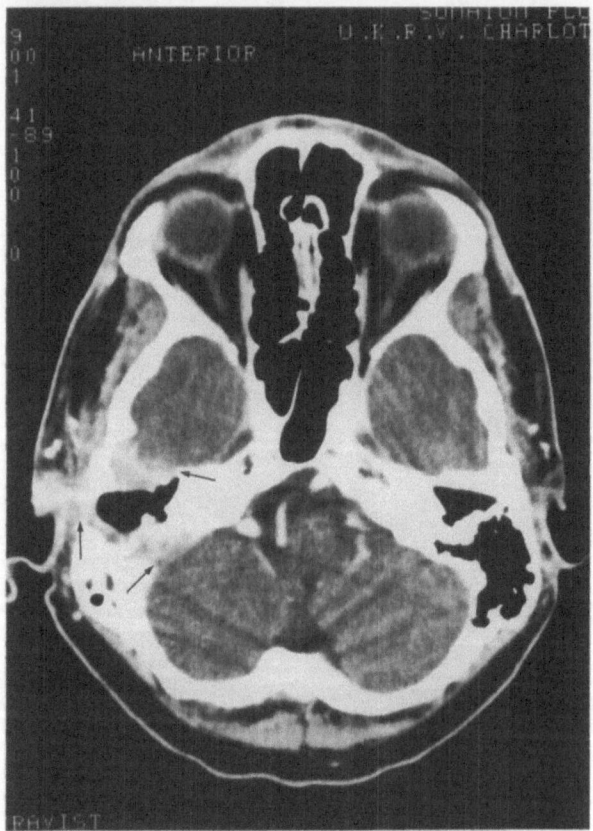

Fig. 3b. Transverse CT slice with soft-tissue windowing technique after i. v. contrast medium administration. Display of the hyperdense, contrast-medium enhanced tumor parts which have projected both periauricularly and into the anterior and posterior cranial fossae (< --)

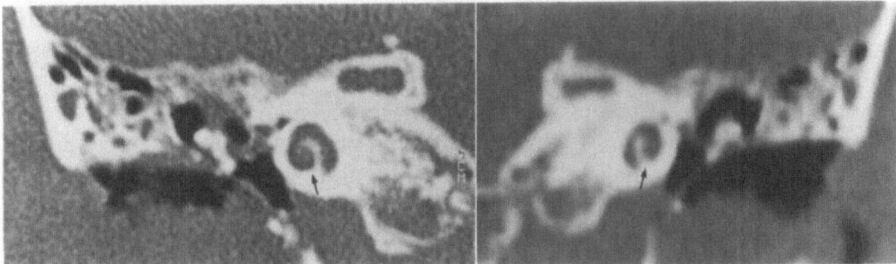

Fig. 3c. The left half shows an enlarged cutout of the coronal primary slice through the left petrosa at the level of the chochlea's spiral canal (< --). Extensive bony destruction with complete obliteration of the auditory canal's floor and an osseus articular fossa resulting from the carcinoma of the auditory canal. Tumor infiltration of the mastoid and the tympanic cavity with initial arrosion of the ossicular chain at the level of the epitympanic recess. The right half shows an ipsilateral, mirror-image, coronal secondary reconstruction with nearly the same scanning plane, in direct comparison

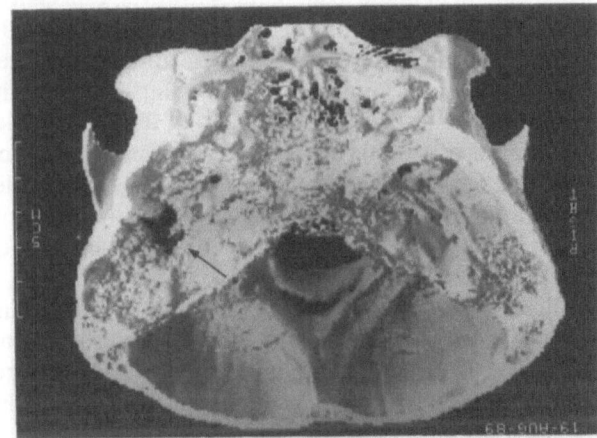

Fig. 3d. Clear, three-dimensional display of extensive bony destruction in the region of the petrosa's anterior wall which reaches into the squamous part of the temporal bone (< --)

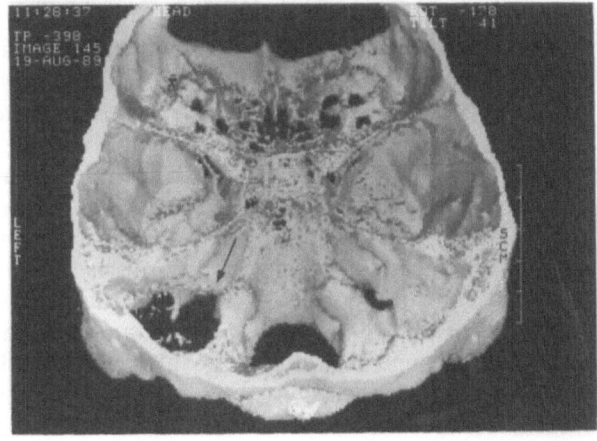

Fig. 3e. Good three-dimensional differentiation of destruction resulting from the tumor in the dorsal part of the left petrosa, the region of the subarcuate fossa, and the condylar part of the occipital bone. Here, the tumor extends beyond the base of the skull suboccipitally (< --)

could be demonstrated in all cases with an axial and in 80% of all cases with a coronal projection. The stapedius muscle with its tendon on the head of the stapes could be imaged axially in 72% of all cases.

Both labyrinthine structures, cochlea and semicircular canals, could be displayed with high resolution. The axial projection plane offered the best conditions for imaging the stapes, the incudomalleolar joint and the processus lenticularis on the long crus of the incus (most often affected in bony destruction of the ossicular chain). The manubrium and long crus of the incus were displayed best in the coronal plane.

A similar differentiation must also be made for extraossicular structures. Thus, the axial plane was found to be advantageous for evaluating the pyramid of the tympanum, tensor tympani muscle, aqueduct of the cochlea, tympanic part of the facial nerve and aditus ad antrum. The coronal plane proved to be better suited for imaging Prussak's space, the lateral epitympanic wall and the facial canal running vertically in the mastoid.

The round and oval windows could be evaluated easily in every examination by displaying them in the axial plane. However, especially for determining the degree of ankylosis in the course of otosclerosis, the coronal plane proved to be better. Here, no partial volume effects were found, and the respective window recess could be imaged without superpositioning. This permits the evaluation of smaller bony arrosions, especially in the area of the semicircular canals, and the demarcation of minute sclerotic and spongiotic, otosclerotic foci (Figs. 2 b + c). These often lead to a narrowing in the spiral canal of the cochlea. Cochlear otospongiosis which usually presents with spongiosis of the labyrinthine capsule's enchondral layer (Fig. 2 a) can also be displayed. Image presentation could be quantified by means of a measured density profile.

These statements are especially applicable for scans of 1 mm slice thickness. Limitations in detail must be made for 2 mm slices, since an increased partial volume effect is present. Here, a superposition of the facial nerve, stapes and perilabyrinthine bone (promontorium) takes place in the oval window, making the differentiation of the structures from one another impossible.

Possibilities with multiplanar secondary reconstruction

The extended possibilities offered by two-dimensional, secondary reconstructions are shown in Figures 4a and b. The right side of each shows an enlarged cutout of a primary coronal scan, whereas the left side is a mirror-image counterpart; i. e., it represents an ipsilateral, coronal secondary reconstruction displayed with nearly the same plane of scanning. Figure 4a shows this scanning technique in the form of a coronal cutout at the level of the cochlea's spiral canal in the healthy, right petrosa of a 42 year-old male patient. One can recognize the external auditory canal, tympanic membrane connected to the manubrium of the malleus, hammer's head and body of the incus with their articulation in the epitympanic recess, the lateral attic wall, and the tensor tympani muscle with its tendon connected to the neck of the hammer. All of these are also recognizable in the mirror-image, coronal secondary reconstruction in the left half of the figure, although with a certain degree of graphic blurring.

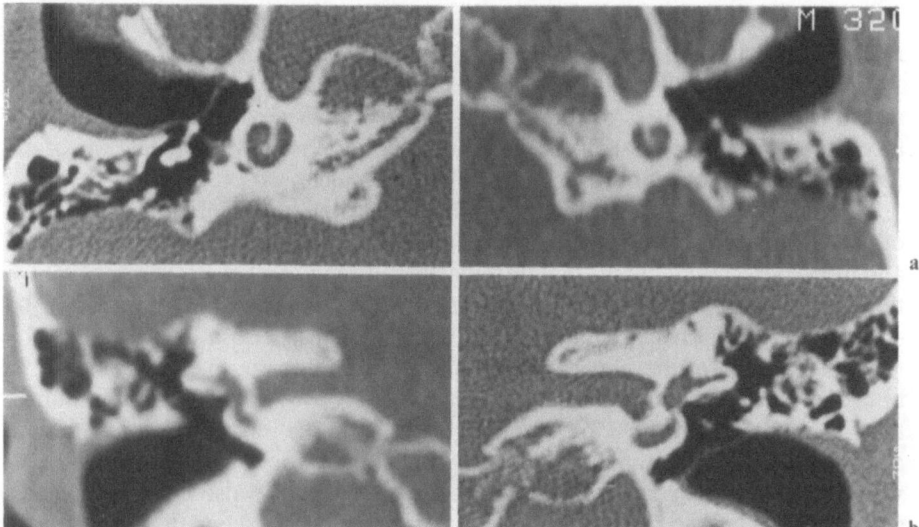

Fig. 4a, b. A comparison of methods. Primary transverse CT slice (enlarged coronal cutout on the right) and secondary reconstruction (performed in nearly the same scanning plane and displayed as a mirror image on the left). Section of a healthy right petrosa at the level of the cochlea's spiral canal (a) and at the level of the oval window's recess (b)

Figure 4b shows an enlarged, coronal cutout at the level of the oval window's recess, bordering on the vestibulum. The external auditory canal with tympanic membrane, internal auditory canal, as well as the anterior part of the lateral semi-circular canal leaving the labyrinth, and the posterior semicircular canal running into the labyrinth from caudal are displayed. From the ossicular chain and within the recess of the oval window, one can recognize only one section on the short crus of the incus at the level of the epitympanic process. In addition, the processus lenticularis on the long crus of the incus as it attaches to the head of the stapes. The coronal secondary reconstruction shown on the left also makes it possible to demarcate even such fine anatomical structures as the stapes within the recess of the oval window, although somewhat obscured.

Figure 3c shows a coronal cutout at the level of the cochlea's spiral canal in a 42 year-old male patient with a carcinoma of the auditory canal. The expanse of the extensive bony destruction can also be realized in the secondary reconstruction. However, this method has its limitations in the assessment of smaller arrosions, e.g. of the auditory ossicles, where graphic blurring is disadvantageous.

The secondary reconstructions shown in Figs. 3 + 4 were produced from primary axial investigations with continuous 1 mm slicing. Secondary reconstruction from primary 2 mm slicing was found to be unsuitable for adequately assessing the fine structures of the middle and inner ear. Restlessness on the part of the patient during and between the scans substantially impairs the image quality of secondary reconstructions.

A high image quality for secondary reconstructions, comparable with that in the figures at hand, could only be accomplished with axial 1 mm slices in half of the 36 examinations. In 10 cases, secondary reconstructions could only be partly assessed due to restlessness of the patient. Another eight reconstructions could not be evaluated, because of algorithmic errors or because access to the data file of the primary axial investigation was impossible due to technical problems.

The three-dimensional display also offered a better spatial orientation in cases of extensive bony destruction. Thus, the breakthrough of a tumor into the middle and posterior cranial fossa and inframastoidally could also be verified with a three-dimensionl display of the base of the skull (see Figures 3 a and b). Figure 3 d shows the bony destruction at the anterior edge of the petrosa brought about by the breakthrough of the tumor into the middle cranial fossa. Figure 3 e shows the breakthrough point into the posterior cranial fossa as well as the obliteration of the condylar part of the occipital bone. The three-dimensional display of finer anatomical structures (e. g. the ossicular chain) is not possible with the present software programs. The absence of soft tissues in the display is also disadvantageous, since determining the real extent of tumor expansion is consequently not possible. High spatial resolution, thinnest slices (1 mm), and the avoidance of motion artifacts with their resulting slice mismatch are of fundamental significance for the quality of multidimensional reconstructions. The increased computer capacity leads to substantial shortening in scan time and in the entire examination time (< 20 minutes). This, together with the comfortable positioning of the patient, results in reduced motion artifacts.

Discussion

Improved diagnostics for clarifying illnesses of the petrosa can be expected thanks to the high spatial resolution of the 1024×1024 pixel display matrix. The HR-CT is today the method of choice for clarifying illnesses of the external auditory canal [15, 31] and inflammatory or tumorous alterations of the middle or inner ear [10, 12, 15, 20, 22, 29]. Further indications include pre- and postoperative follow-ups of an otosclerosis [18, 23, 26], diagnostics of the facial nerve [12, 14, 27], and the question of constitutional abnormalities and deformities of the auditory and vestibular apparatus [5, 12, 16, 24]. HR-CT of the petrosa also offers an additional, preliminary examination possibility prior to cochlea implantation [8, 9, 17]. The superiority of HR-CT in petrosal diagnostics compared with other methods of imaging, especially polytomography with the hypocyclotic blurring technique, is described repeatedly in the literature [1-3, 11-16, 19, 25, 29, 30].

The increased computer capacity leads to substantial shortening in scan time and in the entire examination time. Motion artifacts are therefore reduced during and between the scans. This, together with the excellent resolution of fine detail leads to an improved quality of multiplanar and three-dimensional secondary reconstructions.

Minute anatomical structures, such as the stapes, tympanic membrane, and facial nerve in the entire intrapyramidal course, could be displayed regularly and in a form suitable for evaluation [6, 21]. The facial nerve can be displayed even in the labyrinthine part and in the region of the geniculate ganglion with the branch of the greater superficial petrosal nerve. The claims made by many authors in the past [2, 7, 12, 13] that the tympanic membrane must be pathologically thickened in order to be displayed with CT, were disproved with the use of a 1024 × 1024 pixel matrix. The improved spatial resolution is also evident in displaying the stapes. However, an incomplete display due to possible sectioning phenomena permits no inference that a structure is lacking [5, 13]. On the other hand, the identification of appositional changes can be seen as reliable. In this connection, the potential for better quality coronal secondary reconstruction offers the advantage of a combined soft-tissue/bone display, in contrast to 3D-CT [7]. Furthermore, these high-quality reconstructions provide the only possibility of displaying the findings in a second plane in cases of problems with patient positioning or where additional radiation exposure is to be avoided. This also offers a better spatial orientation for the operating surgeon. In addition, the two-dimensional secondary reconstruction (coronal and sagittal) provides a substantial saving in time compared with the primary investigation in a second plane. On the one hand, this follows from the fact that the secondary reconstruction is performed on a console separated from the running examination program. On the other hand, it follows from the fact that the 16 adjacent, coronal reconstructed slices are produced from the data file of one axial investigation, requiring only 3 minutes. Our experience has shown that saving in time and avoidance of additional patient stress often makes a second primary investigation in the coronal plane unnecessary [7]. However, the loss of detailed information through graphic blurring is disadvantageous for displaying fine bone arrosions, e.g. of the ossicular chain, or minute otosclerotic or spongiotic changes. Here, the primary coronal slice appears to be indispensible.

The three-dimensional display of the petrosa provides clear findings in cases of extensive bony destruction. The danger of finding bony pseudo-defects in the form of pseudoforaminas must be taken into account if the threshold value selected is too high. Selecting too low a threshold value causes increased contour smoothing, in addition to the incorporation of lower-density structures and also artifacts, and leads to a substantial loss in quality of the 3D reconstruction [4]. Detailed internal views of the petrosa or an isolated three-dimensional display of the ossicular chain are impossible with the present software programs. Further disadvantages are the deficient display of soft tissue and the contour smoothing through algorithms. This makes the assessment of the tumor's real expansion and of bony arrosions impossible in cases of tumorous alterations. Therefore, the diagnostics continue to be based on the findings of transverse HR-CT or two-dimensional secondary reconstruction. Although at times advantageous for the quality of secondary reconstructions, adjacent overlapping slices (2 mm slice thickness, 1 mm table feed) should not be used in primary transverse scanning, since there is a loss in detailed information due to partial volume effects. In the same way, the use of non-contiguous slices (table feed > slice thickness) makes it difficult to display the fine structures of the petrosa completely and clearly in the secondary reconstructions. This has been described by several authors [2, 3, 23].

Conclusions

1. The 1024 × 1024 pixel display matrix with improved spatial resolution extends the diagnostic possibilities.
2. Two-dimensional secondary reconstructions of optimal quality can be obtained with high computer capacity and by preparing the thinnest possible, continuous slices (1 mm). The resultant shortening of the entire examination time leads to a further reduction in motion artifacts.
3. The 2D reconstruction offers a substantial saving in time and is frequently sufficient for diagnosis.
4. The 3D-CT permits a clear display of findings demonstrating complex bony destructions.
5. The transverse CT slice remains the basis for diagnosis.

References

1. Chakeres DW, Spiegel PK (1983) A systematic technique for comprehensive evaluation of the temporal bone by computed tomography. Radiology 146: 97-106
2. Fritz P, Lenarz T, Haels J, Fehrentz D (1987) Feinstrukturanalyse des Felsenbeines mittels hochauflösender Dünnschicht-Computertomographie, Teil 1. Fortschr Röntgenstr 147, 3: 266-271
3. Fritz P, Rieden K, Lenarz T (1989) Feinstrukturanalyse des Felsenbeines mittels hochauflösender Dünnschicht-Computertomographie, Teil 2. Fortschr Röntgenstr 151, 2: 171-175
4. Grevers G, Wittman A, Vogl Th, Wiechell R (1989) Untersuchungen zur multiplanaren Darstellung des Felsenbeines. Laryngo-Rhino-Otol 68: 88.91
5. Grevers G, Vogl Th, Markl A, Kang K (1989) Zur Aussagefähigkeit der HR-Computertomographie bei Mittelohrmißbildung. Laryngo-Rhino-Otol 68: 88.91
6. Grobovschek M (1988) Synopsis einer standardisierten, schematischen Analyse der Ossikula und der Tympanonwände, dargestellt mit der hochauflösenden Computertomographie. Digit Bilddiagn 8: 115-127
7. Haas JP, Kahle G (1988) Wie kann heute das Felsenbein radiologisch am besten dargestellt werden? HNO 36: 89-101
8. Harnsberger HRic, Dart DJ, Parkin JL, Smoker WRK, Osborn AG (1987) Cochlear implant candidates: assessment with CT and MR imaging. Radiology 164: 53-57
9. Jackler RK, Luxford WM, Schindler RA, McKerrow WS (1987) Cochlear patency problems in cochlear implantation. Larnygoscope 97: 801-805
10. Johnson DW, Voorhees RL, Lufkin RB, Hanafee W, Canalis R (1983) Cholesteatomas of the temporal bone: role of computed tomographie. Radiology 148: 733-737
11. König H, Kurtz B (1984) Hochauflösende Computertomographie der Felsenbeine. Fortschr Röntgenstr 141, 2: 129-135
12. Köster O (1988) Computertomographie des Felsenbeines. Georg Thieme Verlag
13. Köster O, Böckler R, Lackner K, Koch U (1984) Die hochauflösende Computertomographie des Mittel- und Innenohres. Laryng Rhinol Otol 63: 488-493
14. Köster O, Straehler-Pohl H-J (1987) Hochauflösende Computertomographie bei peripherer Fazialisparese. Fortschr Röntgenstr 146, 1: 7-13
15. Köster O, Straehler-Pohl H-J (1986) Die hochauflösende Computertomographie in der Abklärung knochendestruierender Prozesse des äußeren Ohres. Fortschr Röntgenstr 145, 6: 651-656
16. Köster O, Straehler-Pohl H-J, Kim KH (1987) Hochauflösende Computertomographie bei Mißbildungen des Gehör- und Gleichgewichtsorganes. Fortschr Röntgenstr 147, 1: 39-45

17. Laszig R, Battmer RD, Becker H (1986) Hochauflösende Computertomographie als ergänzende Voruntersuchung zum Cochlear Implant. HNO 34: 429–433
18. Mafee MF, Henrikson GC, Deitch RL, Norouzi P, Kumar A, Kriz R, Valvassori GE (1985) Use of CT in stapedial otosclerosis. Radiology 156: 709–714
19. Mafee MF, Kumar A, Yannias DA, Valvassori GE, Applebaum EL (1983) CT of the middle ear in the evaluation of cholesteatomas and other soft-tissue masses: comparison with pluridirectional tomography. Radiology 148: 465–472
20. Silver AJ, Janecka I, Wazen J, Hilal SK, Rutledge JN (1987) Complicated cholesteatomas: CT findings in inner ear complications of middle ear cholesteatomas. Radiology 164: 47–51
21. Swartz JD (1983) HR-CT of the middle ear and mastoid. Part 1. Radiology 148: 449–454
22. Swartz JD, Berger AS, Zwillenberg S, Popky GL (1987) Ossicular erosions in the dry ear: CT diagnosis. Radiology 163: 763–765
23. Swartz JD, Faerber EN, Wolfson RJ, Marlowe FI (1984) Fenestral otosclerosis: significance of preoperative CT evaluation. Radiology 151: 703–707
24. Swartz JD, Glazer AU, Faerber EN, Capatanio MA, Popky GI (1986) Congenital middle ear deafness: CT study. Radiology 159: 187–190
25. Swartz JD, Goodman RS, Russell KB, Marlowe FI, Wolfson RJ (1983) HR-CT of the middle ear and mastoid. Radiology 148: 455–459
26. Swartz JD, Mandell DW, Berman SE, Wolfson RJ, Marlowe FI, Popky GL (1985) Chochlear otosclerosis (otospongiosis): CT analysis with audiometric correlation. Radiology 155: 147–150
27. Valvanis A, Kubik S, Oguz M (1983) Exploration of the facial nerve canal by HR-CT: anatomy and pathology. Neuroradiology 24: 139–147
28. Vannier MW, Marsh JL, Warren JO (1984) 3D-CT reconstruction images for craniofacial surgical planning and evaluation. Radiology 150: 179–184
29. Virapongse C, Rothman SLG, Sasaki C, Kier EL (1982) The role of HR-CT in evaluating disease of the middle ear. J Comp Ass Tomogr 6 (4): 711–720
30. Virapongse C, Sarwar M, Kier EL, Sasaki C, Pillsbury H (1983) Temporal bone disease: a comparison between HR-CT and pluridirectional tomography. Radiology 147: 743–748
31. Virapongse C, Sawar M, Sasaki C, Kier EL (1983) HR-CT of the osseous external auditory canal. J Comp Ass Tomogr 7 (3): 486–492

Preliminary Results for CT Examinations of Spinal Fractures with a SOMATOM PLUS 3D Software Program

W. VOGEL, W.H. DINGLER, M. SCHÜTZ, H.K. DEININGER

Introduction

CT examinations are a must in cases of severe comminuted fractures and dislocations of the spinal column. Due to the ease of patient positioning as compared to conventional tomography, additional information regarding soft tissue structures, and non-obstructing display of complex multiple layer anatomical structures, CT represents the examination method of choice. Oblique positioning of the patient, which may cause further injury, is often required for a definitive diagnosis with conventional tomography. However, every diagnostic effort must provide information regarding the stability of the vertebral fracture, since all subsequent therapeutic procedures depend upon this data.

Orthopedic surgeons believe that information regarding stability of the spinal column should be obtained not only by focussing on a specific aspect (e. g., verti-

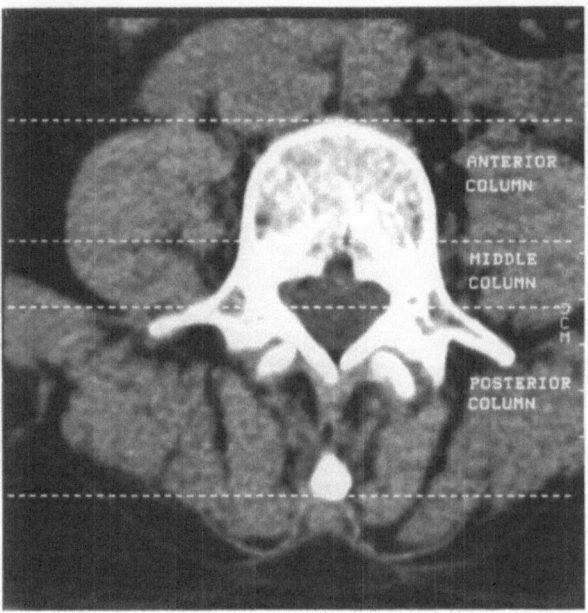

Fig. 1. The three column concept according to Denis and McAfee, shown on an intact lumbar vertebrae

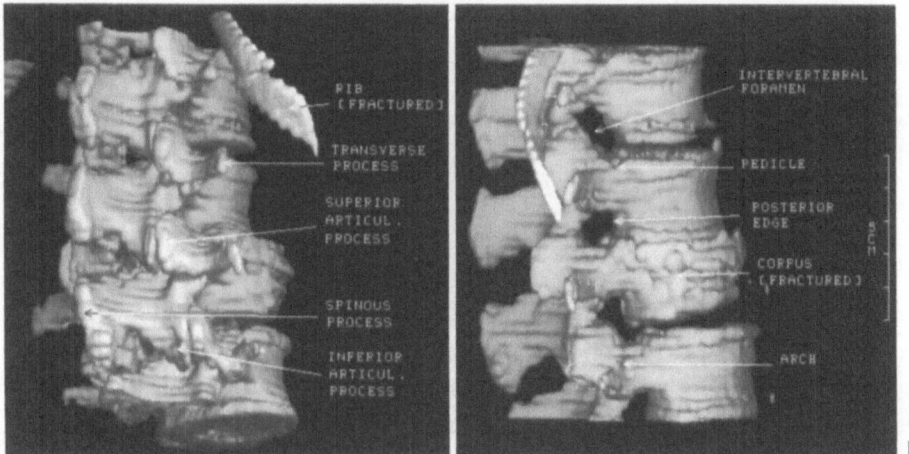

Fig. 2a, b. Rotated 3D overview image postprocessed with "Light". The individual anatomic spinal structures are clearly demarcated

cal or horizontal stability) or an isolated observation of one specific vertebral element [6]. Despite these recommendations, we have decided to adhere to the generally accepted three column spine concept established by Denis and McAffee [1, 7]. Thus, the stabilizing vertebral elements can be delineated and systematically examined (Fig. 1).

The objective of our study was the display and evaluation of spinal column fractures using axial, 2D and 3D methods. We compared the capabilities of these methods, image quality, and diagnostic interpretation of damaged anatomical structures (Fig. 2).

Material and Methods

Thirty-one patients with highly unstable fractures of the cervical, thoracic, and lumbar spine were examined. Patient age ranged from 17 to 62 with an average age of 32 years. There were 19 male and 12 female patients.

Table 1 shows the distribution of fractures according to the spinal column sections as well as the diagnostic methods used.

With the exception of three patients, for whom axial CT slices had been performed during the examination of the cranium, standard x-ray survey exposures in two planes, axial CT slices, and 2D and 3D reconstructions were generated for each patient. For two patients, conventional tomograms were generated for fractures of the cervical spine, thoracic spine, and lumbar spine. We subsequently abandoned this method for reasons of radiation protection.

Contiguous, non-overlapping CT slices were taken with a SOMATOM PLUS computed tomography system. A slice thickness of 2 mm was selected for the cer-

Table 1. Distribution of fractures in particular regions of the vertebral column and their diagnostic imaging

Region Method	Cervical Spine n=14	Thoracal Spine n=11	Lumbar Spine n=6
Plain Radiographs	11	11	6
Conventional Tomography	2	2	2
Axial CT	14	11	6
2D-Reconstructions	14	11	6
3D-Reconstructions	14	11	6

Table 2. Differenciated evaluation of the spinal fractures concerning the involved anatomical vertebral structures

Region Structure	Cervical Spine n=14	Thoracal Spine n=11	Lumbar Spine n=6
Vertebral Body	14	11	6
Posterior Edge of the Vertebral Body	10	9	6
Pedicle	4	6	4
Vertebral Arch	7	8	5
Interarticular Portion	–	–	–
Intervertebral Foramen	4	6	4
Intraspinal Fragments	–	1	1

vical region and 3 mm for the thoracic and lumbar region. The tube current was set to 500 mAs for the cervical region and to 400 mAs for the thoracic and lumbar regions. The standard resolution algorithm was selected.

2D reconstruction was performed in the sagittal and in modified oblique direction in the area of the intervertebral foramen.

3D images were computed using the Siemens SOMATOM PLUS computed tomography system in the "On the Scanner" system described by Herman [5]. We used the first version of Siemens 3D software made available to us in May, 1989. The 3D images were generated using an extraction procedure according to the so-called surface principle, where the threshold selected for bones was set to 150-200 HU. This means that all density values below the threshold are excluded when computing the image. The element matrix for 3D, initially 256 × 256 pixels, was upgraded to 512 × 512 pixels beginning in January, 1990. Earlier examinations were recomputed using the new program version.

The computed 3D images were interactively post-processed as required by the diagnostic findings using the program options "Rotate", "Cut", "Light", and "Roam". "Rotate" allows the object to be rotated along all three spatial axes. The "Cut" function cuts a selected section from the object. The "Light" function changes the gray scale using a virtual light source, which sharpens the three-dimensional image impression. "Roam" is a magnification function.

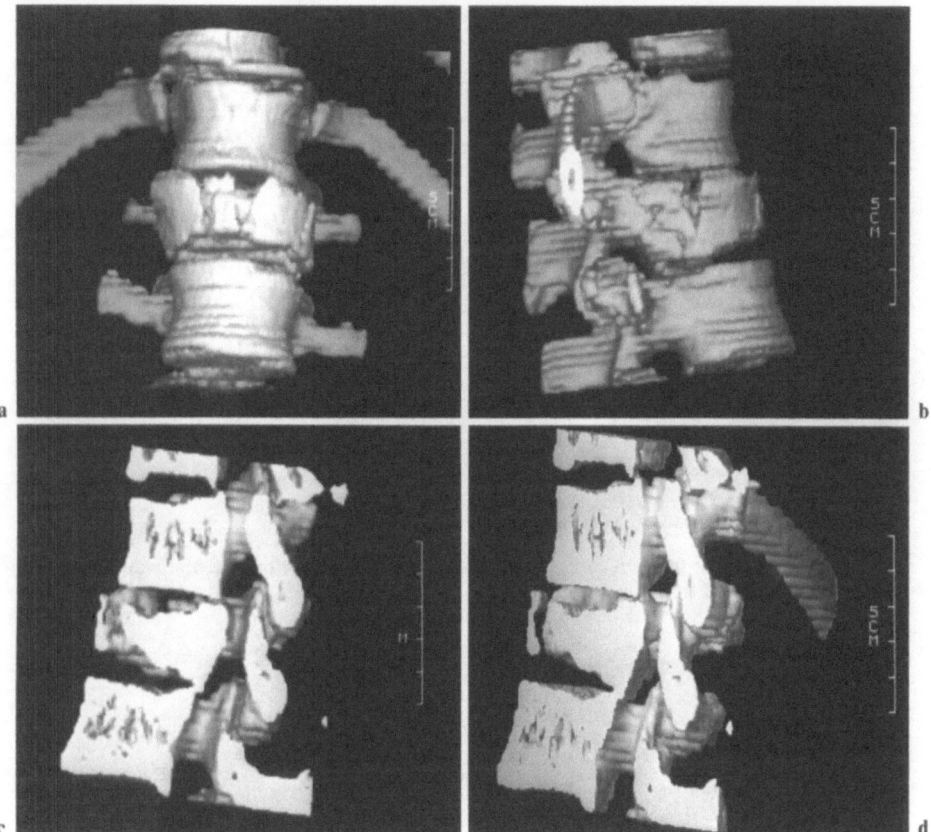

Fig. 3a-d. Burst fracture of L1 (**a**) with constricted intervertebral foramen (**b**). Only after the "Cut", "Light" and "Rotate" subprograms are employed, is there clear evidence of a protrusion of the posterior vertebral wall (**c**). Through image (**d**), a compression of the vertebral arch is shown

After all scans were completed, a systematic comparison of the display and values of the various spinal column regions using axial, 2D and 3D computed tomography methods was performed by two different radiologists. Table 2 shows the vertebral sections from the three examined regions which were included.

Results

When systemically examining the individual sections of the vertebral body, differences affecting the image impression and display of the spinal column sections and vertebral structures could be determined for the three imaging methods.

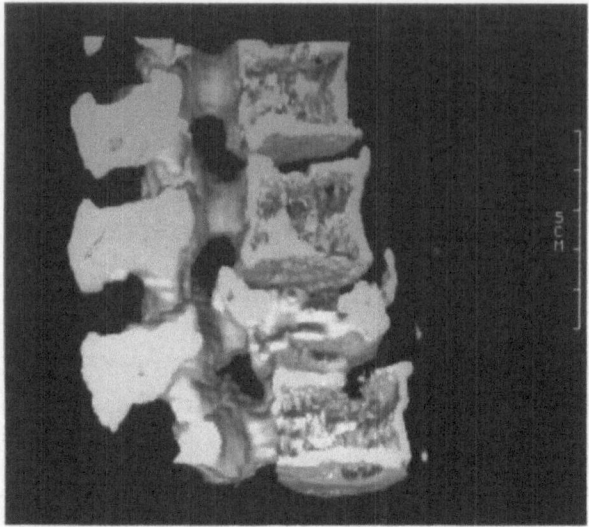

Fig. 4. A lumbar burst fracture with a large fragment at the posterior vertebral wall falsely indicates a constriction of the foramen

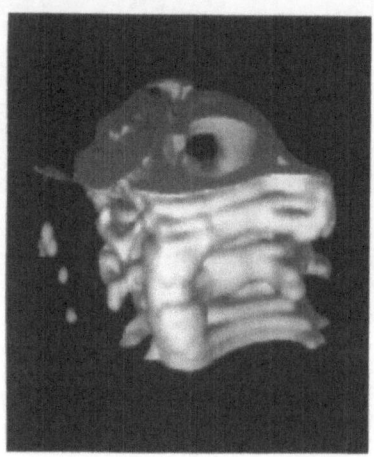

Fig. 5. Tearing of both vertebral arches of C2 without fragmenting of the middle portion of the posterior vertebral wall. For both foraminae, there is no evidence of a constriction or lesion of the arch

Vertebral body

In all the cases we examined, a lesion of the vertebral body was the most important component of the anterior spinal column. The spatial relationship between fractures, particularly with respect to longitudinal extension, were displayed three-dimensionally using 2D and 3D reconstruction (Fig. 3a, b). Lesions in the cervical, thoracic and lumbar regions could be displayed clearly using the Rotate and Light functions as well as the Cut function to some extent. We could not determine any advantage in the 2D display compared to the 3D method, neither with respect to information regarding the fracture nor with respect to improved image impression.

Posterior wall of the vertebral body

Generally, it was not difficult to diagnose the posterior wall of the vertebral body. In one case, 2D and 3D CT methods displayed the pathology of a particularly severe compression/stress fracture in the thoraco-lumbar spine far better than axial slice images. The 3D method provided the most optimal display of the complexities (Fig. 6 a–c).

Peduncle

Lesions could be diagnosed in all cases when imaging with 2D and 3D methods. The methods had a clear advantage over the axial technique. When using the program options Cut and Rotate, fractured and dislocated peduncles from all sections of the spinal column could be displayed three-dimensionally with equal image impression (Fig. 3 d and 5).

Vertebral Arch

Particularly in the cervical region of the spinal column, the 3D method produced higher quality topographic images compared to the 2D method. Even in the thoracic region where the spinal column is obstructed by the ribs this better quality could be demonstrated adequately (Fig. 6 b).

Interarticular Portion

The interarticular portion could be displayed in ⅔ of the cases using the Rotate function. This was especially true in the cervical and lumbar regions where there is no obstruction by ribs. Isolated damage to this vertebral section did not occur in our patient group.

Intervertebral Foramen

3D characteristics are well demonstrated due to the structure of the intervertebral foramen. From a spatial viewpoint, the intervertebral foramen is the connection between the posterior edges of the vertebral body, peduncle, and vertebral arch and is of primary importance for the clinical – neurological phenotype. Using the Rotate, Cut, and Light functions, three-dimensional display of the region was satisfactory in all cases examined (Figs. 4, 5 and 6 c).

Intraspinal Fragments

In the two cases with intraspinal bone fragments, information could be obtained using all three methods. However, 3D provided the best results, since volumetric extension and topographic localization could be displayed more clearly throughout the entire fracture (Figs. 4 and 6 b).

Table 3. Topographic evaluation of spinal fractures. An estimate of the respective presentation in axial-, 2D- and 3D-CT

Method / Structure	Cervical Spine			Thoracic Spine			Lumbar Spine		
	axial	2D	3D	axial	2D	3D	axial	2D	3D
Vertebral Body	++	++	+++	++	++	+++	++	++	+++
Posterior Edge of the Vertebral Body	+++	++	+++	+++	++	+++	+++	++	+++
Pedicle	+	+	+++	+	+	+++	+	+	+++
Vertebral Arch	+	(+)	+++	(+)	(+)	++	+	(+)	+++
Interarticular Portion	+	(+)	++	+	(+)	++	+	(+)	++
Intervertebral Foramen	++	++	+++	++	++	++	++	++	+++
Intraspinal Fragments	+++	++	+++	+++	++	+++	+++	++	+++

(+) poor
+ moderate
++ satisfactory   Improvement of Verification and Spatial Visualisation of the Fracture
+++ optimal

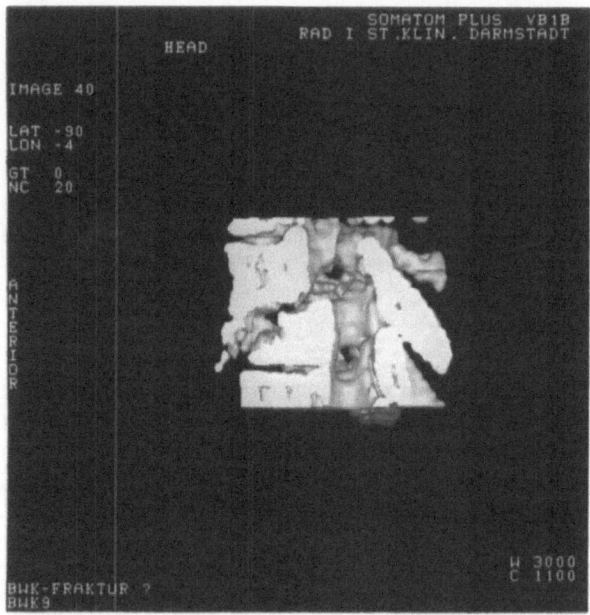

Fig. 6a–c. Image (a) shows the complexity of a severe thoracic luxation/scissor fracture. Image (b) shows that this is in fact a severe displacement of the posterior wall with a separation of arch T8. Intraspinal fractures can be seen. The T8/T9 foramen reveals normal extension, whereas the T7/T8 foramen can only be partially demarcated due to rib superpositioning (6c)

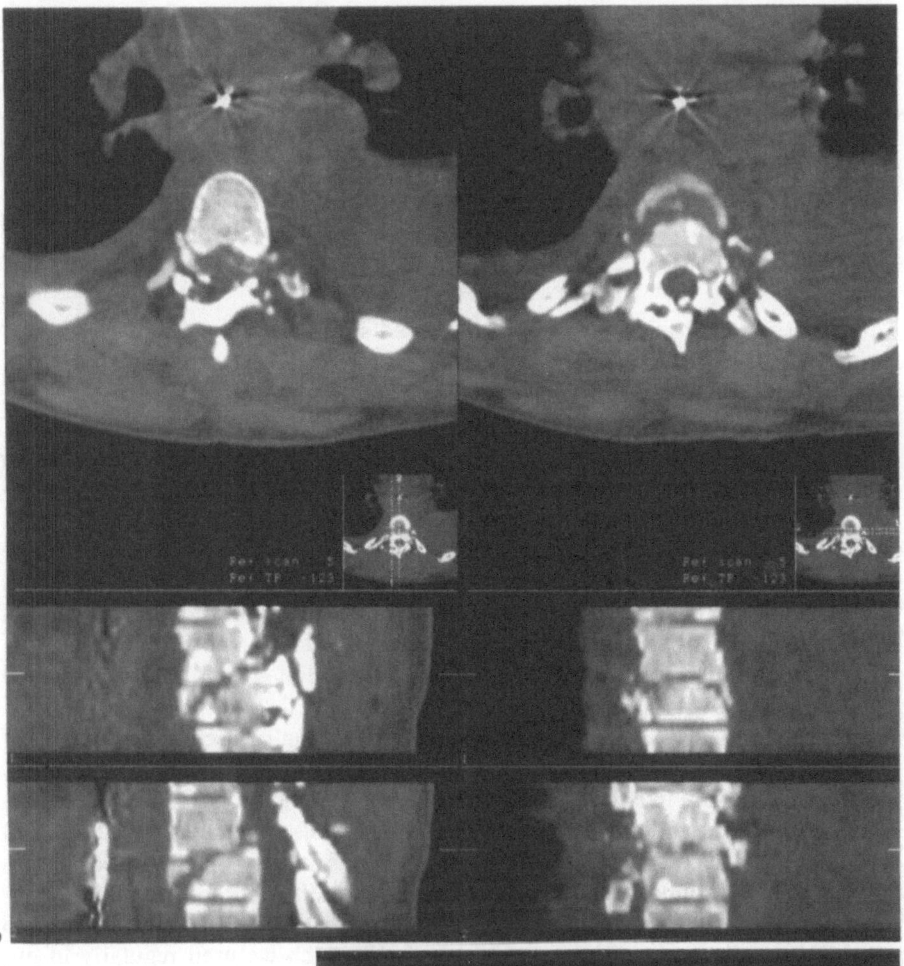

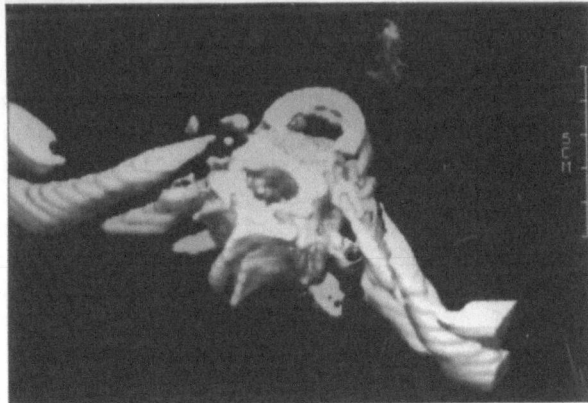

b

c

Table 3 summarizes the results of our examinations and rates the individual methods based on the vertebral elements in the three spinal column portions. A structure which could not be imaged reliably or with poor image impression is rated (+). A method which is clearly superior in displaying a structure is rated +++.

Discussion

Radiological diagnosis of patients with injured spinal columns usually begins by taking survey exposures in two planes. This allows the physician to view the spinal column portions in their entirety. However, the method has its limitations, particularly in the cranio-cervical spine and cervico-thoracic spine. If all technical prerequisites are met, limited information regarding lesions and questions regarding the stability of the fracture mandate the use of CT and its thin slice technique for further clarification. Because contrast can be manipulated easily, CT methods provide non-overlapping images with additional information regarding soft tissue structures (pneumothorax, hematoma, disk prolapse). The stabilizing elements in the central spinal column can be analyzed without the risk of moving the patient, as is necessary in conventional tomography. It should also be noted that up to 16% of the fractures diagnosed as stable using standard radiology had to be reclassified as unstable due to findings during CT examination [9].

In addition to cost and time factors as well as section-by-section acquisition of spinal column lesion data, it should be noted that a single CT image of a complex multi-layer structure like the spinal column is an artificial product which taxes the imagination of the radiologist. The radiologist mentally integrates a multitude of contiguous CT slices to create a three-dimensional image. For torsion fractures and dislocation traumas, axial slices do not provide sufficient information regarding the fracture. For this reason, secondary reconstruction was initiated in order to provide three-dimensional images. This method, which we used regularly in our examinations, attempts to give the impression of spatial dimension. The radiologist can acquire soft tissue information, a disc prolapse for example, and display that information along with the bone structures with very little time expended. The disadvantage of this method is poor detail resolution. In addition, the reconstruction plane is selected interactively. Only one thin slice can be displayed at a time, which means the radiologist must integrate a large number of slices into a spatial structure to obtain complete information regarding the fracture. In addition, when scanning the vertebral arch, pedicle, and intraspinal fragments, the method provides unsatisfactory results compared to the axial CT and 3D methods (Table 3).

The SOMATOM PLUS included surface oriented extraction "on-the-scanner" 3D software, as thoroughly described by Herman [5]. This software allowed us to display even the most complex groups of vertebral segments containing fractures as a juxtaposition of intact and pathologically related anatomical structures, and delimit the structures as required. We obtained satisfactory image quality using the 512×512 element matrix, and therefore agree with the opinion [4] that conventional tomography is no longer necessary now that 3D reconstruction and axial CT slice methods are available.

We were unable to reconstruct problems involving non-existant pathological findings caused by artefacts, e. g., holes in bones [3]. In contrast to lesions of the facial bones or any other flat thin bones, our patient study focussed on solid and compact bone structures.

The advantages of a volumetric 3D method as shown by Drebin [2] do not apply to our study, since the internal surface areas are less important in the evaluation of the stabilizing elements of the central spinal column (one of the main advantages of the volumetric method).

We cannot agree with the criticism that soft tissue information is lost in the 3D procedure by setting a threshold value [3]. Our study primarily required display of bone structures, and 3D image generation was used exclusively based on the findings obtained through existing axial slices.

Summary

Processing axial CT slices into 3D images is a valuable supplement. The radiologist who is no longer confronted with a multitude of CT scans will benefit from three-dimensional display of severe torsion fractures and dislocations which extend over several vertebral segments.

The greatest disadvantage is the long computing time, especially when using the 512×512 element matrix. This means that instant information from 3D images for e. g., multiple trauma, will only be available in exceptional cases.

References

1. Denis F Spinal instability as defined by the three column spine concept in acute spinal trauma. Clin Orthop 189: 65–76
2. Drebin RA, Magid D, Robertson DD, Fishman EK (1989) Fidelity of three-dimensional CT imaging for detecting fracture gaps. J Comp Assist Tomography 13 (3): 487–489
3. Grodd W, Dannenmaier B, Petersen D, Gehrke G (1987) Drei-Dimensionale (3-D) Bildrekonstruktion von Gesichtsschädel und Schädelbasis in der Computertomographie. Radiologe 27: 502–510
4. Hadley MN et al Three-dimensional computed tomography in the diagnosis of vertebral column pathological conditions. Neurosurgery 21 (2): 186–192
5. Herman GT (1988) Three-dimensional imaging on a CT or MR scanner. J Comp Assist Tomography 12 (3): 450–451
6. Louis (1985) Die Chirurgie der Wirbelsäule. Springer, Berlin Heidelberg New York
7. Mc Afee PC, Yuan HA, Fredrickson BE, Lubicky JP (1983) The value of computed tomography in thoracolumbar fractures. An analysis of one hundred consecutive cases and a new classification. J Bone Joint Surg 65 a (4): 461–473
8. Pate D, Resnick D, Andre M, Sartorius DJ, Kursunoglu S, Bielecki D, Dev P, Vassiliadis A (1986) Perspective: three-dimensional imaging of the musculoskeletal system. Am J Roentgenol 147: 545–551
9. Wimmer B (1988) Computertomographie beim Wirbelsäulentrauma. Radiologe 29: 441–446

Conventional CT and 3D of the Normal and Fractured Os Calcis: An Investigation Procedure and a Classification of 21 Calcaneal Fractures

F. P. J. BILLET, W. G. H. SCHMITT, B. GAY, J. LANG

A variety of methods exists to aid in the diagnosis of fractured bones, requiring operative treatment. The complex anatomy of the os calcis can be imaged using high resolution computed tomography. This paper also discusses 3D imaging of the os calcis. 3D images of bone and skin surface are based on multiple conventional CT cross sections. The resulting images, representing the surface in a form similar to anatomic preparations, may facilitate the diagnostic process in regions of interest. The 3D images are not only valuable for surgeons, but also supply information useful to radiologists. The geometrical accuracy of 3D reconstruction from overlapping CT cross sections is compared with contiguous scans of different thicknesses and recon algorithms.

Also major factors, like CT cross sections under different angles necessary to optimize clarification of the fractured os calcis, are presented and illustrated.

The techniques have been performed on 20 patients with 21 fractures of the os calcis, one healthy volunteer and one cadaver. Particular procedures for obtaining cross sections with excellent details as well as good 3D reconstructions are suggested. The 3D image information can be used to define the sizes, shapes and spatial locations of fractures. Moreover 3D makes the extensively described fracture classifications of the os calcis more comprehensible. The utility of this method for investigation of this area of complex skeletal anatomy is demonstrated.

Summary

The complex anatomy of the os calcis is evaluated by contiguous and overlapping CT scans in different planes to arrive at a good investigational procedure for the fractured os calcis. Also a computer program that produces 3D reconstructions from these cross sections is used. Its perspective and value is illustrated in conveying anatomical and traumatical aspects of the os calcis (volunteer, cadaver and 21 fractures). It will have application in the treatment and evaluatation of surgical procedures of the fractured os calcis.

Normal Anatomy

In the middle of the calcaneus lies the facies articularis talaris posterior (f. a. t. p.), approximately 29.0 mm in length and 22.5 mm in width. The f. a. t. p. is moderate-

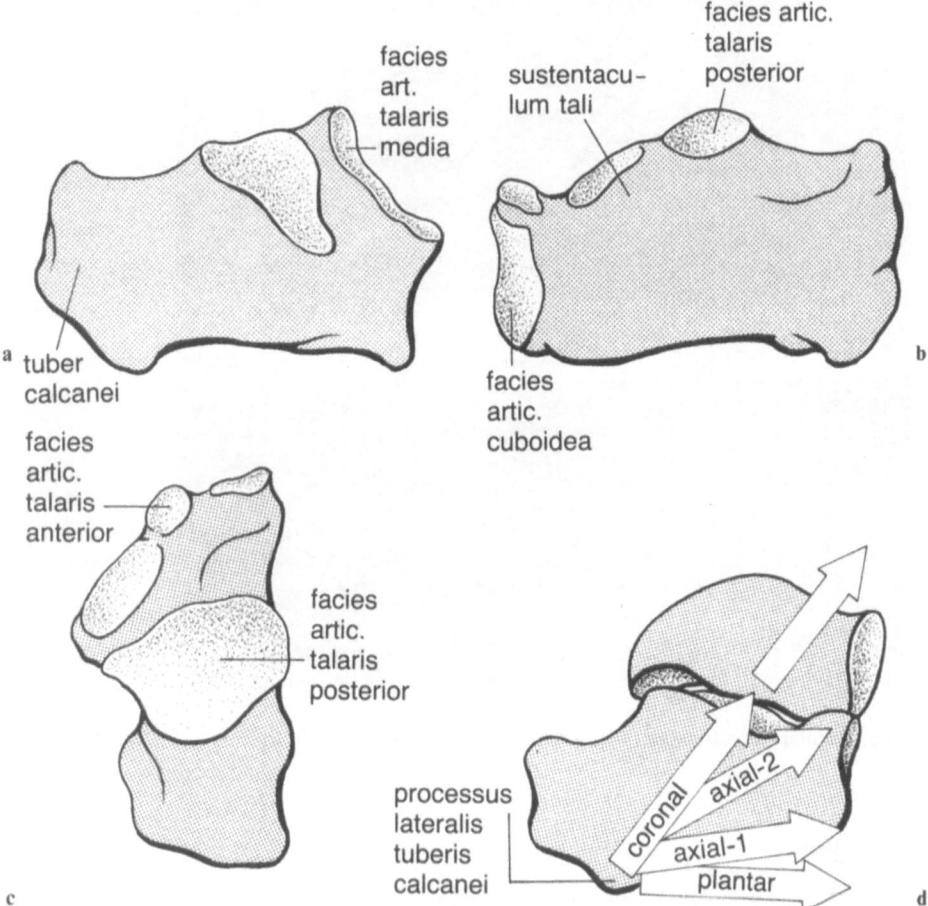

Fig. 1a–d. Normal anatomy of the calcaneus. **a** lateral view, **b** medial view, **c** cranial view, **d** various scanning orientations

ly concave and saddle-shaped. The medial side is 14.0 mm higher than the lateral side. There is a strong and thick cortical strut, extending from the front (we usually name it "Caput Calcanei") to the posterior margin of the f. a. t. p. This angled surface (in relationship to the calcaneus about 40˙degrees) carries the processus lateralis tarsi, which forms a wedge just above it. This angle is of great importance for the fracture mechanism and has been termed "the crucial angle" by Gissane [5]. The mostly oval, sometimes circular facies articularis talaris media lies on the sustentaculum tali and is approximately 20.0 mm long and 12.0 mm wide. The difference in height between the anterior and posterior side is 13.5 mm.

The facies articularis talaris anterior (12.0 mm in length and 8.0 mm in width) is sometimes absent. The angle between the two last facies is 166.0 degrees (see Fig. 1). The mentioned (slightly modified) distances have been measured by Schmidt in his anatomical study about the articulation between talus and calcaneus [12].

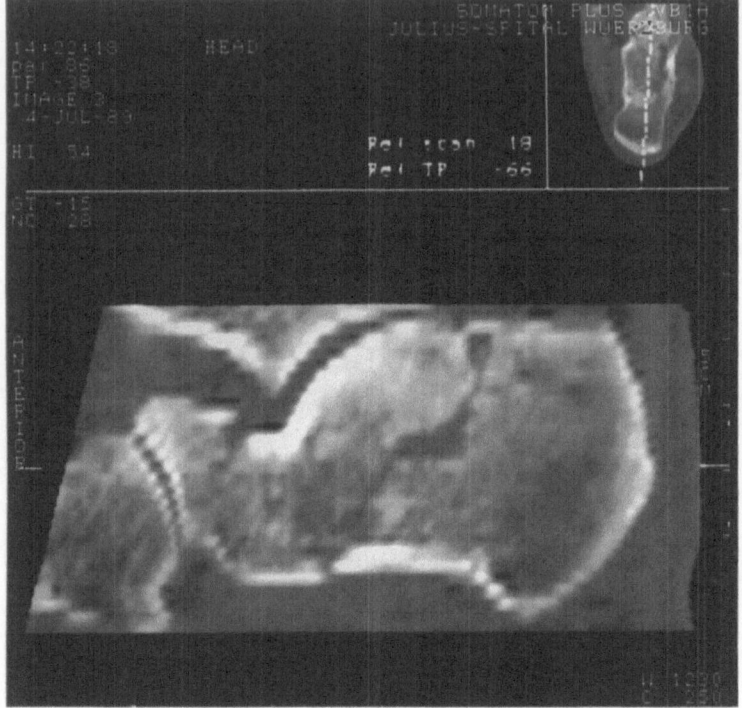

Fig. 2. Sagittal reconstruction of joint depression fracture. The main fracture line is clearly visible

CT Anatomy

The sagittal plane shows the calcaneo-cuboid joint and allows determination of Boehler's angle (see Fig. 2). Also the sulcus calcanei (bottom of the sinus tarsi), the f. a. t. p., the middle and anterior calcaneal facet, and the sustentaculum tali can be demonstrated (see Fig. 3). The subtalar facets, the sinus tarsi and the sustentaculum tali can also be seen in the coronal plane. In addition, it shows the flexor hallucis longus and the peroneal tendons, which are necessary to identify for evaluation of tendon impingement by "burst" injuries [6]. The anterior-inferior aspect of the posterior facet, the width of the body of the calcaneus, the calcaneo-cuboid joint, the peroneal tendons, and also the flexor hallucis longus tendon can be observed rather well in the axial plane (see Fig. 11).

Patients and Methods

All examinations were performed with the SOMATOM PLUS CT system. The foot of a healthy volunteer was scanned to establish the CT appearance of normal calcaneus anatomy in the sagittal plane. (In supine position with flexed knees, a

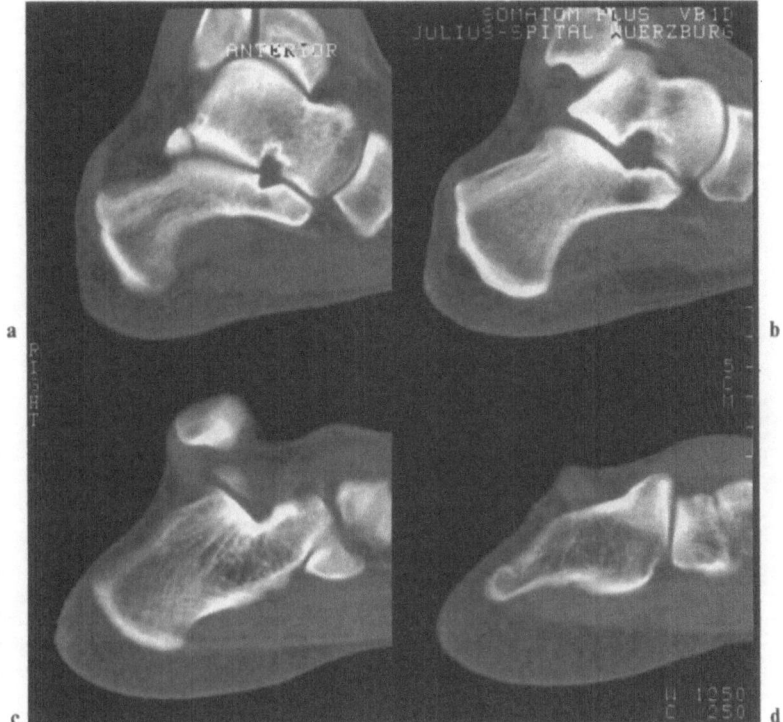

Fig. 3a–d. Sagittal slices, scanned from the inside to the outside. **a, b** Canalus tarsi, posterior facet, the sustentaculum tali with his anterior facet, the sulcus calcanei and the talo-navicular joint are clearly visible. **c** It looks as if the calcaneus had formed a neoarthrotic joint with the os naviculare in this healthy volunteer. Consider the direction of the trabeculae which extends parallel to the mentioned fracture lines. **d** Calcaneal-cuboid joint

maximum endorotation of the foot, and a maximum forward gantry angulation) (see Fig. 3). Also different axial, coronal and 3D images of a normal calcaneus (cadaver) were evaluated. Scan thickness, mAs and recon algorithms were varied in order to obtain the best osseous detail in the shortest time and at the lowest radiation dose (see Table 1). Twenty patients with recent calcaneal fractures underwent a CT examination during a period of 7 months. In one patient, the injury was bilateral, so a total of 21 fractures were examined. Thirteen calcanei were scanned in two different planes. The other 8 patients underwent a single plane examination. Section thickness was either 5 mm or 2 mm, contiguous. Also, 5 mm slice thickness and 3 mm table increments were used (see Table 2). The foot was relaxed in slight dorsoflexion and inversion. The toes were taped to the table with adhesive plaster (patient in supine position). The visualized area covered the whole calcaneus and at least a part of the talus, the os cuboideum and naviculare. See for the scan directions Fig. 4. Line 1–2 corresponds with axial 1 and line 1–3 with the axial 2 scan direction. Line 3 represents the coronal and line 4 the plantar plane.

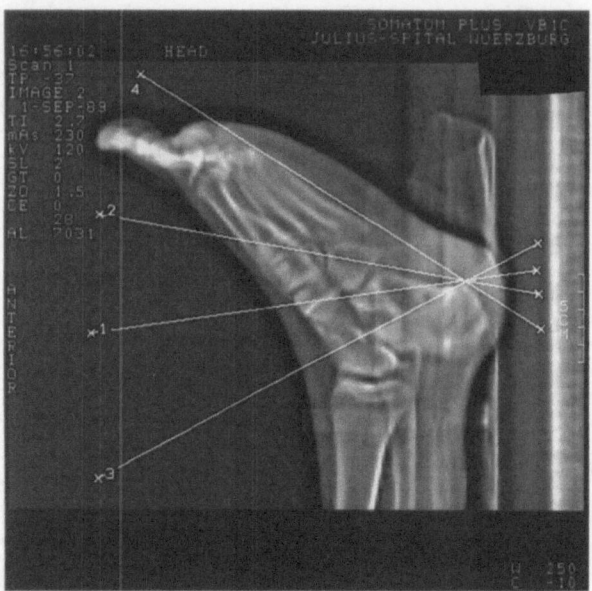

Fig. 4. Topogram. Starting point is the processus medialis or lateralis tuberis calcanei. The first line goes to the upper margin of the calcaneal-cuboid joint. The second line is parallel to the bottom of the calcaneal body. The third line is pointed to the roof of the sinus tarsi. The fourth line is parallel to the sole of the foot

So far the results confirm our suggestions, we recommend a low mAs mode (340 mAs/standard for 2 mm scans and 510 mAs/high for 5 mm scans) that provides good image quality (see Fig. 5). The different sections were compared to 3D images that were reconstructed from the different scans of each calcaneus (see Fig. 6). Then, the fractures were classified and the fracture symptoms evaluated (see Table 3).

All patients were operated on, so the radiological diagnosis could be verified. All diagnoses were correct. In addition, the surgical findings were reviewed and compared to the cross sections and 3D reconstructions once more. So the use of one particular scan direction (in combination with 3D images) to enable diagnosis of calcaneal fractures precisely, could be defined as a 5/3 mm scan (high mode at 340 mAs) in the axial 2 plane.

For scanning the calcaneus in the (2/2 mm) axial 1 −, (5/5 mm) coronal- and (5/3 mm) axial 2-plane respectively, you need approximately 30, 18 and 25 scans.

Fracture Mechanism

Most fractures of our series had been sustained in falls. This trauma assists in explaining fracture mechanisms. The two more frequent fracture types ("tongue-type" and the "joint depression type") each have a typical fracture mechanism.

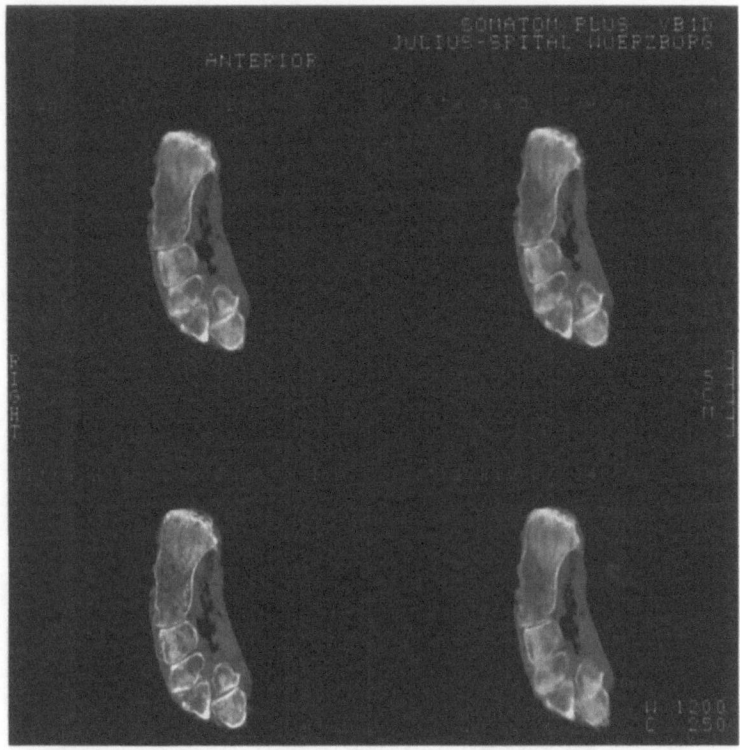

Fig. 5. Comparison of different modes and scan techniques at 340 mAs. Consider that a 3D reconstruction of the 2 mm scans in a high or ultrahigh mode will not show any difference in quality

Tongue-Type

Although it happens almost simultaneously, the action of the fracture mechanism has to be divided in a first and a second stage. When the tuber calcanei strikes the ground, a fracture line usually runs from the processus medialis tuberis calcanei laterally towards the front (first stage). This fracture represents the main fracture line [1, 9, 13]. During the first stage, a rotation of the calcaneus takes place, so that the direction of the main forces are changed in the second stage (see Fig. 9a–c). In the second stage, vertical compression of the talus on the calcaneal body results in a shearing fracture of sustentaculum tali on the medial side and the "wedge" of the processus lateralis drives into the crucial angle on the lateral side (Essex-Lopresti called this the inner and outer route). The force that follows the outer route has to be separated into two momenta "F3 and F2". The first "F3", perpendicular to the posterior margin of the f. a. t. p., knocks off a tongue-type fragment. The second momentum "F2" opposes the force "Fr", splitting the floor of the joint into two parts (see Fig. 9b–c and 15).

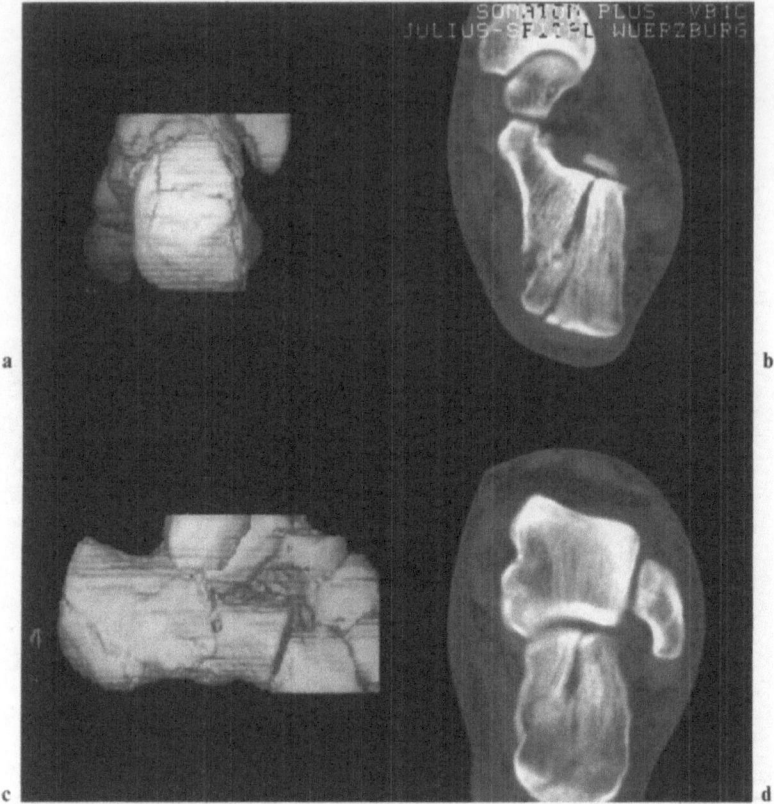

Fig. 6a-d. Tongue-type fracture (2/2 mm, axial 1 and 5/5 mm coronal). **a** 3D image (seen from behind), compared with an axial image **(b)** **c** 3D image (lateral view), compared with a coronal image **(c)** Notice that image **a** discloses the "tongue-type fracture" more distinctly. As a 3D disadvantage should be mentioned in this context that only image **d** could exclude "tendon impingement"

Joint depression

In the first stage, the calcaneus hits the ground in a flat position (see Fig. 10a-c). Now the two opposite forces meet each other in a parallel manner. The main fracture line extends its way towards the f. a. t. p. At the end of the second stage, rotation will take place, because the torso falls down. At that time, the momentum "fa2" on the outer route is not strong enough to cause a tongue-type fracture.

Before the patient falls down, the force of the talus on the inner route will cause a shearing fracture of the sustentaculum tali. The force on the outer route causes the so called joint depression. In addition, you are frequently confronted with an inversion of the foot just before the trauma sets in. This inversion can cause a fragmentation of the lateral side (lambda fracture). Broadening of the calcaneal body laterally can be responsible for tendon impingement (see Fig. 10c and 12-14).

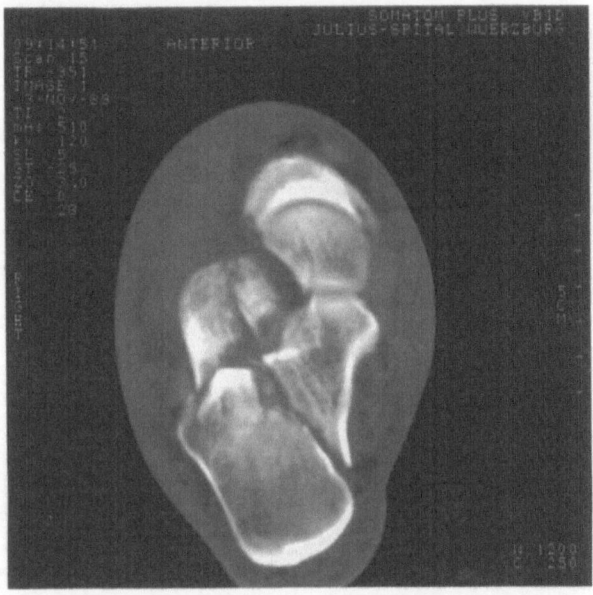

Fig. 7. Joint depression fracture with medial overlap. (axial 5/3 mm scan). Notice the "main fragment" on the lateral side

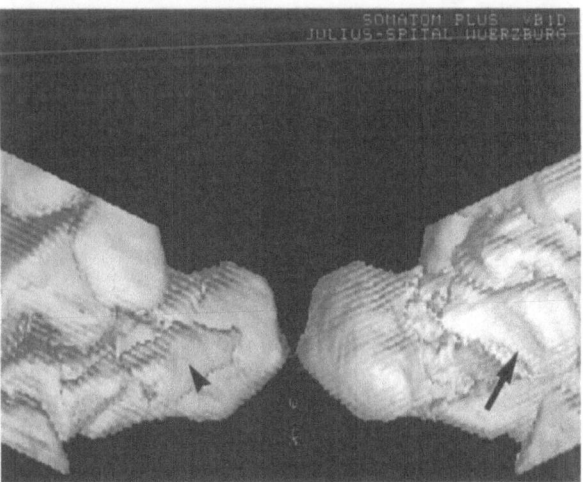

Fig. 8. Joint depression fracture. 3D images (2/2 mm) seen from lateral and medial, respectively. *Arrowhead:* typical small shell-like fragment, covering the lateral block. *Arrow:* shearing fracture of the sustentaculum

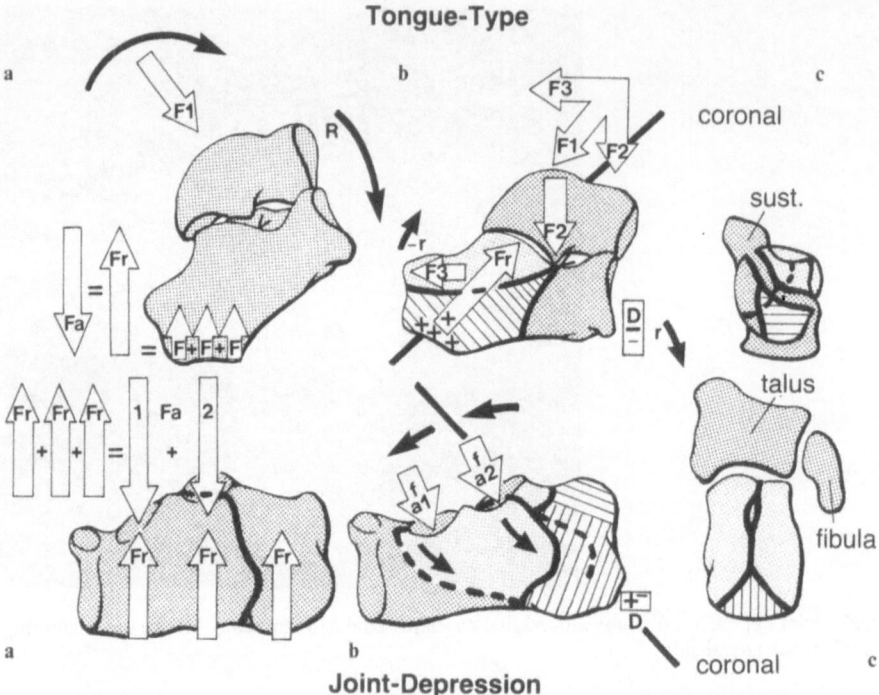

Fig. 9a–c *(above)*. Mechanism of the tongue-type fracture (right foot) in a fall. **a** Beginning of stage 1. During this very short period, a rotation of the calcaneus takes place. F(action) = F(reaction). Open arrow points at the crucial angle. **b** Beginning of stage 2. The calcaneum is in a flat position. The normal distance between the caput calcanei and the ground is diminishing. The momenta "F3 and F2" will cause the typical tongue-type fragmentation and the so called main fracture. **c** Double projection of coronal slice, seen from behind (see for slice direction the black stripe in Fig. 9b). Shearing fracture of the sustentaculum at the front and typical tongue fragmentation at the back

Fig. 10a–c *(below)*. Mechanism of joint depression. **a** The calcaneum has landed in a flat position and during the two stages no relevant rotation will take place. 2F(action) = 3F(reaction). Tendency to form a main fracture line. **b** End of stage 2. Shearing fracture of the sustentaculum. The "axe" on the crucial angle gives the main fracture line a finishing touch. **c** Coronal slice, seen from behind. An inversion of the foot can be responsible for a so called lambda fracture

Fracture classification

Fractures involving the subtaloid joint: After the trauma the body of the calcaneus moves forward (widening and shortening with medial overlap) and the tuber rotates in an upward direction by contraction of the achilles tendon (fragment no. 1). It is relatively seldom seen as a single intra-articular fracture with involvement of the f. a. t. p., but without any dislocation. This fracture is described in the classification of Essex-Lopresti as a Boehler's Type 1. While it cannot be detached from the main fracture line, we propose to call it "the main fragment". If there is a dislocation, it has to be classified as Type 3a (see Fig. 7).

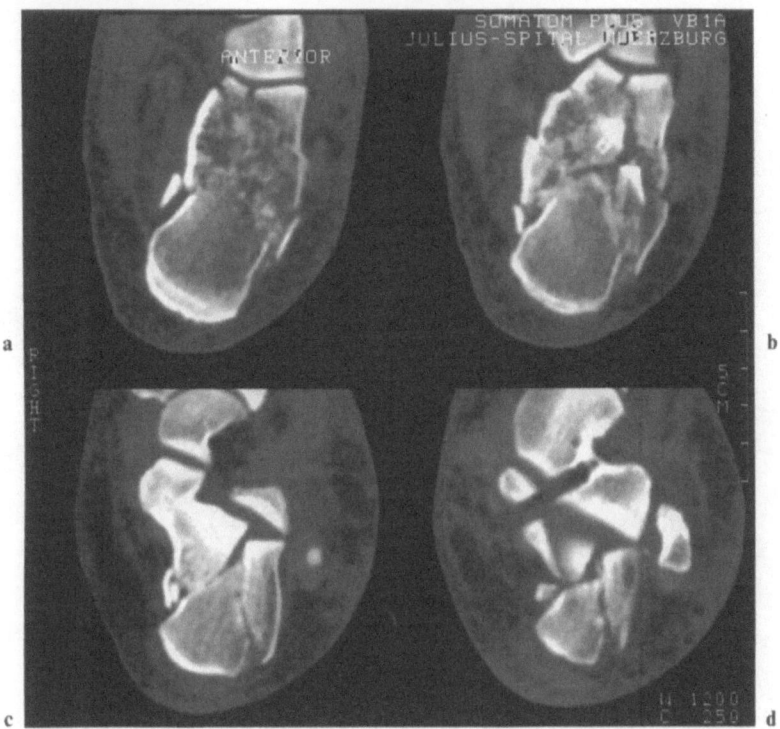

Fig. 11a-d. Comminution: Boehler's Type 5a (2/2 mm axial 1). **a** Comminution in caput calcanei with intra-articular fracture from calcaneo-cuboid joint. **b** widening of calcaneal body. **c** lambda fracture (split posterior facet). **d** moderate "tendon impingement"

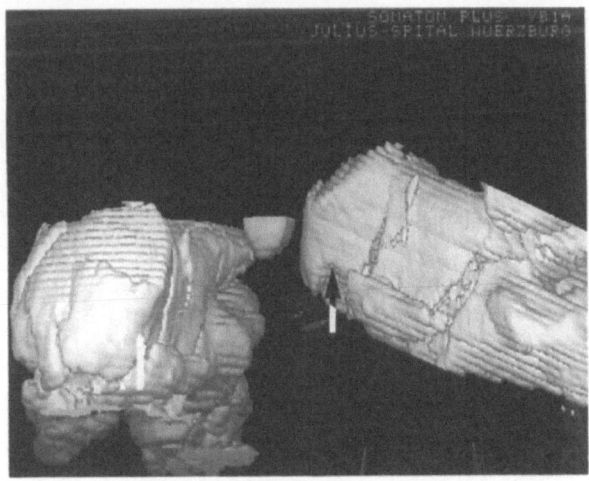

Fig. 11e. 3D image (2/2 mm), seen from the back and a lateral point of view, respecitvely. Combination of joint depression and a big fragment at the back of the calcaneus *(see arrow)*

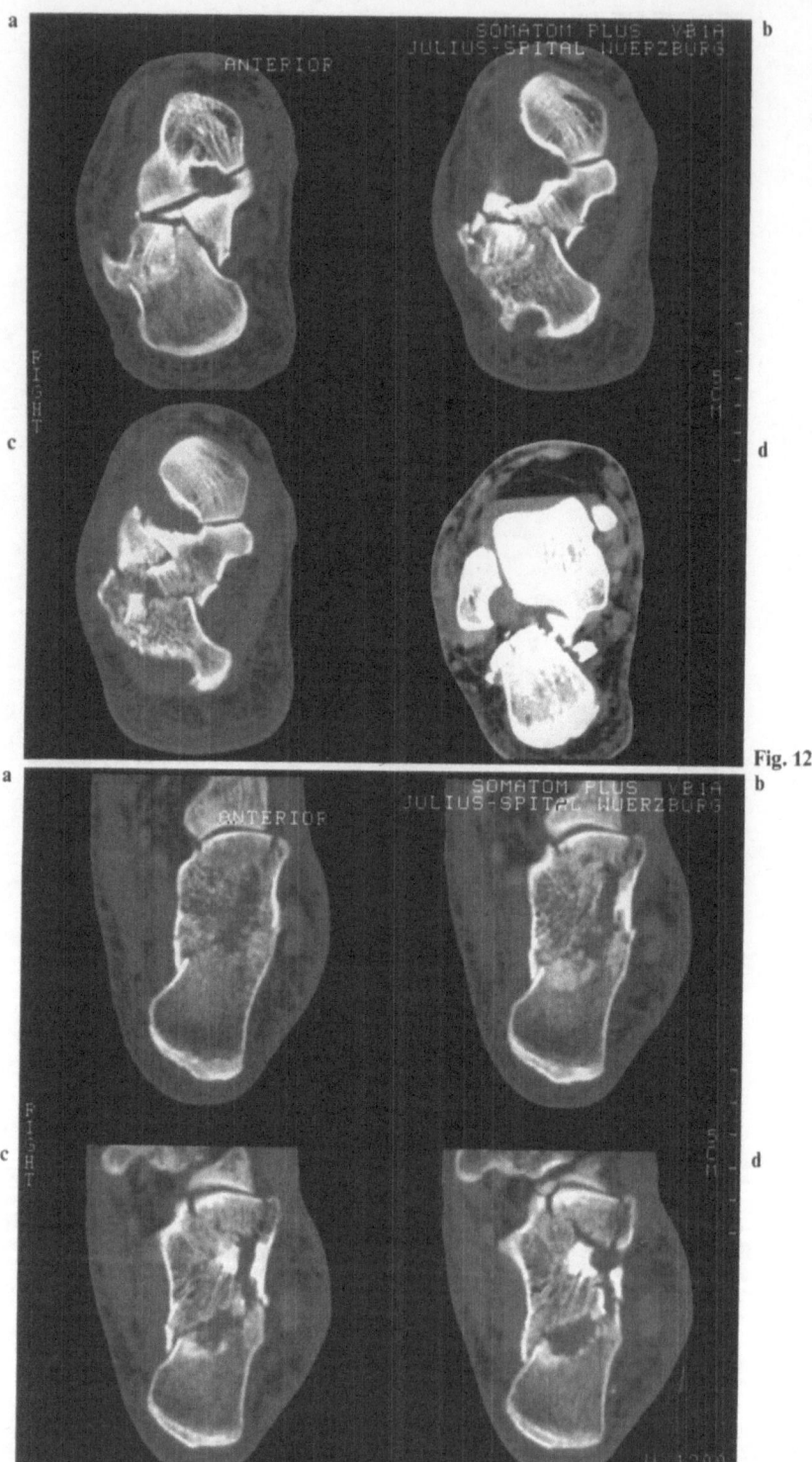

Fig. 12

Fig. 13

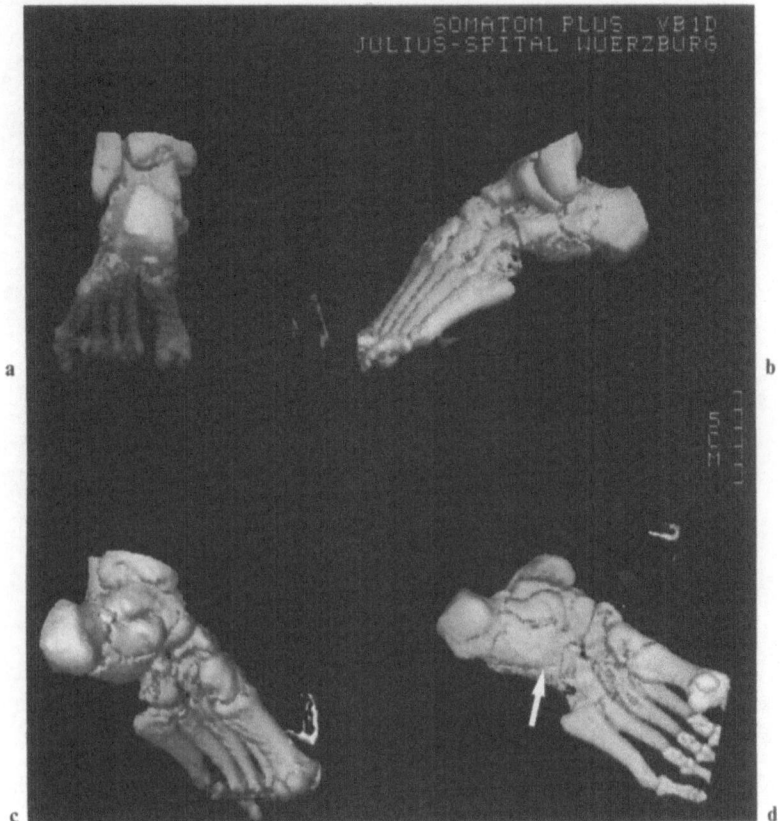

Fig. 14a–d. Joint depression (3D images, reconstructed from plantar 5/3 mm scans). **a** view from behind, excluding a tongue-type fracture. **b** typical small shell-like fragment covers lateral block. **c** shearing fracture of sustentaculum. **d** intraarticular involvement of calcaneal-cuboid joint

Fig. 12a–d. Joint depression (2/2 mm, coronal). **a** intraarticular fragment. **b** shearing fracture of sustentaculum. **c** comminution from calcaneal body. **d** moderate "tendon impingement"

Fig. 13a–d. Joint depression with Y-fracture in caput calcanei (2/2 mm, axial 1)

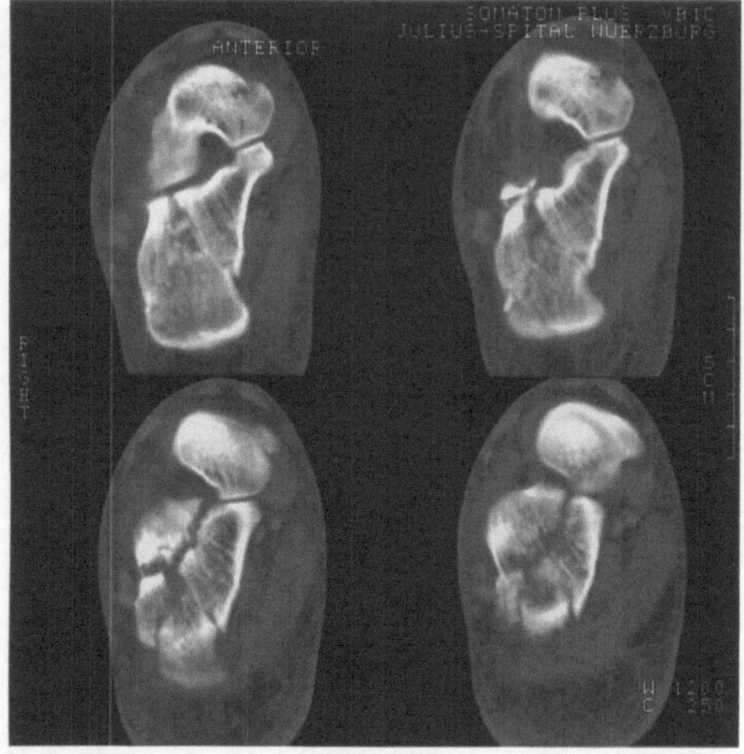

Fig. 15. Tongue-type fracture, scanned backwards in coronal direction. Lambda fracture through body of calcaneus

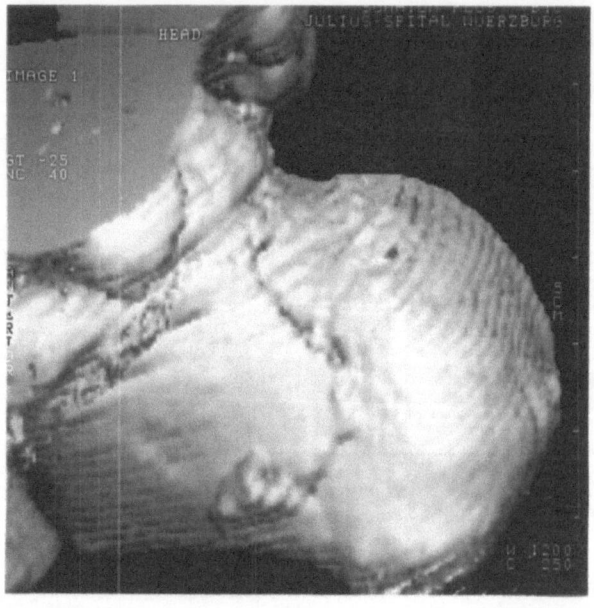

Fig. 16. Cranio-medial dorsal view of 3D image, showing the main fracture line (reconstruction from 2/2 mm scans)

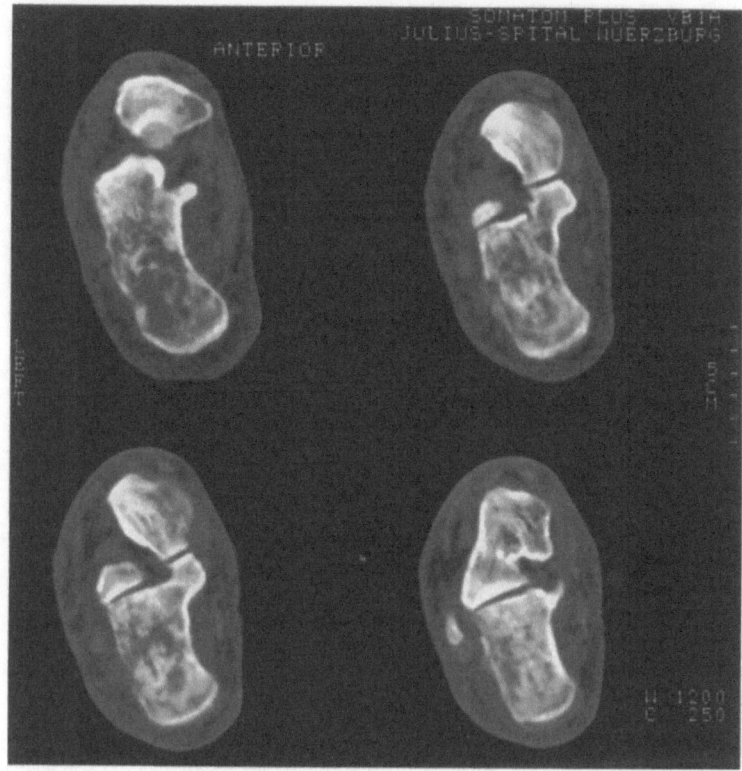

Fig. 17. Pathological fracture: metastasis from colon carcinoma (coronal 2/2 mm)

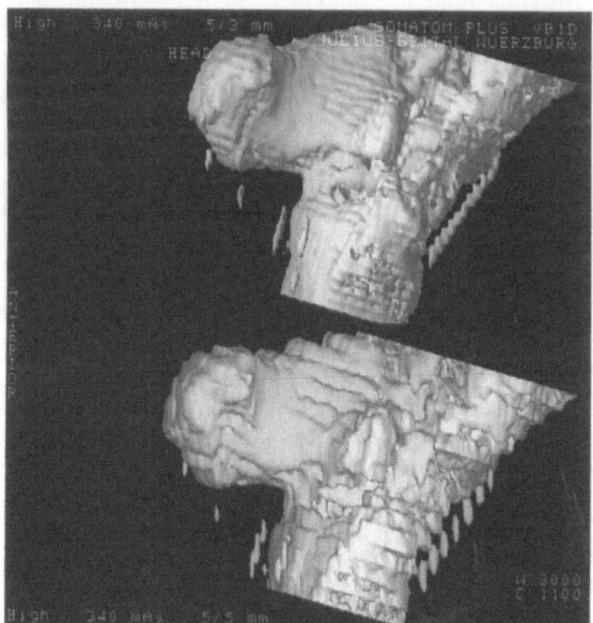

Fig. 18. Cadaverfoot; a comparison between two 3D images, reconstructed with 5/3 and 5/5 mm

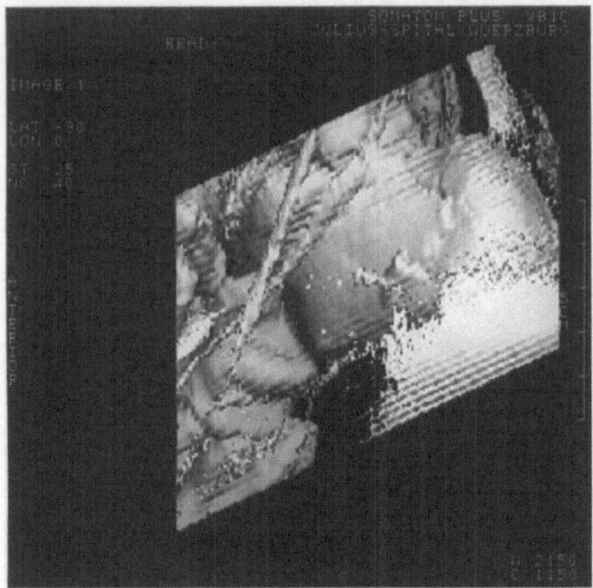

Fig. 19. 3D image, showing the peroneal and achilles tendons (medial view)

Fragmentation of the "tongue" shaped piece of bone, out of the upper posterior part of the calcaneus, has already been mentioned (fragment no. 2). In combination with the appearance of the main fracture line and the shearing fracture of the sustentaculum, it should be classified as Boehler's Type 2a, without the main fracture line as Type 2b (the last tpye has been described by Malgaigne in 1843). For a better understanding it is important to know that the upper part of the shearing-fracture corresponds with the upper part of the main fracture line.

Other subsidiary lines of cleavage (fragment no. 3-5) are the small shell-like fragment that covers the lateral block (Type 3b) and the Y-fracture through the caput calcanei that causes a fragmentation on the front (Type 3c) and on the lateral side from the caput calcanei (Type 3d). Boehler's Types 3b-d usually occur in combination with joint depression.

Palmer was probably the first to describe this small lateral shell-like fragment [11]. Anatomically speaking, it corresponds with the trochlea peronealis (see Fig. 8). Dividing the form of the fractures in "lambda and Y" is advocated by Vollrath c. s. [14].

The undisplaced sustentaculum tali can include a smaller or even bigger part of the f. a. t. p. The deltoid and talocalcaneal interosseous ligaments connect it rigidly to the talus [10]. It must not be considered as a fragmentation, but rather as a stable part of the calcaneus. A sustentaculum tali fracture alone was classified by Essex-Lopresti as Boehler's Type 4 (if the f. a. t. p. is involved, it is Boehler's Type 1 or 3a).

If more than 5 fragments in combination with depression of Boehler's angle, intra-articular fragmentation and widening of the calcaneal body exist, one should

Table 1. Cadaverstudy

usefullness/image-quality		axial	coronal	3D
2/2 mm,	high, 340 mAs	+ +/+ +	+/+ + +	+ +/+ + +
5/3 mm,	high, 340 mAs		+ +/+ +	+ + +/+ +
5/5 mm,	high, 510 mAs		+ +/+ +	+ +/+
5/5 mm,	ultra-high, 340 mAs	+/+ +		
1/1 mm,	ultra-high, 340 mAs	+/+ + +		
2/2 mm,	ultra-high, 340 mAs	+ +/+ +		
2/2 mm,	standard, 340 mAs	+ +/+ +		+ +/+ + +
2/2 mm,	smooth, 340 mAs	+ +/+		

+ = moderate   + + = good   + + + = excellent

Table 2. Technique

Modes	Axial 1*-2**	Plantar	Coronal
Pat. 1	2/2 mm, 510 mAs*		5/5 mm, 510 mAs
Pat. 2	2/2 mm, 510 mAs*		5/5 mm, 510 mAs
Pat. 3	2/2 mm, 510 mAs*		5/5 mm, 340 mAs
Pat. 4	2/2 mm, 510 mAs*		
Pat. 5	2/2 mm, 340 mAs*		5/5 mm, 340 mAs
Pat. 6	2/2 mm, 510 mAs*		5/5 mm, 510 mAs
Pat. 7	2/2 mm, 510 mAs*		5/5 mm, 340 mAs
Pat. 8	5/5 mm, 510 mAs**	5/5 mm, 510 mAs	
Pat. 9		5/5 mm, 340 mAs	5/5 mm, 340 mAs
Pat. 10			2/2 mm, 510 mAs
Pat. 11	2/2 mm, 510 mAs*		2/2 mm, 510 mAs
Pat. 12		2/2 mm, 340 mAs	2/2 mm, 340 mAs
Pat. 13	3/5 mm, 510 mAs*		5/5 mm, 340 mAs
Pat. 14		3/5 mm, 340 mAs	
Pat. 15	2/2 mm, 340 mAs*		2/2 mm, 340 mAs
	2/2 mm, 340 mAs*		2/2 mm, 340 mAs
Pat. 16	5/3 mm, 340 mAs**		
Pat. 17	5/3 mm, 340 mAs**		
Pat. 18	5/3 mm, 340 mAs**		
Pat. 19	5/3 mm, 340 mAs**		
Pat. 20	5/3 mm, 340 mAs**		

talk about comminution (Boehler's Type 5). We suggest that it should be indicated precisely if the comminution mainly took place in the caput calcanei with impaction of the calcaneo-cuboid joint (Type 5a), in the calcaneal body with impaction of the posterior facet (Type 5b), or only in the tuberculum calcanei (Type 5c) (see Fig. 11). Also the combination of the above types, for example Type 5a and b, can occur. In four patients (about 20%), we found a relative broad piece of bone at the back of the calcaneus, cut off in the frontal plane (see Fig. 11e).

Fractures not involving the subtaloid joint: The appearance of a shell-like fragmentation of the medial or lateral calcaneal tubercle is seen in comminution, but it can also occur as a single fracture. Relatively seldom, an intra-articular fracture of the calcaneo-cuboid joint will occur as a single fracture (Table 3).

Table 3. Classification of the patients

Cases	Non-/Intra-Articular	Fracture-Types	Classification
Pat. 1	+	fracture med.-/lat.-tubercle	non-thalamic
Pat. 2	+ACC/ACTp	"joint-depr."	Boehler-3c
Pat. 3	+ACTp	"joint-depr."	Boehler-3a
Pat. 4	+	lat.-tubercle	non-thalamic
Pat. 5	+ACTp	"tongue-type"	Boehler-2a
Pat. 6	+ACTp	"tongue-type"	Boehler-2a
Pat. 7	+ACTp	"main-fragm."	Boehler-1
Pat. 8	+ACC/ACTp	comminution	Boehler-5a/b
Pat. 9	+ACC/ACTp	comminution	Boehler-5a/b
Pat. 10	+	burst-fract.	pathological
Pat. 11	+ACTp	"joint-depr."	Boehler-3a
Pat. 12	+ACC/ACTp	comminution	Boehler-5a/b
Pat. 13	+ACTp	"joint-depr."	Boehler-3a
Pat. 14	+ACC	comminution	Boehler-5a
Pat. 15	+ACTp	"joint-depr."	Boehler-3a.
	+ACTp	"joint-depr."	Boehler-3a.
Pat. 16	+ACC/ACTp	comminution	Boehler-5a/b
Pat. 17	+	med.-tubercle	non-thalamic
Pat. 18	+ACTp	"joint-depr."	Boehler-3a
Pat. 19	+ACC	burst-fract.	non-thalamic
Pat. 20	+ACTp	"joint-depr."	Boehler-3a

ACC = calcaneo-cuboid joint   ACTp = posterior facet (f. a. t. p.)

Discussion

CT is an excellent method to investigate the fractured calcaneus. 3D images do not provide new data, but make the anatomy of the fractured calcaneus more comprehensible for our clinical colleagues. 3D is very helpful in classifying the calcaneal fracture. An exact classification is important for the surgeon. The classification we mentioned incorporates the findings of Boehler [3], the classification of Essex-Lopresti (thalamic/nonthalamic) and the injury mechanism of Palmer (shearing fracture). Almost all fracture types can be retranslated into this classification, attaching special importance to the differentiation of comminution (impaction of caput, calcaneal body or tuber calcanei). Because the number of fragments is difficult to judge by a single CT plane examination, we recommend a multiplanar contiguous CT examination (2 mm scans parallel to the body of the calcaneum, axial 1) in combination with coronal 5 mm scans, running from the processus lateralis or medialis tuberculi to the roof of the sinus tarsi.

If a 3D software program is available, we think that a single plane examination (overlapping 5/3 mm scan technique in axial 2 direction) in combination with 3D reconstructions may be allowed. We suggest a standard mode/340 mAs for the 2/2 mm, a high mode/340 mAs for the 5/3 mm scans, and a high mode/510 mAs for the 5/5 mm scans.

We also choose for the overlapping scan technique in the single plane examination as a possible solution to the time problem: The calcaneus is relatively long in the axial 2 plane.

Furthermore, the overlapping scan technique diminishes the so called "stair stepping", caused by slight movements of the leg [2], and 3D images at 5/3 mm provide a good quality (see Fig. 18).

A 2D sagittal reconstruction always has to be made in order to mark Boehler's angle. A decreased Boehler's angle, which is the classical radiological sign for evaluating the severity of a calcaneus fracture, can be misleading if multiple overlapping fragments obscure the reference point in conventional radiology or if the tuberosity fragment is tilted [7, 8]. For these last circumstances, it should be mentioned that the coronal and axial 2 plane should make an angle of 45 and 20 degrees, respectively, with the base of the body of the calcaneus (line 2 in Fig. 4).

Futuristic is 3D presentation of tendons (see Fig. 19).

Acknowledgement: We thank Mr. R. Brandl (Siemens) for photographic work and technical assistance.

References

1. Bauer GW, Mutschler W, Heuchemer Th, Lob G (1987) Fortschritte in der Diagnostik der intraartikulären Calcaneusfrakturen durch die Computertomographie. Unfallchirurg 90: 496–501
2. Billet FP, Schmitt WG, Gay B, Hoffmann M, Huber M (Work in progress) 3D-Rekonstruktionsprogramme in der Computertomographie als diagnostischer Gewinn in der Traumatologie? Roentgenpraxis
3. Boehler L (1931) Diagnosis, pathology and treatment of fractures of the os calcis. J Bone Joint Surg 13: 75–89
4. Essex-Lopresti P (1952) Fractures of the os calics. The mechanism, reduction technique and results in fractures of the os calcis. Brit J Surg 39: 395–419
5. Gissane W (1947) J Bone Joint Surg 29: 254
6. Guyer BH, Levinsohn EM, Fredrickson BE, Bailey GL, Formikell M (1985) Computed Tomography of Calcaneal Fractures: Anatomy Pathology, Dosimetry and Clinical Relevance. Amer J Roentgenol 45: 911–919
7. Heger L, Wulff K (1985) Computed Tomography of the Calcaneus: normal anatomy. Amer J Roentgenol 145: 123–129
8. Heger L, Wulff K, Seddiqi MSA (1985) Computed Tomography of Calcaneus Fractures. Amer J Roentgenol 145: 131–137
9. Heuchemer Th, Bargon G, Bauer G, Mutschler W (1988) Vorteile in Diagnose und Einteilung der intraartikulären Kalkaneusfraktur durch die Computertomographie. Fortsch Roentgenstr 149: 8–14
10. Herzenberg JE (1986) CT of Calcaneal Fractures. Amer J Roengenol 146: 644–645
11. Palmer I (1948) The mechanism and treatment for the fractures of calcaneus. Open reduction with use of cancellous grafts. J Bone Joint Surg 30: 2–8
12. Schmidt H-K (1978) Untersuchungen über die Form der unteren Sprunggelenkflächen beim Menschen. Verh Anat Ges 72: 449–451
13. Slaetis P, Kiviluoto O, Santavirta S, Laasonen M (1979) Fractures of the Calcaneum. J Trauma 19: 939–943
14. Vollrath T, Eberle Ch, Grauer W (1987) Computertomographie intraartikulärer Kalkaneusfrakturen. Fortschr Roentgenstr 146: 400–403

Discussion

J. Hodler, Zurich: Three-Dimensional Imaging: Technical Aspects

C. Zwicker, Berlin: Evaluation of Three-Dimensional CT in Orofacial Surgery

F. Astinet, Berlin: High Resolution CT of the Petrosa with Two- and Three-Dimensional Reconstruction

F. P. Billet, Würzburg: Conventional and 3D of the Normal and Fractured Os Calcis: An Investigation Procedure and a Classification of 21 Calcaneal Fractures

Kramann, Homburg:
Recently a highly sophisticated modelling and shaping tool has been developed by the manufacturing industry. It is made by light stimulation of phosphor polymerization. A milling machine is not needed. The bones can be shaped automatically in the machine. This technique is called stereolithography. Is there any likelihood of combining this with CT?

Hupke, Erlangen:
As far as I know there are no such investigations under way.

Hodler, Zurich:
3D reconstruction is useful in fractures of complex bones such as scapula or spine. Interactive capabilities will be necessary as 3D CT will be really useful for planning of e. g. arthroplasties.

Billet, Würzburg:
In fractures of the calcaneus CT scans in one plane in combination with 3D will save time. The real scan time of one axial plane is about six minutes, for scanning in two planes, you need twice as much, i. e. about 12 minutes. You save time when you combine 3D with only one plane and you can define the size and shape and in particular the location of the fragments.

Astinet, Berlin:
For reconstruction of the temporal bone 2-dimensional reconstructions are really a saving of time, because you need just only 2 or 3 minutes for the whole temporal bone in a second plane. We underestimate the importance of 2D reconstructions, which can be done without undue demands on the patient, or further radiation.

2D reconstruction can be of a high quality and standard. 3D in the temporal bone is not important for diagnosis.

Fuchs, Zurich:
3D reconstruction may not be especially important for the diagnosis, but this is currently a problem of interaction between the radiologist and the surgeon. The radiologist does not quite understand all the time what the surgeon actually wants and has in mind when planning the operation, on the other hand the surgeon does not know from the radiologist what he can actually get. There is a lot of mutual learning to be done. 3D imaging might be important for computer design, for the modelling of a prosthesis or bone replacement in reconstructive surgery.

Riemann, Frankfurt:
We still have a great deal to learn about 3D reconstruction. The problem is that the 3D should be less distorted by artefacts.

v. Engelshoven, Maastricht:
What we need is a very quick interactive system without films. Then we can, together with the surgeon, look at all the separate projections on the screen, but the present system is too slow.

Dixon, Cambridge:
I agree that the best method is to view the examination with the surgeon and only do the projections that he is interested in.

Hupke, Erlangen:
We know that the programme takes a relatively long time for the routine use, and the software group is working on this topic.

Kalender, Erlangen:
In future systems we will not be using films, but real time interactive displays for multiplanar and 3D imaging.

Fuchs:
Do you plan a surface smoothening program in order to eliminate those disturbing steps on the surface?

Hupke:
The 3D final image can only be as good as the incoming 2D images, and with developments such as spiral scanning in the 2D imaging, we will end up with better 3D images.

Fuchs:
What about eliminating the artefacts due to metal implants?

Kalender:
We have high quality original images already, but they need to be continuous, because 3D is a volume display. Spiral CT is the initial step. The more severe problem of metal artefacts is a very complicated problem. We have made some progress there, but I am not optimistic with respect to e. g. dental fillings or metal in a very complex anatomical region.

Kloswijk, Rotterdam:
Did any of the authors consider steroscopic presentation of these 3D imaging?

Vock, Bern:
With the old SOMATOM DRH software it was possible to choose the angle for 3D reconstructions. With the light pen or with the mouse we cannot choose the angle so precisely and it is difficult to get a 3D movie of the reconstructions. We need new software to do that.

Rienmüller, Munich:
With these new technologies today we can see more than we were used to see. How can we get this new information into the clinical use? The only method is that after treatment e. g. of the calcaneus fracture, we repeat the CT study to analyze the postsurgical results in order to obtain optimal treatment.

Schmitt, Würzburg:
With the SOMATOM PLUS equipment is it now possible to visualize in 3D the ventricular system in the brain, a low density system?

Hupke:
With a so-called editor program the region of interest can be selected and e. g. the ventricular system displayed. This program has been developed, is now in the testing phase and will soon be commercially available.

Kalender:
When doing ventricular volume determinations, we have had to use quite sophisticated statistical techniques like region growing to get good results, and I assume that you will find Magnetic Resonance Imaging preferable.

Fuchs:
What about segmentation of particular structures, e. g. the patella?

Hupke:
It will be possible with this program to do segmentation of e. g. the patella or the hip joints. Structures can be worked out with a program which has a region drawing unit and segmentation etc.

Fuchs:
When will this program be available?

Hupke:
It is being tested and should be available in 2 or 3 months.

Fuchs:
What is the price tag?

Hupke:
It's included in the 3D program.

Fuchs:
I have a question concerning the radiation dose to the lens in your investigation of the skull and the facial fractures. Did you measure it?

Zwicker:
This investigation should be done with reduced mAs values. We have not measured the dose, but we use 60 mAs, – about tenth compared to the conventional transverse scan – so the dose is the same as in conventional CT of the orbit. However, radiation is a problem in 3D CT.

Hupke:
When you recalculate the dose it is of the same order as that for a normal head scanning including the orbita at 60 mAs.

Vock:
The diagnosis is made on conventional CT scans, so two scans will be performed thus doubling the dose.

Zwicker:
The diagnosis is usually made from the plain films. But if further imaging is needed, we use 3 DCT. If localization of fragments is needed a conventional 2D CT with 5 mm slice thickness is performed. For orbital fractures we obtain images with 5 mm slice thickness. Only if the surgeons need a 3D CT for visualization of fragments do we do a 3D scan. Normally we prefer the 2D CT with 5 mm slice thickness.

Fuchs:
Do you see a future in computer designed prostheses, e. g. interaction with 3D imaging?

Kalender:
We supply data formats, but we do not engage ourselves in the design or manufacturing of individual prostheses.

Dynamic Studies

Chairmen: J. v. Engelshoven, A. K. Dixon

The SOMATOM PLUS in the Mediastinum: Preliminary Observations

A. K. DIXON, C. D. R. FLOWER

Introduction

The mediastinum has been one of those anatomical sites for which CT has brought about a large change in radiological practice. Once the hidden areas of the thorax [Heitzman 1981], most of the individual structures can now be rendered visible. Indeed CT of the mediastinum is widely performed, either as part of a CT study of the thorax (e. g. staging for teratoma) or as a study in isolation (e. g. thoracic aortic dissection). The anatomical and technical problems which arose with second generation machines [Dixon et al. 1981, Husband and Kelsey Fry 1981] were replaced by a variety of artefacts produced by modern machines which became available in the early 1980s. The versatility of these machines allowed the evaluation of a wider range of clinical problems. This in turn led to a variety of diagnostic pitfalls which have slowly (and often painfully) been learnt [Godwin et al. 1982, Gallagher and Dixon 1984].

Now come yet more modern machines with much improved resolution and, in particular, shorter data acquisition times. The capability for dynamic sequence studies is considerably improved: the Siemens SOMATOM PLUS can yield up to 110 images per 12 s (at minimum 0.7 s data acquisition time), whereas the Imatron can yield images with data acquisition as short as 50 ms [Lipton et al. 1984]. Such welcome advances in technology inevitably lead to a reassessment of the technique of mediastinal CT which has been established over more than ten years. These exciting technical possibilities have led to a new and complex range of diagnostic pitfalls.

Addenbrooke's Hospital is a large teaching hospital with close to 1000 inpatient beds. It lies geographically close to Papworth Hospital which houses the East Anglian Regional Cardiothoracic Unit and there are extensive CT referrals from that centre. A Siemens SOMATOM II was installed by a local charity in 1981 and approximately 3000 body CT examinations were performed annually until November 1989 when the original body CT system was replaced by a SOMATOM PLUS. This report details some of our initial observations about the use of the new machine for the study of the mediastinum. In particular, differences between this unit and the SOMATOM II (which is representative of many systems currently installed in this country) will be highlighted. The technical possibilities will first be addressed, followed by the applications and findings in a range of clinical problems.

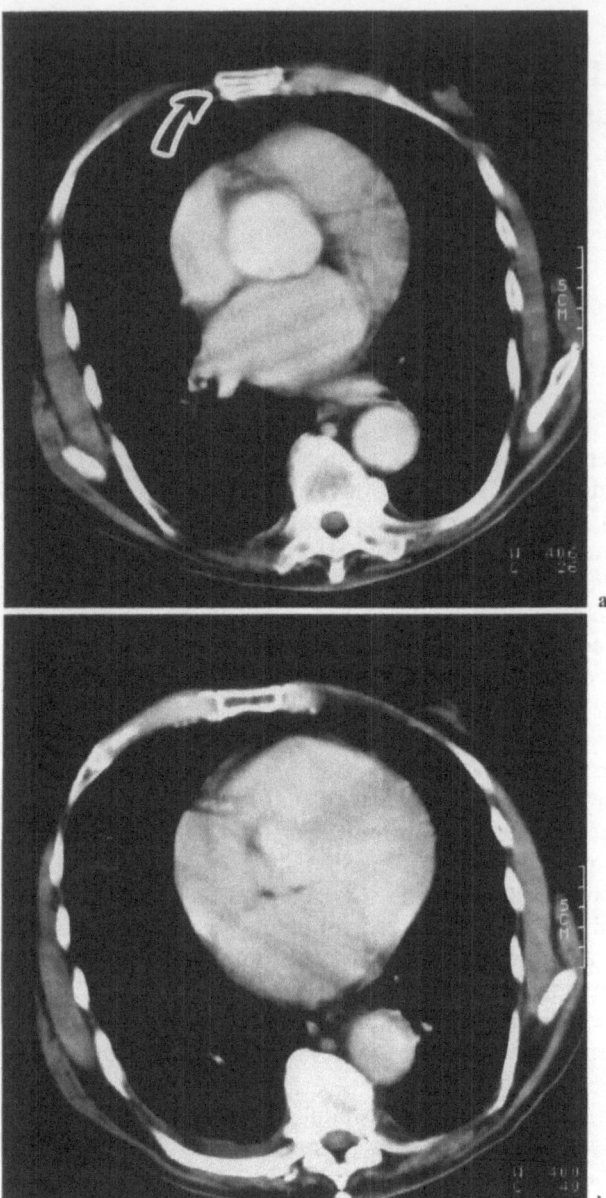

Fig. 1a, b. A very elderly dyspnoeic patient with possible aortic dissection who might well have been unable to cooperate with a slower CT system. **a** Dynamic sequence post-bolus image with no attempt to control respiration. Despite obvious movement of the sternum (arrow) there is remarkably little overall artefact. Aorta (both ascending and descending) appears normal. Very slow circulation, dilated cardiac chambers and mild heart failure have led to a relatively low peak concentration of contrast medium. **b** Image through the hearth of the same patient. Some artefact from the edge of the aorta runs across the large left atrium. Remarkable clarity of aortic root (with a fleck of calcium on one cusp)

Technical Options

Continuous Exposure: up to 12 Seconds (Dynamic Multiscan)

Initially this might seem to be the optimal method of studying many mediastinal problems. The tube exposes continuously during 12 rotations, theoretically allowing up to 110 images to be processed at a single anatomical position. Fit patients might reasonably be expected to maintain a full inspiration for this length of time. However the very patient for whom such a study is needed (e. g. one in pain following aortic dissection) is likely to find a prolonged inspiration difficult, especially following a bolus of contrast medium. The lack of table incrementation (currently impossibe during such a series of images) is another important constraint. More work is required to assess the utility of this technique which has only recently become available to us. However it is possible that a major role within the mediastinum may be the dynamic assessment of physiological movement such as cardiac motion, changes in calibre of the trachea in tracheomalacia or closure of the upper airways in sleep apnoea [Stein et al. 1987] rather than the evaluation of the aorta and other mediastinal structures following bolus contrast enhancement.

Rapid Sequence with Table Incrementation Without Control of Respiration (Dynamic Screening or Sequence)

Here the images can be obtained quickly (scan time: 1 or 0.7 s) with rapid table movement. The table increment has to be standard and the cycle time depends on the increments selected. The patient breathes normally throughout the procedure. This technique allows a large volume of tissue to be studied. Some images will be slightly degraded by respiration artefact; others will not (Fig. 1). Provided that breathing is *gentle,* supposedly contiguous images will appear approximately anatomically contiguous. However none of the images will be at full inspiration.

Rapid Sequence with Table Incrementation with Control of Respiration (Dynamic Screening or Sequence)

Cooperative patients may be able to suspend respiration while images are obtained during a rapid sequence with table incrementation. The green/red light system will warn the patient to stop breathing during the exposures. However it is difficult for many patients to control their respiratory cycle at these speeds and some images are likely to be obtained during inspiration and some during expiration. Thus supposedly contiguous images may not appear so anatomically and some of the images may be degraded by respiratory artefact. Again, none of the images will be obtained at full inspiration (s. Fig. 2).

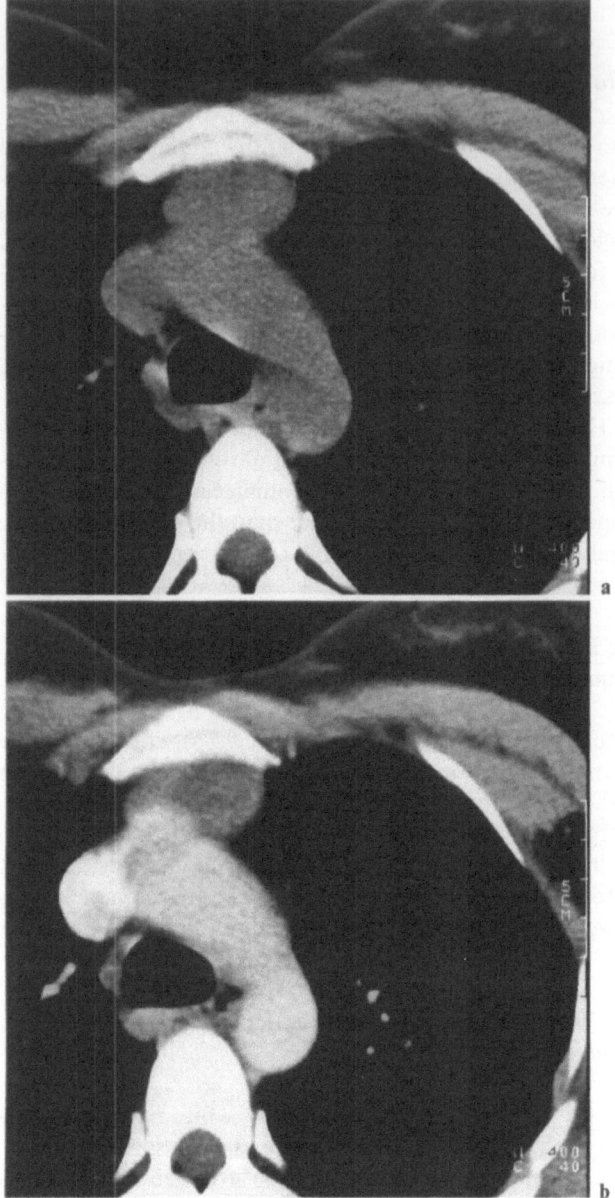

Fig. 2a–c. A young female patient in whom an anterior mediastinal mass was discovered as an incidental finding during the CT evaluation of a shoulder problem. There were no symptoms referable to the chest. She returned for further CT evaluation. **a** Reference image before dynamic sequence. Respiration suspended on the red light. **b** Dynamic sequence: image obtained during a bolus of 50 ml urographic contrast medium (15 grams iodine). Respiration suspended on the red light. **c** Image obtained much later, at comfortable suspended *inspiration*. Note how the anterior mediastinal soft tissue has altered in shape on this image. The exact nature of the mass is not yet established; it may yet prove to be normal thymus

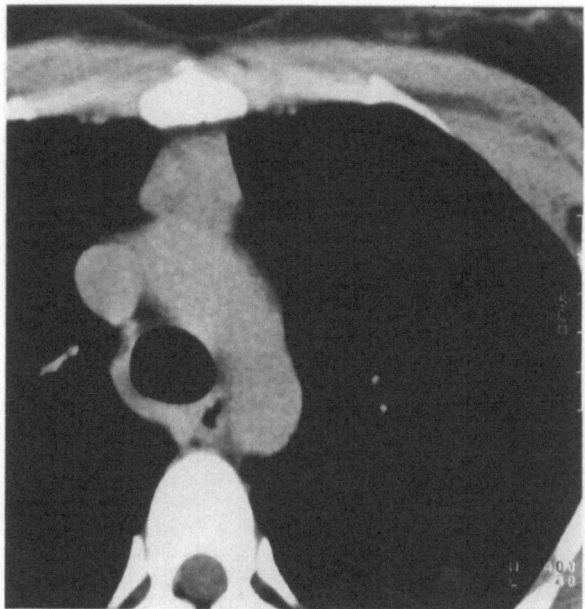

Fig. 2c

Sequence Obtained with Table Incrementation and each Image Obtained at Full Inspiration (Autosequence)

Here the sequence of images is obtained more slowly, with the patient instructed to complete a full respiratory cycle between each data acquisition. This allows larger table increments and also provides images at full inspiration free from respiratory artefact. However, the benefits of rapid examination techniques possible with this machine are not fully exploited; indeed such techniques are analogous to those previously employed with slower systems. Furthermore, as most such studies involve contrast enhancement, large volumes of contrast medium are needed to maintain an adequate intravascular concentration for the duration of the study.

The Patient

The choice of technique will depend, in part, on the well being and cooperation of the patient. Patients with language problems, the deaf and those who are breathless or otherwise too ill to cooperate pose particular problems. Relatively fit patients can understand and cooperate with the system of exposure lights: the reference image acts as a trial exposure. In our practice, a series of unenhanced images is usually obtained before a dynamic series is attempted; such a series, which may answer the clinical question, also gives the patient (and the radiographer!) extra confidence. It is perfectly possible for a cooperative patient to hold their breath for ten seconds to allow a single study at one anatomical level and for some ex-

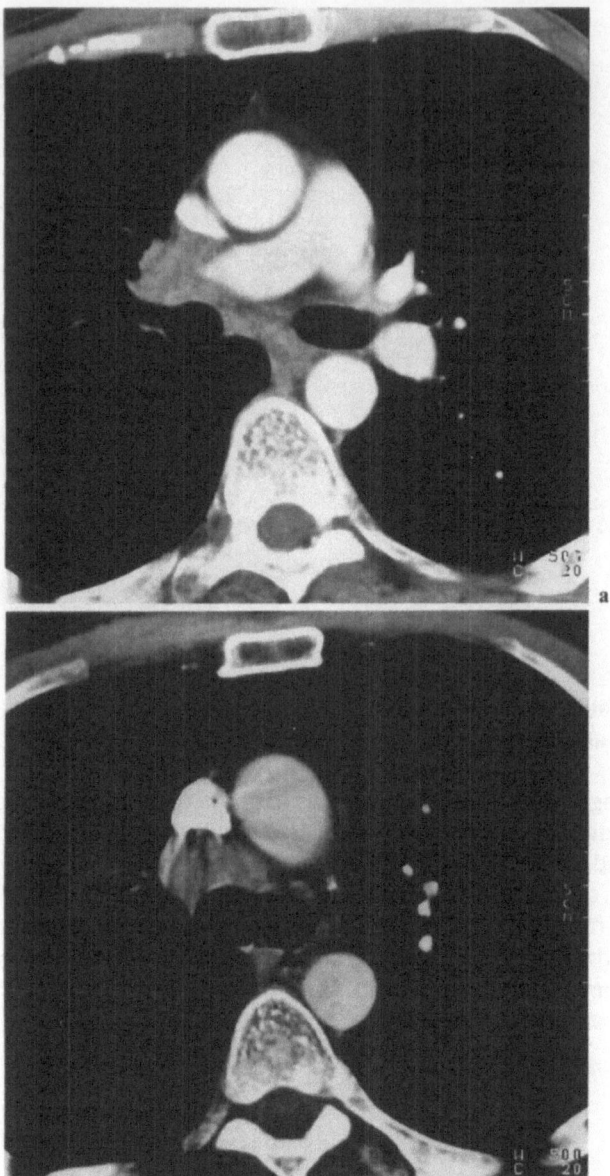

Fig. 3a, b. A female patient with extensive tumor tissue at the right hilum which is causing marked compression of the right pulmonary artery. **a** Image from a dynamic sequence obtained at the end of a bolus injection of 50 ml contrast medium. Excellent delineation of vascular structures. **b** The first image of the dynamic sequence obtained during the second half of the bolus injection. The pre-carinal nodes can be identified. The aorta has started to opacify. The dense contrast medium in the superior vena cava is causing considerable streak artefacts, especially across the ascending aorta

aminations of the mediastinum (e. g. for suspected dissection or cardiac studies) this may be optimal. It is worth noting that the venous return may be fractionally slower under these circumstances and that contrast medium may not circulate to the left heart quite as quickly as expected.

Few patients, however fit, can suspend inspiration under these circumstances for much more than twenty seconds and if a dynamic sequence series with table incrementation is to be used, a run of about 5-6 images is the most that can be obtained during a single breath hold. Therefore, if rapid table incrementation is used, it is probably better to obtain the images whilst the patient breathes regularly with minimal respiratory excursions.

The inevitable anxiety of the patient over the study, the sense of claustrophobia, the noise of the machine and the effects of the contrast medium all tend to distract the patient and can prevent a perfect examination. Time spent giving clear and precise instructions is well invested. In some ways it is easier for the cooperative patient to only have one thing to worry about: either the instructions over the intercom or the lights.

If the patient is a child, very old or very uncooperative it is usually best to aim for very gentle respiration throughout the procedure with no special instructions at all. So long as movement and respiratory excursions are kept to a minimum, the short exposure times often yield surprisingly good data (s. Fig. 1). The pros and cons of sedation for paediatric patients will not be considered apart from noting that the reduced examination time (compared with previous systems) should reduce the need for such premedication.

Contrast Medium

The widespread discrepancies in opinion on indications for enhancement and variation in the manner in which the contrast medium is administered suggest that there is no ideal technique for all examinations: the 'optimal technique' will vary according to the clinical problem as well as from machine to machine. As described above, the SOMATOM PLUS has posed a number of new dilemmas in this latter regard.

Before considering the beneficial aspects of the improved technology, a few minor details will be considered: firstly access to the patient's antecubital fossa. Despite the larger gantry aperture of the SOMATOM PLUS, access is considerably more difficult than with the Siemens SOMATOM II, which had a dual table top. Furthermore the new gantry is wider from front to back and the shoulder rest, although comfortable for the patient, occasionally limits arm abduction. Because of the depth of the gantry, the overhead lighting in our unit did not adequately illuminate the antecubital fossa for the purposes of venepuncture and a portable angle-poise lamp was required. Despite this, it is still difficult for the radiologist to observe the antecubital fossa *during* the injection without being almost within the gantry aperture (and thereby receiving an unnecessarily high radiation dose).

We do not use a pump injector, having believed that we could retain control of the procedure by using hand injections. This philosophy was based on our experi-

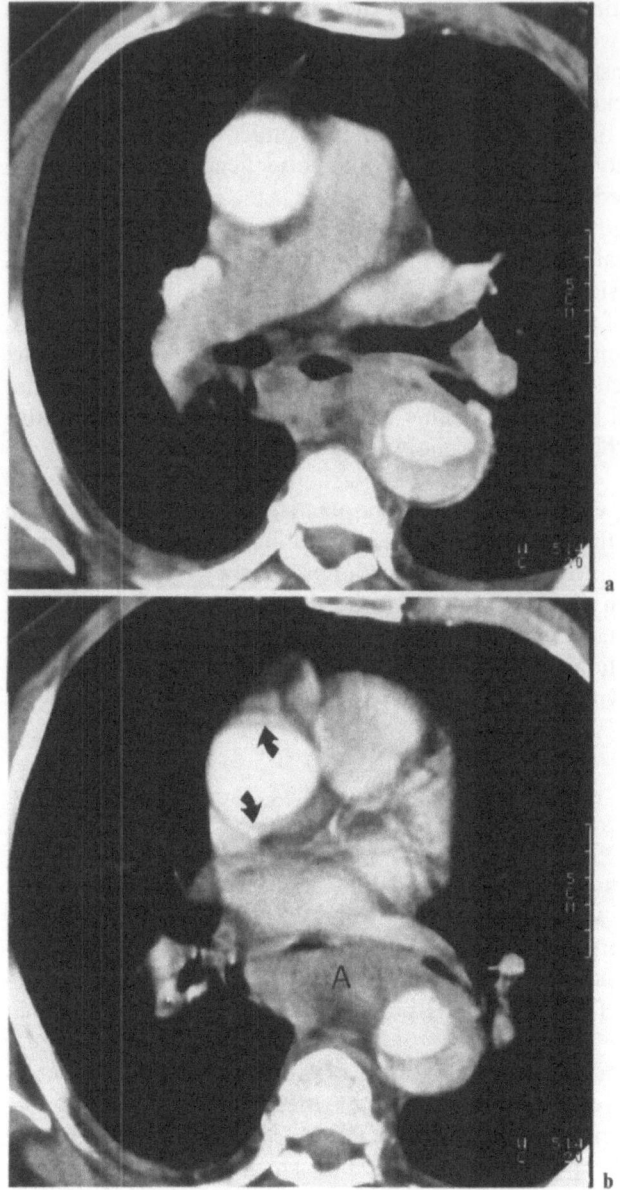

Fig. 4a–c. An elderly male patient with severe chest pain due to an extensive type B dissection within a very tortuous descending aorta. A small amount of posterior mediastinal haemorrhage has also occurred. A dynamic sequence has been obtained with control of respiration by the red light system. The sequence was started towards the end of a bolus of 50 ml contrast medium (15 grams iodine). **a** Excellent opacification of the ascending (normal) and descending aorta. Note the two lumina in the descending aorta confirming the type B dissection. **b** More caudally, the tortuous descending aorta is distorting the oesophagus and left atrium. The two lumina are again seen although the cranial portion of the transversely orientated descending aorta (A) has not opacified. Of particular interest are the artefacts (arrows) on the anterior and posterior margins of the normal ascending aorta caused by aortic compliance

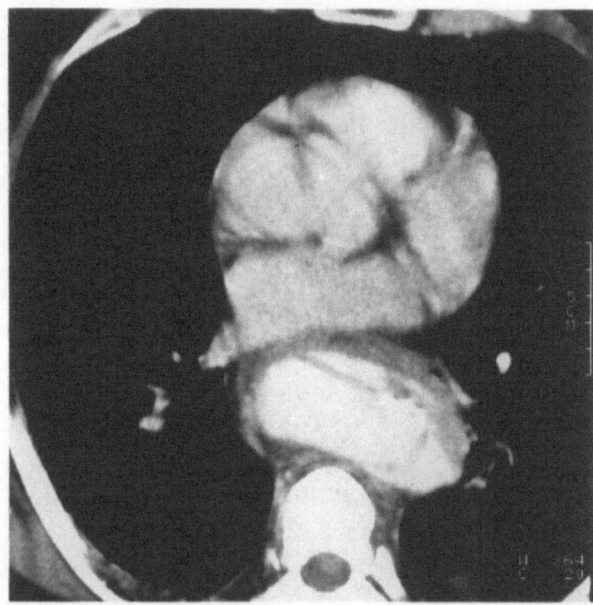

Fig. 4c. More caudal still. The intimal flap in the descending aorta is well demonstrated. Again cardiac and aortic wall motion are causing some artefacts in the region of the ascending aorta

ence with the Siemens SOMATOM II when we tended to use contrast medium for problem solving rather than as a routine. There might be greater use for a pump injector should this policy alter. However part from the cost of the injector itself, there would also be the increased cost of the inevitably larger quantities of contrast medium used. Furthermore when larger quantities of contrast medium are used, the case can often be made for non-ionic agents, with yet further cost!

Our initial experience with the SOMATOM PLUS suggests that most diagnostic problems within the mediastinum remaining after a routine pre-contrast series of images can be solved using a bolus of 50 ml of urographic contrast medium (c. 16 grams of iodine). So long as the timing of images is carefully selected in relation to the injection, the series can be obtained during peak vascular opacification with excellent results (s. Fig. 3). This is in contrast to our work with the SOMA-TOM II where 100 ml of contrast medium was often required in order to maintain peak opacification for the duration of the series of images.

Clinical Problems

Aortic Dissection

The precise examination technique (and method of contrast medium administration) for suspected aortic dissection with the SOMATOM PLUS has not yet been finalised in our hospital. Although the 3 level single slice dynamic technique pro-

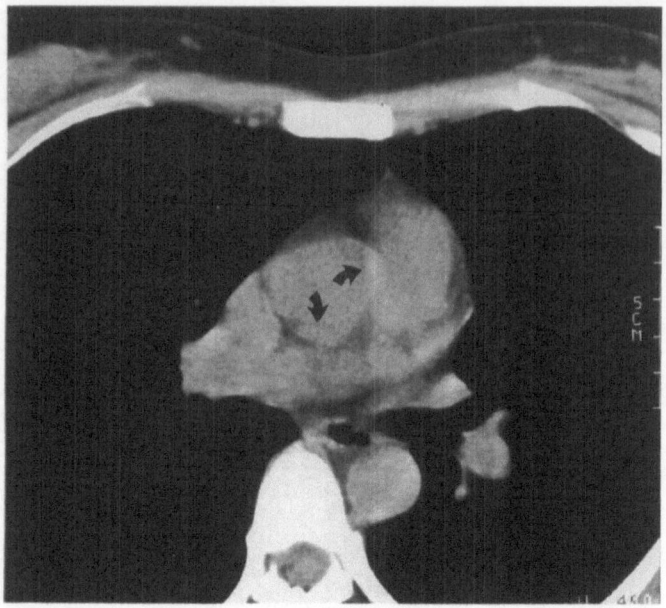

Fig. 5. An unenhanced 1 s image in a young female patient with normal thoracic CT findings. Note the artefacts (arrows) caused by the pulsatility (compliance) of the ascending aorta

posed by Thorsen et al. (1983) carries many theoretical advantages and can be performed either with the dynamic serio or multiscan modes, it has the singular disadvantage of not fully assessing the cranio-caudal extent of a dissection which is of importance to a surgeon. Furthermore, it employs a large volume of contrast medium (c. 120 ml) which may 'ration' the amount of contrast medium available for an angiogram should this latter test be considered necessary because of an equivocal CT result or for better anatomical information. Hence we usually attempted a dynamic series with table incrementation with the SOMATOM II with slices selected in accordance with the findings of a limited series of pre-contrast images (many dissections are evident on such images as a high attenuation crescent). Such a series should always include one slice through the common carotids, several slices through the ascending (and descending) aorta, one through the aortic root, one through the pericardium/descending aorta and one close to the origins of the renal arteries. We have adopted this protocol using the SOMATOM PLUS, without making any attempt at controlling respiration. To date, the results have been very satisfactory (s. Fig. 4) although the number of patients studied is still small. It seems inevitable and desirable that 'spiral' imaging techniques will become available in the future on the SOMATOM PLUS. Such techniques allowing 12 second continuous exposure (dynamic multiscan) with continuous table movement would be invaluable for the mediastinum.

Many of the pitfalls associated with the diagnosis of aortic dissection still pertain with the more modern system. Those resulting from anatomical mimics, such as the superior pericardial recess [Godwin et al. 1982], will still be present even though the true anatomical nature of such structures may be better delineated. Streak artefacts across the aorta, either resulting from high attenuation contrast medium in the superior vena cava (see Fig. 3b) or caused by moving edge artefact [Gallagher and Dixon 1984], are still troublesome, although again more easily recognised. One new problem created by the very short data acquisition times is that of aortic wall motion. On slower systems the aortic outline would be obtained during approximately 2 to 5 heartbeats and any aortic wall movement (compliance) would be averaged out to give a slightly blurred aortic outline. Now, if the data acquisition happens to straddle the maximal change in cross-sectional area between end-diastole and end-systole, quite troublesome artefacts can result which can superficially simulate a dissection (s. Figs.4b and 5). They are quickly recognised as such. Interestingly this observation comes at a time of renewed interest in aortic compliance as a measurement of cardiovascular status which hitherto has been measured in vivo by magnetic resonance [Mohiaddin et al. 1989, Lancet 1990]. It would be easy enough to develop techniques addressing this feature on the SOMATOM PLUS using the dynamic multiscan mode (without the need for intravenous contrast medium).

The Anterior Mediastinum

Despite some debate about the value of CT in the management of myasthenia gravis [Moore 1989] and allied conditions, there are still numerous referrals for the study of the anterior mediastinum. One of the key factors when assessing this region is the overall shape and outline; concavity of the interface with adjacent lung has long been regarded as a reassuring sign. The outline greatly depends on the phase of respiration. Therefore examinations obtained at full inspiration usually provide the optimal assessment of the anterior mediastinum. This raises problems when trying to evaluate a lesion by dynamic post-enhancement techniques. As stated above, it may be better to sacrifice speed in order to obtain a full inspiratory effort (s. Fig. 2).

The Mediastinum for Nodes

The common referrals in our practice are patients with known lymphoma or carcinoma of the bronchus. Occasionally patients are referred with an unknown diagnosis to see whether there are any nodes of sufficient importance to warrant biopsy. According to the various clinical problems, the relative importance of the discovery of a lymph node varies. In the patient with disseminated non-Hodgkin's lymphoma (who is anyway going to be treated with chemotherapy), the presence of a node of equivocal significance (e. g. 1.5 cm in long axis) will not affect management in any substantial way; the region of the node will, anyway, be reassessed following chemotherapy. However the presence of such a node in a patient with carcinoma of the bronchus who is being evaluated before possible thoracotomy may affect management quite profoundly. Accordingly we have long practised different techniques based on the likely management and therapeutic implications with slightly wider slice intervals (1.5 cm) for patients with lymphoma than those being evaluated for carcinoma of the bronchus (1 cm intervals down to the carina, wider intervals below).

Whatever the clinical indication for CT, our initial sequence is an unenhanced series of thoracic images obtained at a comfortable inspiration. Interpretation of mediastinal structures is much more difficult when they are affected by movement artefact (more common after enhancement and when attempting rapid examination techniques) or compressed together by expiration. We admit that this philosophy may have been determined by lengthy experience using a slower CT system where it was difficult to obtain more than eight images at peak vascular enhancement. Nevertheless our initial experience with the SOMATOM PLUS has not led to a substantial change in this philosophy. The excellent artefact-free anatomical detail available on a routine unenhanced autosequence obtained at inspiration is an invaluable start point to any thoracic CT examination. Such a series may be so normal or so definitely abnormal that no further images are necessary. If uncertainty persists, or better anatomical delineation is required, the unenhanced series will allow a tailor-designed set of enhanced images to be obtained. For example, the aortico-pulmonic window can be a particularly troublesome area; enhancement is usually needed to exclude nodes at this site. It may be particularly difficult to separate small nodes from the left pulmonary artery which, because of its arching course through the sequence of axial slices, may cause partial volume effects. Post-contrast enhanced images obtained at narrow collimation may be required to sort out such problems [Zerhouni E, personal communication].

Whenever changing from a 'leisurely' Autosequence of images obtained at inspiration to a Dynamic sequence with breath-holding in accordance with the exposure light, a reference image is essential. There can be quite a marked change in the anatomical position of various structures between inspiration and suspended gentle respiration.

With this 'problem solving' use of enhancement, the rapid capabilities of the SOMATOM PLUS (e. g. 10 slices in 35 s in Dynamic sequence mode) allow a reasonable volume of tissue to be examined during peak vascular enhancement with a relatively small dose of contrast medium. Inevitably techniques vary from centre to centre. In some institutions the CT staging of a patient with carcinoma of the bronchus begins with a dynamic CT study of the liver using a large dose of contrast medium. Then, when that is finished, the mediastinum is examined as quickly as possible when a reasonable vascular concentration persists [Gamsu G, personal communication].

References

1. Anonymous (1990) Magnetic resonance and the revival of arterial sclerosis. Lancet editorial 335: 139-140
2. Daily PO, Trueblood HW, Stinson EB, Wuerflein RD, Shumway NE (1970) Management of acute aortic dissections. Ann Thorac Surg 10: 237-247
3. Dixon AK, Hilton CJ, Williams GT (1981) Computed tomography and histological correlation of the thymic remnant. Clinical Radiology 32: 255-257

4. Gallagher S, Dixon AK (1984) Streak artefacts of the thoracic aorta: pseudodissection. J Comput Assist Tomogr 8: 688–693
5. Godwin JD, Breiman RS, Speckman JM (1982) Problems and pitfalls in the evaluation of thoracic aorta dissection by computed tomography. J Comput Assist Tomogr 6: 750–756
6. Heitzmann ER (1981) Fleischner lecture: computed tomography of the thorax: current perspectives. Am J Roentgenology 136: 3–12
7. Husband J, Kelsey Fry (1981) Computed tomography of the body. Macmillan, London
8. Lipton MJ, Higgins CB, Farmer D, Boyd DP (1984) Cardiac imaging with a high-speed cine-CT scanner: preliminary results. Radiology 152: 579–582
9. Mohiaddin RH, Underwood SR, Bogren HG et al. (1989) Regional aortic compliance studied by magnetic resonance imaging: the effects of age, training and coronary heart disease. Br Heart Journal 62: 90–96
10. Moore NR (1989) Imaging in myasthenia gravis. Clinical Radiology 40: 115–116
11. Stein MG, Gamsu G, de Geer G, Golden JA, Crumley RL, Webb WR (1987) Cine CT in obstructive sleep apnoea. Am J Roentgenology 148: 1069–1074
12. Thorsen MK, San Dretto MA, Lawson TL, Foley WD, Smith DF, Berland LL (1983) Dissecting aortic aneurysms: accuracy of computed tomographic diagnosis. 148: 773–777

New Clinical Perspectives in CT: Initial Results of Dynamic Contrast Medium Studies with Continuous Rotation Scanning of the Heart, Liver, Pancreas and Kidney

K. ENGELHARD, G. LASEK, O. BARTELS, J. DREXLER

Abstract

Two new CT techniques, dynamic multiscan and dynamic sequence, are introduced using examples from initial heart, liver, pancreas and kidney examinations. Dynamic multiscan provides reconstructed CT images at 0.1 sec intervals, permitting improved assessment of the perfusion phase in liver processes and aortocoronary bypass studies. Dynamic sequence allows the examination of a single anatomical region by using rapid scan sequences with table feed. A single bolus administration of contrast medium is sufficient to display the enhancement of a mass in numerous tomographic planes, as demonstrated in the pancreas and kidney. Both methods raise hopes for improved early diagnosis of smaller masses in parenchymal organs. The decisive advantage of the new technology is the high economy made possible by the tremendous saving in contrast medium dosage.

Key Words

Dynamic multiscan – dynamic sequence – organ perfusion – heart – liver – pancreas – kidney.

Introduction

The goal of dynamic CT is to provide the greatest number of images within the shortest time interval. Not only the morphology but also the role of pathological alterations or the function of an organ should be displayed during contrast medium enhancement. Short examination times and rapid scan rates permit the dynamic imaging of the contrast medium enhancement resulting from its influx into the vessels and the interstitium [4, 8, 9, 10].

An improved diagnosis can be expected from the following [2, 12, 16]:
1. Higher scan rate
2. Shorter scan times
3. Higher tube rating
4. The possibility of reconstructing numerous organ or lesion slices with one contrast medium bolus in the shortest time interval.

Material and Methods

Terminology

1. Dynamic Multiscan

This technique is only possible in CT scanners with continuous rotation measurement systems. Data are accumulated from several sequential rotation cycles for as long as 12 seconds. The reconstruction of over one hundred 1 second images temporally displaced by 0.1 sec is thus possible. This splitting into shortest time intervals allows the almost uninterrupted imaging of an organ in the perfusion phase. Short scan times of 1 or 0.7 sec permit the elimination of motion artifacts.

2. Dynamic Sequence CT

Dynamic scan cycles with table feed (dynamic sequencing) represent a further development to the serio CT examination-technique already known. This examination technique permits rapid scan sequencing with table feed (cycle time: 3.5 sec, concurrent image reconstruction). An organ or its parts can be displayed in the perfusion phase with a single contrast medium bolus (30 ml).

Examination technique

Our first studies comprised 20 patients, whereby 9 examinations were performed on the liver, 5 on the heart, 2 on the pancreas and 4 on the kidney. The hepatic foci revealed four cases of hemangioma, two cases of focal nodular hyperplasia (FNH), and one case each of liver adenoma, focal, nonadipose liver degeneration and primary hepatocellular carcinoma. Diagnoses were established by observing the clinical course of the illness, by scintigraphic scan, liver biopsy and autopsy. Cardiac studies comprised three patients with aortocoronary bypasses and two patients with normal findings. A normal pancreas finding and a caudal pancreas carcinoma were also examined. Four patients with kidney lesions demonstrated two cases each of hypernephroma and angiomyolipoma. The diagnosis of renal masses was verified surgically. Independent of the scanning technique and after determining the pulse rate, each patient received a manual bolus administration of non-ionic contrast medium (40 ml within 5 to 10 sec) via a large-bore cannula (17 gauge). After initial contrast medium administration and dependent on pulse rate (delay time), scan begin for both methods was determined as follows: The influence of cardiac output in bolus administration can be taken into account by using the circulation time (in heart beats), according to Schad [23].

Cardio CT examinations were approximated by tipping the gantry caudal to the longitudinal axis of the heart (Fig. 1).

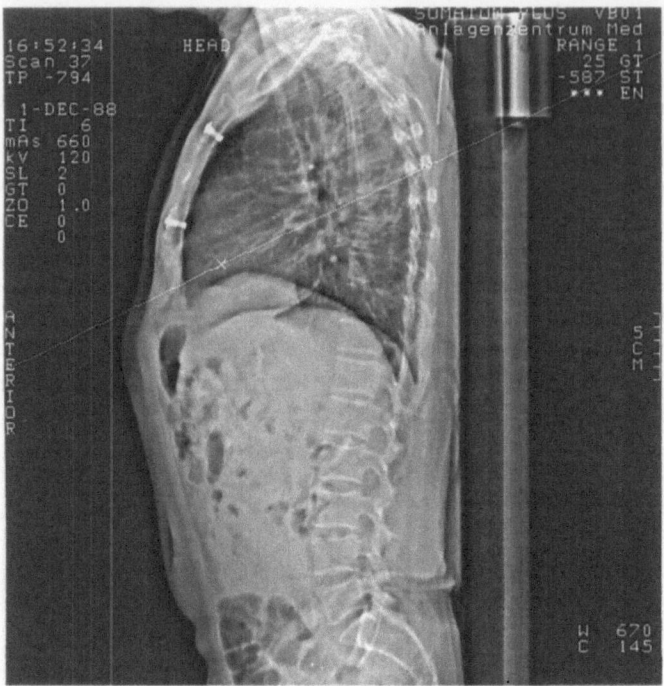

Fig. 1. Lateral tomogram with changing position

Table 1. Circulation times (t) [sec] in heart beats (n)

Arm - right ventricle	4
Arm - left ventricle	11
Arm - thoracic artery	12
Arm - abdominal artery	13
Arm - brain	13
Arm - iliac arteries	15

with $t = n \cdot 60/f$ [sec]
f = heart frequency [min-1]

Results

Liver. A more exact analysis of the perfusion stage in hepatic processes could only be performed for hemangiomas, FNH and adenomas in the examined cases. The four hemangiomas were examined in dynamic multiscan with rapid scan sequences of 0.2 to 0.3 second per scan cycle. The total scan time for a full rotation lasted 8 or 12 seconds. This was followed by a late scan in the same scanning plane after 8 and 20 minutes in the case of hemangiomas. A focal reduction was recognizable in all four cases after bolus contrast medium administration (Fig. 2, "iris-diaphragm phenomenon"). It began from 5 to 7 sec after administration and

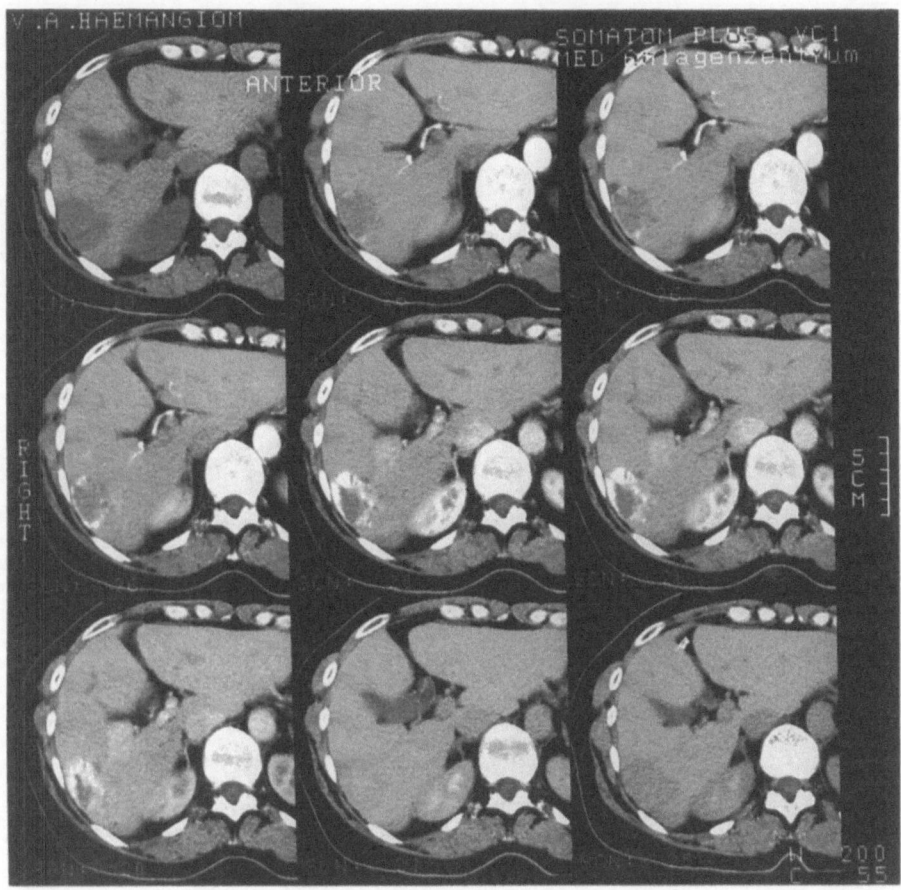

Fig. 2. Hemangioma of the right liver lobe. Distinct "iris-diaphragm phenomenon" with marginal hypervascularization and focal uniformity within 9 seconds. Scan sequence of 0.2 sec

in each of the four cases reached a total or near uniformity of the foci to the surrounding hepatic tissue after 9 sec. A tuberous, garland-like hypervascularization in the marginal regions of the lesions could be displayed in three of the four cases. The hemangiomas studied were hypodense with respect to the surrounding hepatic tissue about 2 to 8 minutes after administration. A late scan after 20 min provided no additional information. The rapid scan sequencing offered no improved display of FNH in a fatty liver than that with the conventional, slower scan times. The second case examined demonstrated a rapid contrast medium enhancement (approx. 50 HU) in the entire isodense region during the first 10 to 15 sec (Fig. 3). The examined adenoma revealed a diffuse, homogeneous contrast enhancement 20 sec after administration. A uniform contrast reduction with the renewed display of a homogeneous, hypodense area was seen after 25 sec. A substantially improved analysis of contrast enhancement behavior could not be substantiated in one case of primary hepatocellular carcinoma and one of nonadipose focal liver degeneration.

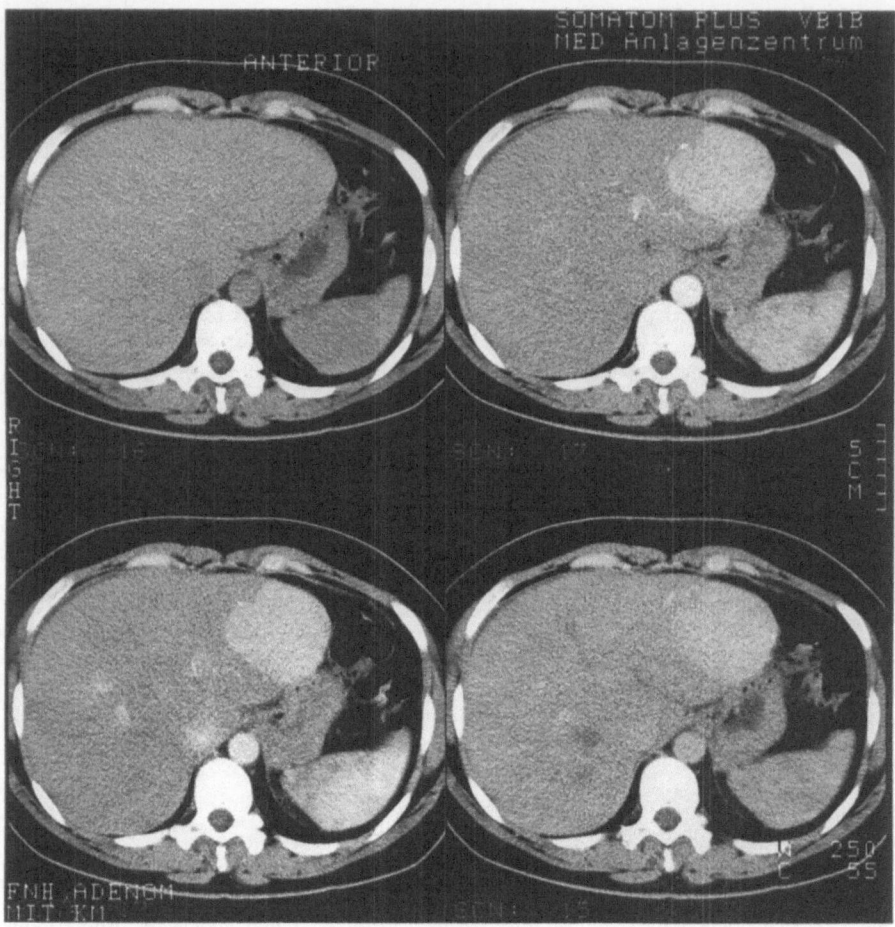

Fig. 3. FNH of the left liver lobe. Distinct differentiation to the homogeneous contrast medium enhancement of the lesion. Scan sequence of 0.2 sec

Heart. An improved morphological display of normally pathological alterations could be visualized in the examination of cardiac studies by eliminating motion artifacts of cardiac and respiratory phases. Even without EKG triggering, the ventricles, ventricular septum and myocardial-wall thickness could be displayed with higher definition and without the blurring artifacts. An artifact-free, functional examination of the aortocoronary-bypass could be performed on 3 patients, since the short scan times of 0.7 or 1 sec permit the elimination of artifacts caused by cardiomotility and respiratory motion (Fig. 4). The display of all bypasses demonstrated patency as far as blood flow is concerned. Especially those to the right coronary artery which were previously difficult to visualize could now be displayed artifact-free (Fig. 5).

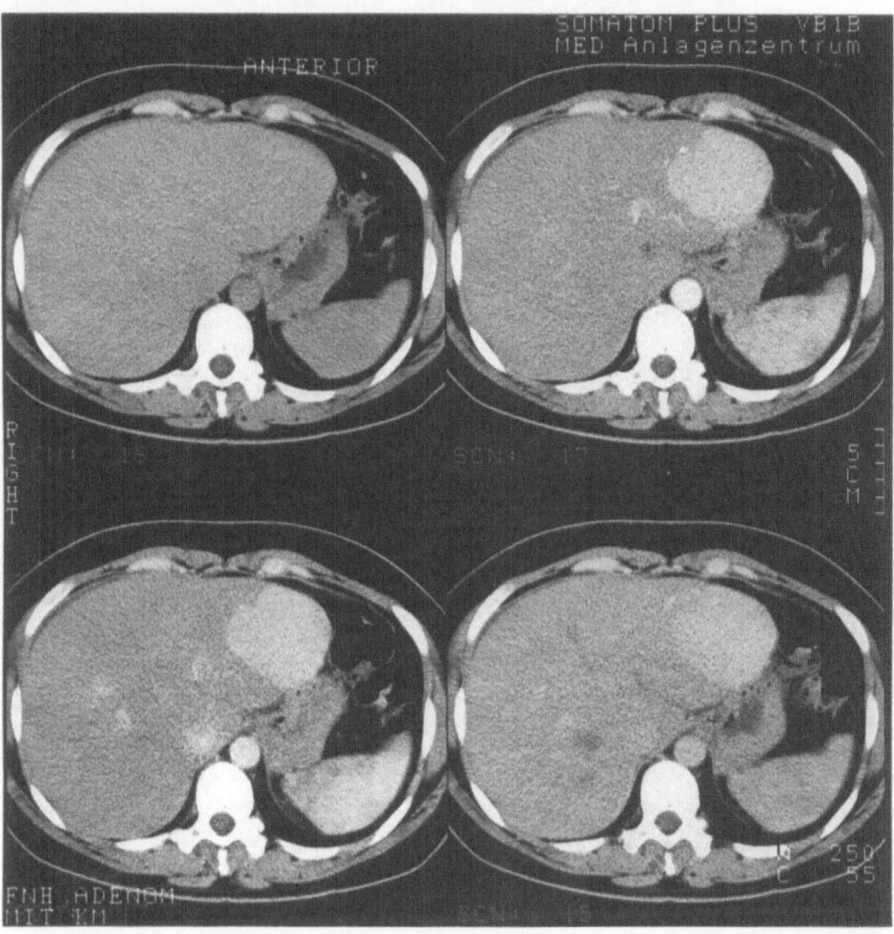

Fig. 4. Bypass to the interventricular branch of the left coronary artery. Density accentuation in the punctiform region of the cross-sectional bypass. Artifact-free border to the ventricular septum and both ventricles. Scan sequence of 0.1 sec

Pancreas. A 5 mm slice thickness and a 5 mm table feed was used for both pancreas studies. This was followed in one case by bolus administration in the slice of interest (dynamic multiscan), in another case by a rapid scan sequences (dynamic sequence) through the entire organ during a contrast medium bolus. The conventional contrast medium bolus technique provided no additional information in a pancreas with normal findings. A homogeneous contrast medium enhancement was found with rapid visualization of the splenic vein. The enhanced perfusion took place somewhat undulatory with density values of about 45 HU. After six minutes the pancreas returned to the original values of 35 HU. The entire pancreas could be displayed with a single, 30 ml contrast medium bolus in a patient with a small caudal pancreas carcinoma (cycle time of 3 sec, 5 mm slice thickness, 5 mm table feed) (Fig. 6). Compared to conventional contrast medium studies an

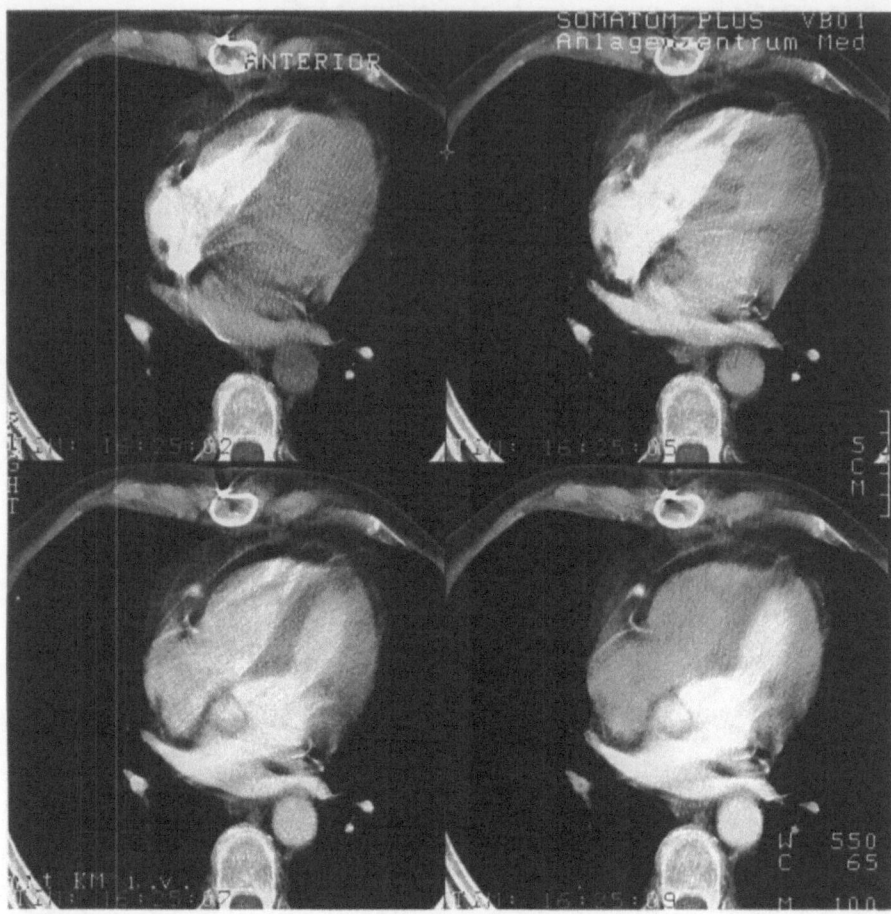

Fig. 5. Bypass to the right coronary artery. Sharp and artifact-free display of the density accentuation in the cross-sectional bypass. Distinct differentiation of the ventricular septum and the wall of the left ventricle. Scan sequence of 0.1 sec

exceptional display of both the arterial and venous structures could be obtained. The hepatic arteries, celiac trunk and splenic artery as well as the splenic vein, vena cava, portal vein and renal veins could be clearly differentiated from the tumor and the residual parts of the organ. A hypodense region indicating a necrosis in the enlarged, tumor infiltrated tail of the pancreas could be demarcated clearly. Both the tumor and the residual parts of the organ could be displayed in all slices with more rapid sequencing.

Kidney. With the sequencing technique a clear differentiation of the renal medulla and cortex in numerous slices was possible in the four cases with kidney tumors. The rapidly appearing and undesirable homogeneous enhancement of the renal medulla and the early elimination into the renal pelvis found previously in the conventional serio CT studies could therefore be avoided in diagnostics (Fig. 7).

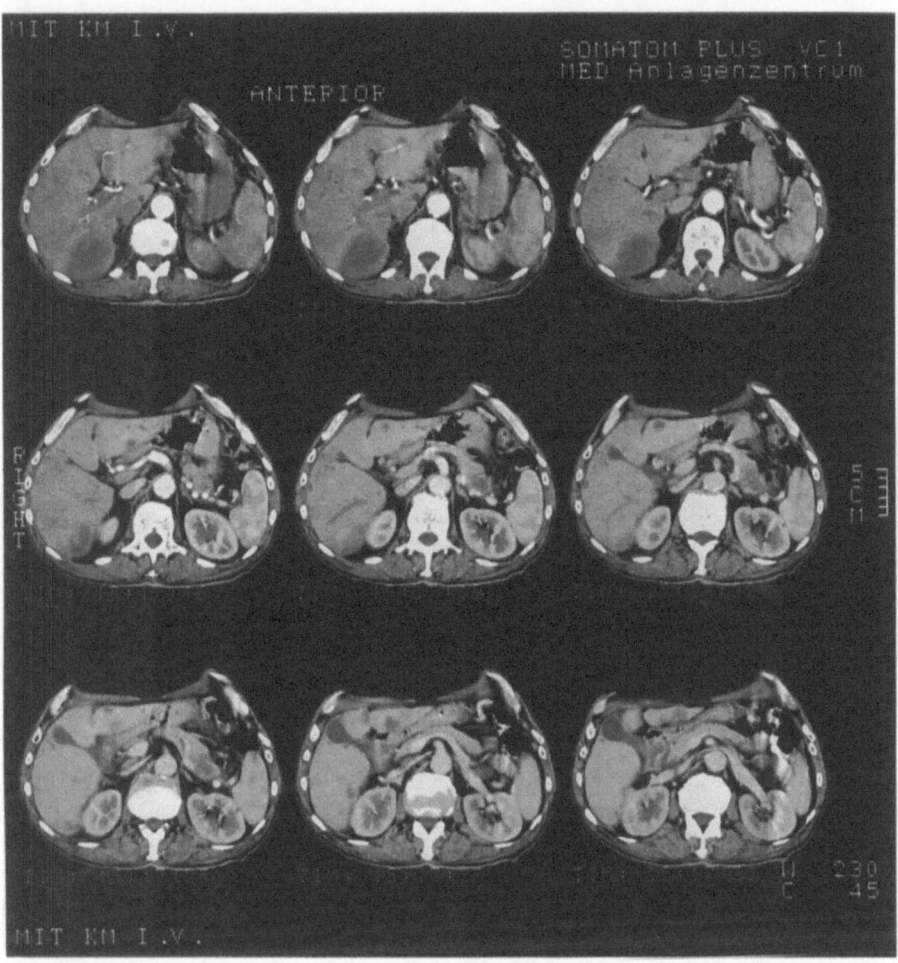

Fig. 6. Dynamic sequence of a carcinoma in the tail of the pancreas. Display of the entire tumor and of the residual pancreas with a 30 ml contrast medium bolus. Clear differentiation of all epigastric arteries and veins in the vicinity of the tumor

Discussion

With dynamic multiscanning it is now possible, for the first time to accurately display the state of perfusion in liver processes during the first 60 seconds in most rapid scan sequences. As experimental studies have shown, this technique also permits the visualization of interstitial contrast medium enhancement in pathological processes. The vascularization of hepatic masses has been examined adequately by displaying the arterial and venous phases of the liver. The rapid interstitial contrast medium enhancement during the first circulation time, on the other hand, could not be displayed previously with CT units. Nuclear medical examinations of laboratory animal livers have shown that the 50% passage time of a sub-

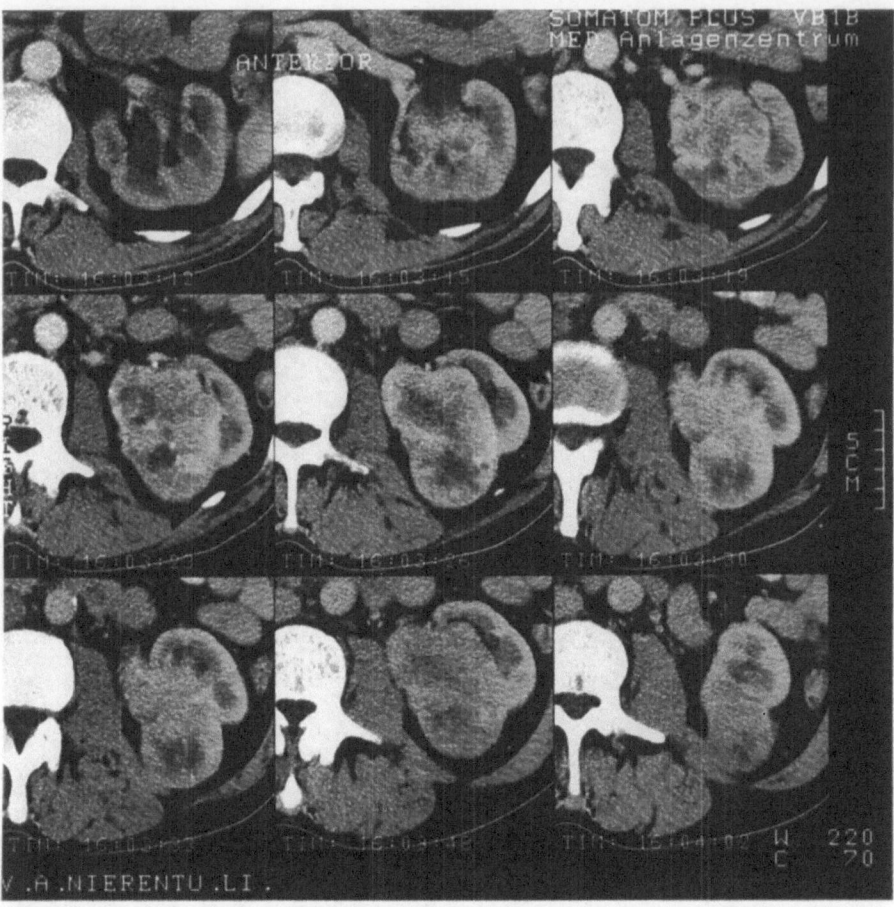

Fig. 7. Dynamic sequence of a hypernephroma. Display of the entire tumor during the early perfusion phase with a 30 ml contrast medium bolus. Sharp demarcation of the renal medulla and cortex in all slices

stance diffusing fully from the interstitium through the capillary wall into the extracellular space demonstrates a half-time of 2 seconds [18]. This explains why early interstitial contrast medium enhancement in tissues and pathological processes is not visualizable with conventional scanners of the 3rd generation. Further studies must now be performed to determine the suitability of early interstitial contrast medium enhancement for differentiating pathological processes, as compared to the later phases in the so-called steady state [1, 2, 4, 9, 12, 18]. The multiscan technique, however, at least offers a method for imaging such rapid diffusion processes [1, 2, 4, 8, 9, 12, 18]. The decisive advantage over conventional CT is the nearly uninterrupted imaging of the first 20 seconds of contrast medium enhancement. If our first liver studies of hemangiomas and FNH are compared with the common, slower contrast medium studies, the stage of perfusion ("iris-diaphragm phenomenon", homogeneous contrast accentuation and uniformity to the surrounding hepatic tissue) is now seen in higher detail for improved documentation [2, 3, 7, 13, 16, 20]. As far as differential diagnosis and accuracy of diagnosis are concerned, a clear diagnostic gain is not attainable. Even though scans display the contrast medium stage more impressively, further studies are required to provide evidence that small masses could be diagnosed and differentiated more readily. A most definite advantage is the reduced motion artifacts in dynamic contrast medium studies due to the short scan times.

The significance of the conventional cardio CT (without EKG triggering) is based on the morphological display of myocardial and pericardial illnesses in noninvasive examinations of aortocoronary bypasses [3, 5, 10, 14, 19, 21]. The patency of bypasses can now be tested with substantially reduced amounts of contrast medium (30 ml) instead of the large amounts required previously (100 to 150 ml per bypass study). Together with the short scan times the reduction in motion artifacts, even without EKG triggering, permits an unobjectionable identification of the perfused bypass. In contrast to previously, even patients with a manifested cardiac insufficiency can therefore be subjected to a bypass examination.

With the dynamic sequencing technique, a pathological process or an organ part can be displayed in continuous slices during the enhancement phase of a single bolus contrast medium administration. As seen in the pancreas, an improved differentiation of the tumor's hypodense region with a good display of epigastric vessels can be attained [2, 11, 22]. The clear differentiation of the renal cortex and medulla is evident in numerous slices so that the previously disturbing scanning enhancement of the organ and the early elimination become unimportant. The pathological process can thereby be recognized in numerous slices during the early phase of enhancement [1, 15, 24]. Whether smaller renal lesions can be identified with this technique remains undecided.

We believe at present that the decisive advantage of the new techniques appears to be the high economy. Whereas dynamic contrast medium studies thus far require a minimum of 100 to 150 ml contrast medium per study, a reduction of 30% per organ study is possible with the new techniques. The enormous costs resulting from very expensive contrast media can thereby be reduced appreciably.

In the same way, the saving of contrast medium for high-risk patients seems to be worth mentioning.

We believe that a further examination of the method is well deserved, especially with reference to the improved early diagnostics of pancreas and liver tumors.

References

1. Baert AL, Wilms G, Marchal G, De Mayer P, De Sommer F (1980) Contrast enhancement of the bolus technique in the examination of the kidney. Radiologe 20: 279–287
2. Clark LR, Jakobs NM, Zeman RK et al. (1985) Enhanced pancreatic CT imaging utilizing a geometric magnification technique. Radiology 20: 531–538
3. Claussen C, Lochner B (1983) Dynamische Computertomographie. 1st revised edition. Springer, Berlin Heidelberg New York
4. Dean PB, Kivisaari L, Kormano M (1978) The diagnostic potential of contrast enhancement pharmacokinetics. Investigative Radiology 12: 533–540

5. Dueber C, Thelen M (1986) Welche Rolle spielt die Kontrastmittelgabe in der CT-Diagnostik am Herzen heute? In: Wolf KJ, Zeitler E (eds) Neues im Kontrastbild Herz und grosse Gefässe. 1st revised edition. Schering, Berlin, pp 139–144
6. Foley D (1989) Dynamic hepatic CT. Radiology 170: 617–622
7. Freeny PC, Marks WM (1986) Hepatic hemangioma: Dynamic bolus CT. AJR 147: 711–719
8. Fuchs WA, Vock P, Haertel M (1979) Pharmakokinetik intravasaler Kontrastmittel bei der Computer-Tomographie. Radiologe 19: 90–93
9. Gardeur D, Lautrou J, Millard JC, Berger N, Metzger J (1989) Pharmacokinetics of contrast media: Experimental results in dog and man with CT implications. J Comput Assist Tomogr 4: 178–185
10. Heuser L, Lackner K, Hauser H (1982) Validität der Computertomographie bei der Darstellung offener und verschlossener aortokoronarer Venenbrücken (ACVB) RÖFO 137: 619–626
11. Kloeppel R, Schulz H-G, Lieberenz S (1985) Zweijährige Erfahrung mit der dynamischen Computertomographie des Pankreas. Radiol Diagn 26 (1): 31–39
12. Kormano M, Dean PB (1976) Extravascular contrast material: The major component of contrast enhancement. Radiology 121: 379–382
13. Kurtz B (1988) Leberdiagnostik I: Dynamische CT-Studien. In: Claussen C, Felix R (eds) Quo Vadis CT? 1st revised edition. Springer, Berlin Heidelberg New York, pp 151–159
14. Lackner K, Landwehr P, Krahe T, Thurn P (1988) Konventionelle Cardio-CT. In: Claussen C, Felix R (eds) Quo Vadis CT? 1st revised edition. Springer, Berlin Heidelberg New York, pp 103–111
15. Lackner K, Koischwitz D, Molitor B, Vogel J, Schmidt S (1984) Treffsicherheit in der Diagnostik renaler Raumforderungen: Computertomographie, Sonographie, Urographie, Angiographie. RÖFO 140: 363–372
16. Luening M, Wolff H, Herolpsheimer F, Jordan O (1985) Dynamische Computertomographie – Eine Hilfe zur artdiagnostischen Differenzierung von Leberraumforderungen. Radiol Diagn 26: 501–515
17. Mathieu D, Bruneton JN, Drouillard J, Pointreau CC, Vasile N (1986) Hepatic adenomas and focal nodular hyperplasia: Dynamic CT study. Radiology 160: 53–58
18. Metzger H, Küpper K, Feller A (1985) Experimentelle Untersuchung zur KM-Dynamik der Leber mittels schneller Sequenz-CT. In: Digitale bildgebende Verfahren. – Integrierte digitale Radiologie. 4th Radiological Symposium in Graz, Austria. Schering, Berlin, pp 534–540
19. Sandring KH, Luening M, Heublein B, Geissler W (1983) Computertomographische Beurteilung der Durchgängigkeit aortokoronarer Bypässe. Dt Gesundh-Wesen 38: 59–62
20. Schild H, Kreitner KF, Thelen M et al. (1987) Fokal-noduläre Hyperplasie der Leber bei 930 Patienten. RÖFO 147: 612–618
21. Schlolaut KH, Lackner K, Becher H, Grube E, Orellano L (1986) Treffsicherheit der Kardio-CT und Echokardiographie in der Diagnostik raumfordernder Prozesse des Herzens. RÖFO 145: 527–535
22. Ward Ellen M et al. (1983) Pancreatic carcinoma CT. Characteristics of 100 cases. Radio Graphies 3 (4)
23. Wegener OH (1981) Ganzkörper-Computertomographie. Karger, Basel Munich Paris, pp 4–32
24. Wimmer B, Hauenstein KH (1988) Grenzen der computertomographischen Differentialdiagnostik bei fokalen Leberveränderungen. Radiologe 28: 356–361
25. Zeman RK, Cronan JJ, Rosenfield AT, Lynch JH, Jaffe MH, Clark LR (1988) Renal CT of vascular invasion and tumor vascularity. Radiology 167: 393–396

Dynamic CT in Transplanted Hearts

R. RIENMÜLLER, B.E. KEMKES

In the postsurgical care of patients after heart transplantation a number of various clinical studies and imaging modalities are used for early recognition of deteriorated myocardial function as sequels of rejection, coronary arthero-sclerosis, systemic hypertension, drug toxicity and denervation [1, 2, 3].

Previously in a long term follow up study of transplanted hearts we could show that using a suitable MR-method of evaluating the morphology and function of the heart the number of angiographic studies and biopsies may be reduced from one to two years control period [4–8].

Prior condition is that the MR-examination performed every six month reveals unchanged, normal endiastolic volume and unchanged left ventricular muscle mass (mostly increased) accompanied by typical wall thickness changes over the cardiac cycle without regional or global irregularities.

In this MR-study we found that the extent of left ventricular muscle mass of transplanted hearts does not correlate with the degree or time of systemic hypertension, or time of posttransplantation period. However, there was linear correlation with the number of passed rejection episodes per patients, showing that increasing numbers of rejection episodes correlate with the decrease of left ventricular muscle mass [7].

Owing to implied methodological grounds, patients with acute rejection and/or implanted pacemakers cannot be studies by MR presently.

Considering our experimental MR-results in dogs with transplanted hearts we found (as others too) that at the time of acute rejection there is a wall thickness increase of the ventricles caused by edema. The intracavitary volumes remain unchanged.

In contrast to MR, CT may be used in the evaluation of transplanted hearts without the mentioned handicaps. If compared with conventional CT-machine, the new CT (SOMATOM PLUS) allows shorter exposure times of 1.0 s and 0.7 s respectively (Fig. 1). That way the image quality of fast moving parts of the body as the heart improved dramatically especially in regard to the visualization of the myocardial wall. The dynamic scan mode (Fig. 2) characterized by a continuous exposure of 8 to 12 seconds with additional image reconstruction at arbitrary defined times permity, i. e., the visualization of contrast agent flow through the heart chambers and vessels as well as through the myocardium. The excellent CT delineation of the left ventricular myocardial wall and the visualization of the left ventricular cavity of the own and of the transplanted heart (at the neck) in an anesthetized dog (Fig. 3, 4) demonstrate the improvement in image quality. It also confirms that the exposure time is the most important determinant in imaging the

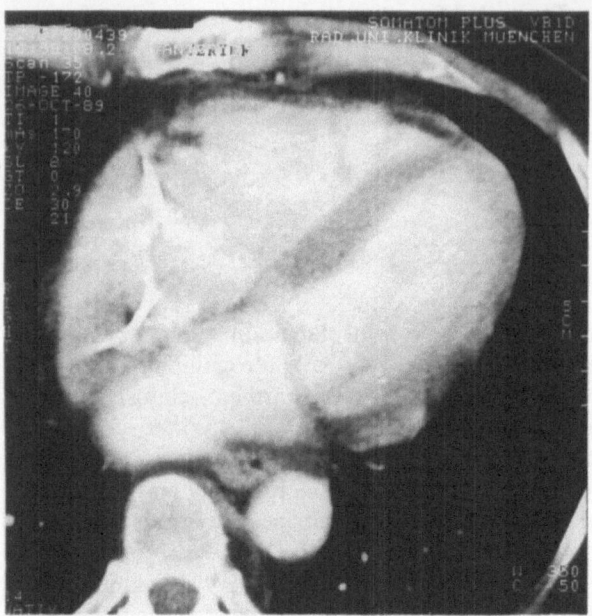

Fig. 1. Transversal CT image selected from dynamic CT-study through the midportion of the left ventricle after intravenous contrast agent application with good delination of the interventricular septum, of the posterolateral wall and mitral valves as well. Notize the wires of the pacemaker in the right atrium

moving parts of the body. Because of severe anemia the left ventricular cavity may be separated from the myocardium even without intravenous contrast agent application (Fig. 5, 6).

Our CT experience in the evaluation of transplanted hearts in man using SO-MATOM PLUS is until now limited to four patients. At the time of their CT studies, no signs of acute rejection were present.

The CT studies were first performed as native scanning from the diaphragma to the aortic arch followed by intravenous contrast agent application of 40 ccm and repeated scanning again from the diaphragm to the aortic arch. In this second CT study we selected that CT level, the left ventricle was shown in its largest circumference. At this level we repeat the CT study after additional application of 40 to 60 ccm of contrast agent followed by dynamic mode of CT scanning for a period of 8 seconds. The CT image reconstruction succeeded in steps of 0.5 seconds from the beginning to the end of the exposure time. Afterwards we selected the CT image with the best delineation of the left ventricular myocardial wall and calculated the left ventricular muscle mass using the two axis method and the formula of a rotating elipsoid.

The mean value of 134,5 g of left ventricular muscle mass is similar to the amount of left ventricular muscle mass (151 g ± 41,8) of transplanted heart determined by MR.

Although this results are only preliminary it may be postulated, that in case of patients with pacemakers a CT study of the heart may be performed obtaining re-

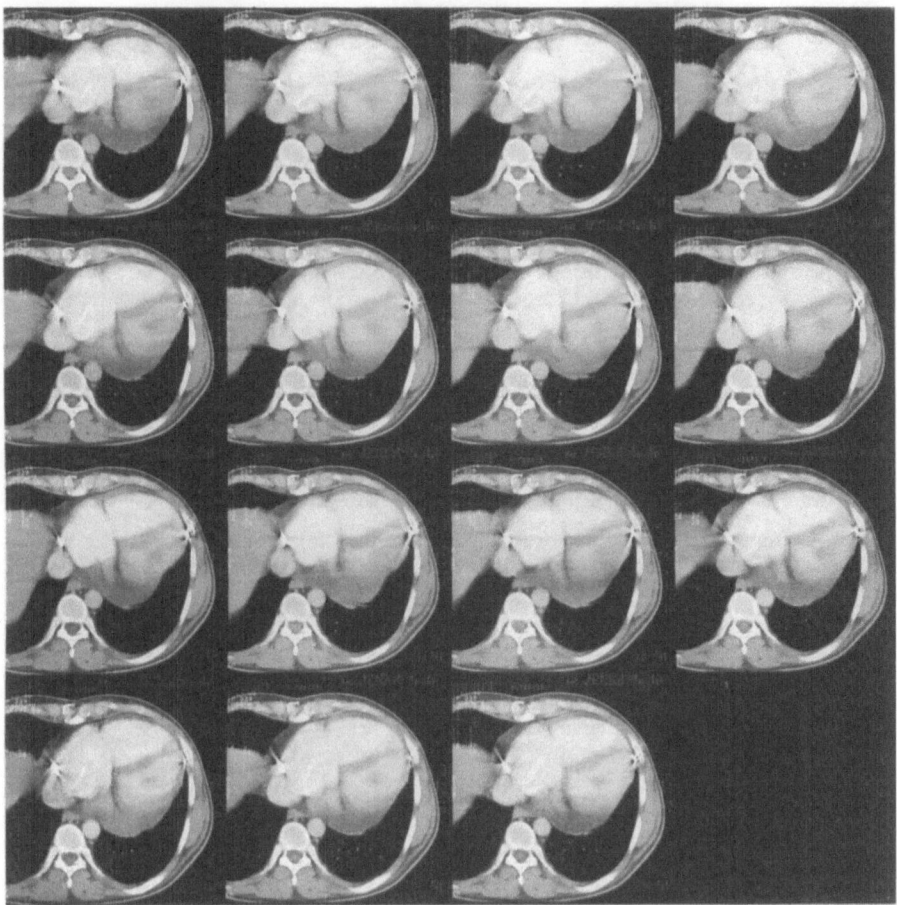

Fig. 2. Dynamic CT-study after intravenous contrast agent application of a patient after orthotopic hearttransplantation through the midportion of its heart (without ECG-gating) showing continous increase of CT density of the left ventricle over the time (from the left uppercorner to the right lower corner)

sults comparable to those of MR. Further more because of the simplicity of the CT study and the shortness of the exposure time, even patients with suspected acute rejection may be studied. It seems reasonable to assume that in this situation an increase of wall thickness would be found.

Summary

Based on our preliminary experimental and clinical results in the CT evaluation of transplanted hearts and based on our daily experience in CT studies of the hearts with various pathology, SOMATOM PLUS is presenting a real progress in image

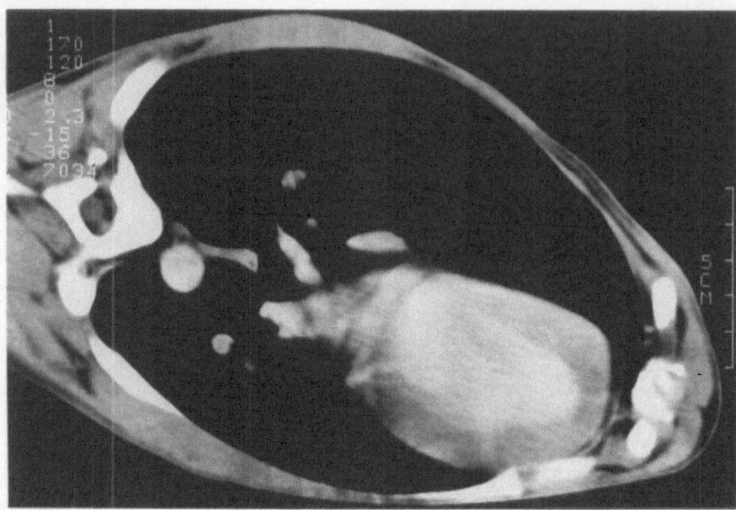

Fig. 3. CT transversal scan through the midportion of the left ventricle of a dog (selected from a dynamic CT-study) after intravenous contrast agent application with excellent delineation of the myocardial wall

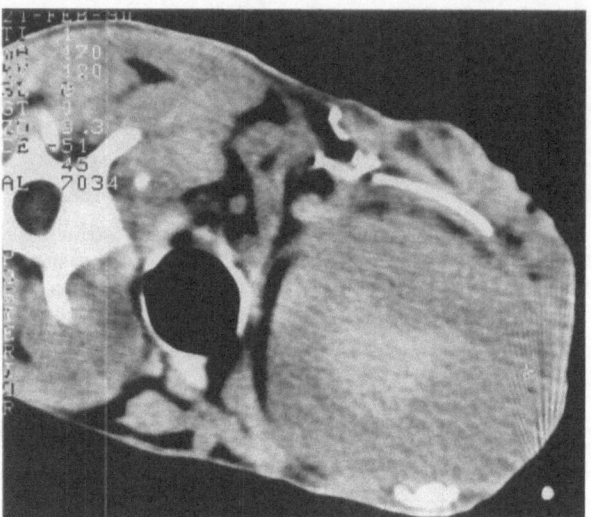

Fig. 4. CT transversal scan through the midportion of the heterotropic transplanted heart in the same dog as in Fig. 3 (subcutaneously at the neck) after intravenous contrast agent application with good delineation of the ventricular cavity

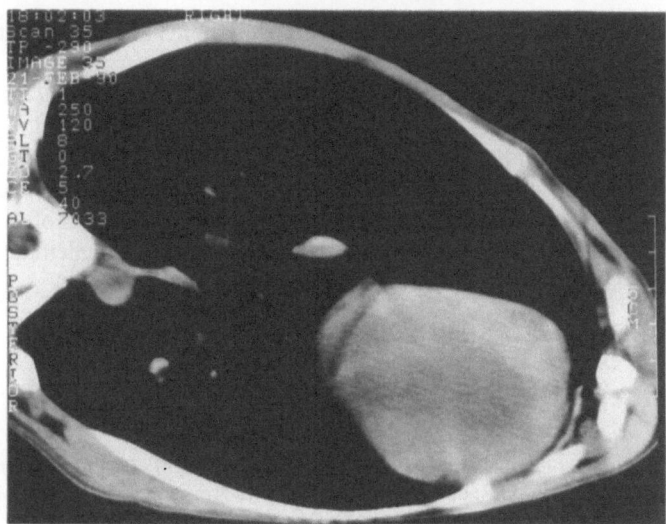

Fig. 5. CT transversal scan as in Fig. 3 however without contrast agent application. The delineation of the myocardial wall from the left ventricular cavity is caused by severe anemia in this animal

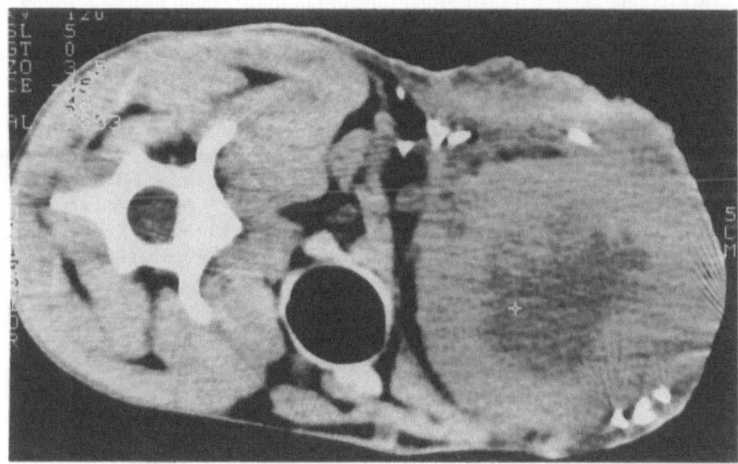

Fig. 6. CT transversal scan as in Fig. 4. Explanation the same like in Fig. 5

quality and that way in diagnostic statements if compared to conventional computed tomographic machines.

It also demonstrates clearly the importance of the factor of exposure time in imaging fast moving organs as the heart or flowing blood.

For the evaluation of additional functional parameters of the heart some improvement of the software should be introduced as the possibility of retrograde gating if dynamic mode is used, further the techniques of fast contour tracing for the delineation of myocardial walls and cavities to calculate volumes and muscle mass and a 3D reconstruction program as well.

References

1. Guthaner DF, Schnittger J, Wright A, Wexler L (1987) Diagnostic challenges following cardiac transplantation. Radiologic Clinics of North America Vol 25, No 2, March (367–376)
2. Kemkes BM, Reichenspurner H, Osterholzer G, Angermann C, Schad N, Erdmann E, Rienmüller R, Gokel JM (1986) Hemodynamic results after orthotopic heart transplantation. Transplantation Proceedings, Vol XVIII, No 4, Supp 3, pp 31–34
3. Kemkes BM, Weiler A, Schütz A, Kugler C, Wenke C, Anthuber M, Angermann C, Spes C, Erdmann E, Rienmüller R (1989) Komplikationen nach orthotoper Herztransplantation. Ein Erfahrungsbericht von 100 Transplantationen. Herzmedizin 12: 6–17
4. Rienmüller R, Brunnhölzl W, Gärtner Ch, Kemkes BM, Erdmann E (1987) MR bei transplantierten Herzen. In: Lissner J, Doppman JL, Margulis AR (Hrsg) MR'87, 2. Internationales Kernspintomographie-Symposium. Schnetztor Verlag GmbH, Konstanz, S 69–77
5. Rienmüller R, Lloret JL, Kemkes BM, Erdmann E, Gärtner Ch, Hacker H, Tiling R (1988) MR-evaluation of left myocardial function in transplanted hearts: A follow-up study. Radiology, Volume 169 (P), p 110
6. Rienmüller R, Gärtner Ch, Schütz A, v. Scheidt W, Kemkes BM (1989) What is the role of magnetic resonance after heart transplantation – can it replace repetitive cardiac biopsy. Am Heart (in press)
7. Rienmüller R, Gärtner Ch, Lloret JL, Schütz A, Tiling R, Kemkes BM, v. Scheidt W (1990) MR-Ergebnisse einer 4-jährigen Studie in der postoperativen Nachsorge herztransplantierter Patienten. In: Lissner J, Doppman JL, Margulis AR (Hrsg) MR'89, 3. Internationales Kernspintomographie-Symposium. Deutsche Ärzte-Verlag, Köln, S 166–175
8. Rienmüller R, Gärtner Ch, Schütz A, Keming K, v. Scheidt W, Kemkes BM (1990) Welche Bedeutung hat die Kernspintomographie in der Nachsorge herztransplantierter Patienten? Thorac Cardiovasc Surg, Suppl Vol 38, pp 23

Dynamic CT of Malignant Liver Tumors and Liver Transplants

C. Zwicker, M. Langer, F. Astinet, R. Langer, R. Felix

Introduction

Contrast medium supported computed tomography has proved itself in the diagnostics of liver tumors. The high specificity and sensitivity of this method has been demonstrated in such benign focal masses as hemangiomas or focal nodular hyperplasias (FNH). However, malignant tumors of the liver are more difficult to differentiate because of only slight distinctions in contrast medium behavior. One reason for constantly improving liver transplantations is the timely diagnosis of postoperative complications. Follow-up controls after liver transplantation should not, if possible, be invasive and should demonstrate complications early to allow the initiation of sufficient therapeutic measures.

One goal of this prospective study with the rapid SOMATOM PLUS scanner is to distinguish specific diagnostic criteria for malignant tumors based upon the contrast medium behavior. Further, determining the value of CT for the postoperative follow-up controls after liver transplantations.

Patients and methods

Thirty-nine patients demonstrating malignant hepatic tumors were evaluated and twenty-eight after undergoing liver transplantation. Each examination was made with the SOMATOM PLUS and the following examination routine:

1. Native study: 10 mm slice thickness and interscan distance. 1 sec scan time at 120 mAs and 120 kV.
2. Angio-CT without table feed: Bolus administration of 80 ml Ultravist 370 (Schering AG) at a rate of 4 ml/sec via a computer-assisted pump (Ulrich Corp.). Scan begin 12 seconds after starting the injection (p. i.) with 8 scans and 3 sec interscan time during the arterial perfusion. This was followed by respiratory triggered individual scans (10 sec interscan time) during the first minute as well as 2, 3, and 5 minutes p. i.
3. Dynamic CT with table feed: Continuous application of 100 ml contrast medium at a rate of 1 ml/sec. Scan begin 30 sec p. i. Scan parameters as in native series.

All Angio CT studies were analyzed quantitatively with time-density curves. The density measurements in tumor patients were made in the aorta, liver and vascularized parts of masses. The time-density distributions after liver transplantation, on the other hand, were measured in the aorta, liver and portal vein. The time to peak and maximum enhancement were evaluated and compared with initial values in the native study. Measurements were normalized to the aortic maximum in order to minimize the effects of circulatory factors (cardiac output, reduced cardiovasculatory system, peripheral venous passage). Therefore, in determining the time until maximum enhancement of the liver or tumor, the respective time interval of the aorta had to be subtracted from the measured values. The following quotients were determined for tumor patients:

1. Time (T): $\dfrac{\text{max. enhancement of tumor} - \text{max. enhancement of aorta}}{\text{max. enhancement of liver} - \text{max. enhancement of aorta}}$

2. relative max. enhancement (D): $\dfrac{\text{max. enhancement of tumor}}{\text{max. enhancement of liver}}$

Furthermore, four qualitative criteria were established for qualitative analysis:
− : unable to demarcate the limits of the tumor
(+): satisfactory ability to demarcate the limits of the tumor
+ : reliable ability to demarcate the limits of the tumor
+ + : very good ability to demarcate the limits of the tumor

A very good image quality (+ +) was defined in the demarcation of the peripheral and central parts of the hepatic artery and portal vein after liver transplantation. Classifying the ability to demarcate the central parts of the vessels alone provided a qualitatively good image (+). However, without sufficient information concerning the patency of the central vessels, the image quality could be classified as poor (−).

Results

Eight of the nine hepatocellular carcinomas (HCC) revealed a mean $T = 0.33 \pm 0.2$ sec. The density elevation was reduced to 1/3 the time of the surrounding liver and the slightly elevated maximum of $D = 1.20 \pm 0.4$, due to the arterial hypervascularization (Fig. 1). Angio CT, with a very good capability for demarcating the limits of the tumor (89%), was superior to all other methods (Table 1). One HCC with reduced vascularization was displayed as a hypodense mass during all phases of the Angio CT.

Each of ten patients with cholangiomas or gallbladder carcinomas demonstrated a substantially slower density elevation with an average time of $T = 3.1 \pm 1.8$ sec and a reduced maximum enhancement of $D = 0.7 \pm 0.2$ compared to the liver. The image quality was classified as very good in 70% of the cases with angio CT and 40% with dynamic CT (Table 2).

Eighteen patients demonstrated reduced vascularization (Fig. 2) and two revealed hypervascularized metastases. A considerable spread in time was found with a mean $T = 2.3 \pm 2.7$ sec. The density of these filia demonstrated a mean value

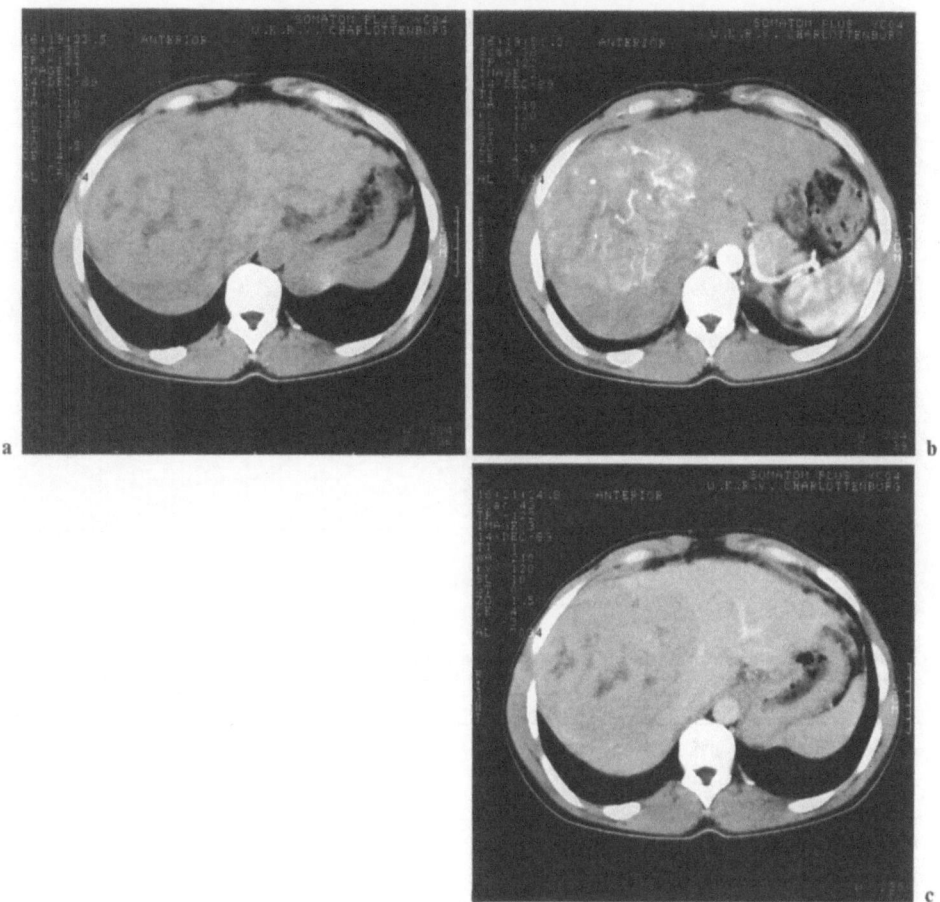

Fig. 1a–c. Hepatocellular carcinoma (HCC) in the right lobe of the liver. **a** precontrast CT: hypodense tumor, **b** angio CT, arterial phase: hypervascularization of HCC, **c** angio CT, parenchymal phase: hypodense tumor

Table 1. Diagnostic information for hepatocellular carcinomas

	native study	Angio CT	Dynamic CT
−	22	0	0
(+)	44	0	34
+	34	11	44
+ +	0	89	22

n=9, all values in %

Table 2. Diagnostic information for tumors of the bile ducts and gallbladder

	native study	Angio CT	Dynamic CT
–	10	0	0
(+)	20	0	10
+	70	30	50
+ +	0	70	40

n = 10, all values in %

Table 3. Diagnostic information for hepatic metastases

	native study	Angio CT	Dynamic CT
–	5	0	0
(+)	25	0	0
+	70	15	15
+ +	0	85	85

n = 20, all values in %

Table 4. Diagnostic information for liver transplantations

	Angio CT	Dynamic CT
+ +	79	47
+	18	50
–	3	3

n = 28, all values in %

of D = 0.55 ± 0.3. The filia could be displayed very well in 85% of the cases with angio CT and dynamic CT. The dynamic study should be applied for the evaluation of all lesions, however, since the entire organ volume is examined (Table 3).

Angio CT, with 79%, was seen to be superior to dynamic CT (47%) for demarcating even peripheral vessels in postoperative control examinations after liver transplantations (Table 4). Both examinations could answer the clinically critical question as to the patency of the central portal vein and hepatic artery in 97% of the cases (Fig. 3).

The mean aortic maximum of 237 HU was reached after 25 ± 16 seconds. The liver maximum of 46 ± 14 HU was reached 25 seconds after that of the aorta. The portal vein demonstrated the highest mean density elevation of 93 ± 33 HU after an average of 13 ± 7 seconds.

A triangular hepatic infarction, a recent, hyperdense, postoperative hemorrhage, two arterioportal fistulas and seven periportal lymphedemas were verified. The fistulas could only be displayed with angio CT during the arterial and early venous phase of the portal vein.

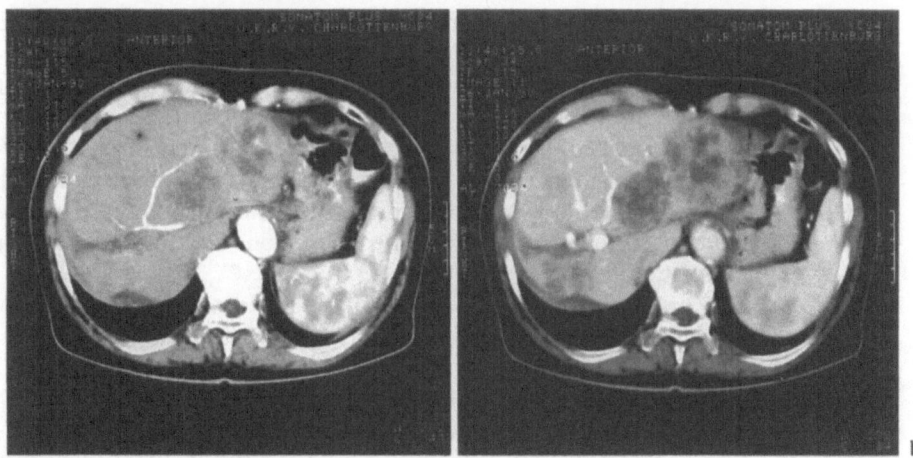

Fig. 2a, b. Left lobe of the liver, demonstrating metastases of a colon carcinoma following right lobectomy. **a** angio CT, arterial phase: no arterial hypervascularization, **b** angio CT, venoportal phase: hypodense tumors in the left lobe of the liver. Tumor borders are easy to demarcate

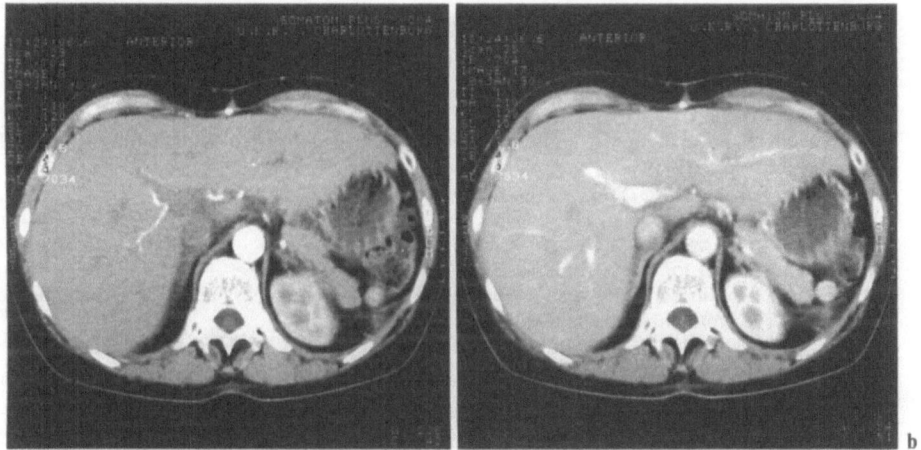

Fig. 3a, b. Condition after liver transplantation. Good visualization of hepatic arteries. **a** hepatic arteries, **b** hepatic portal veins

Discussion

Due to the arterial hypervascularization present in hepatocellular carcinomas, our results permitted a differentiation of hypovascularized cholangiomas in most cases [1]. However, the quantitative analyses of a tumor's contrast medium behavior alone should not be considered as the basis for differential diagnosis, since exceptions can be found (one case of HCC with reduced vascularization). Further morphological criteria must be taken into consideration for clarification. HCCs are often found in combination with a cirrhosis of the liver and an elevated α-1-feto-protein level. Cholangiocarcinomas, however, are generally located in the hilum of the liver and lead to an obstruction of the intrahepatic bile passages. Moreover, the differentiation of isolated, hypovascularized fila from cholangiomas and hypervascularized metastases from hepatocellular carcinomas is problematic [4]. Whereas angio CT is the method of choice for classifying hepatic tumors, dynamic CT should be employed to search for focal hepatic lesions and to describe their expansion and quantity.

Angio CT is superior to dynamic CT in clarifying time-dependent perfusion behavior and displaying the peripheral, vascular twigs after liver transplantation. However, the question as to the patency of central parts of the hepatic artery and the portal vein can usually be answered with a dynamic examination as well [5]. Only angio CT is effective for demonstrating arterioportal fistulas [2], in accordance with Grabbe's findings (1985). We find, as did Letourneau (1987), that CT is a very good method for diagnosing postoperative complications. Bolus contrast medium administration leads to a further improvement in diagnostics [3]. Additional, detailed, clinical investigations are required to determine the value of angio CT and time-density curves in graft rejection.

References

1. Araki T, Itai Y, Furui S, Tasaka A (1980) Dynamic CT densitometry of hepatic tumors. Amer J Roentgenol 135: 1037-1043
2. Grabbe E, Jend HH (1982) Arteriovenöse Fisteln in der Leber. Fortschr Röntgenstr 136, 4: 386-390
3. Letourneau JG, Day DL, Maile CW, Crass JR, Ascher NL Frick MP (1987) Liver allograft transplantation: postoperative findings. Amer J Roentgenol 148: 1099-1103
4. Majewski A, Hendrickx P, Brölsch C, Wiese H (1983) Computertomographische Densitometrie primärer Lebertumoren. Fortschr Roentgenstr 138: 8-14
5. Schurawitzki H, Barton P, Stiglbauer R, Karnel F, Gritzmann N, Mühlbacher F (1988) CT vor und nach Lebertransplantation. Fortschr Roentgenstr 149, 4: 349-353

Diagnosis of Hepatic Hemangiomas Using Rapid Dynamic CT

J. Gaa, M. Schütz, H. K. Deininger

Summary

Hemangioma, the most frequent benign tumor of the liver, can be diagnosed non-invasively with dynamic computed tomography (CT). The specificity of CT in evaluating hemangiomas is between 55 and 90% and is dependent on the respective system and examination methods. The short scan times and fast scan cycles of the SOMATOM PLUS permit the improved evaluation of the focal circulatory behavior in liver lesions. During the enhancement phase of fast CT sequencing, a strong, nodular enhancement was displayed on the lesion border in 17 of 20 hemangiomas. In our experience the peripheral, nodular density accentuation seems to be nearly pathognomic for hemangiomas and makes further examination unnecessary even in oncology patients.

Introduction

Hemangioma, with an incidence of 0.4–7.3%, is the most frequent benign tumor of the liver. The foci, which are generally detected sonographically, can be easily diagnosed in the absence of malignant underlying disease. The necessary differential-diagnostic demarcation to liver metastases is often very difficult with existent malignant disease. Dynamic computed tomography (CT) plays an important role in differentiation and in assessing the effects of intrahepatic masses (Araki et al. 1980, Foley 1989, Freeny and Marks 1986, Itai et al. 1981). Modern computer tomography scanners with continuously-rotating measurement systems provide improved spatial resolution and image quality. Additionally, shortest scan times permit even more rapid scan rates and thereby a better evaluation of the perfusion behavior for a process. A report on initial practical experience in diagnosing liver hemangiomas with rapid dynamic computed tomography follows.

Patients and Methods

Sixteen patients demonstrating 20 liver hemangiomas were examined prospectively with a dynamic CT. The mean age of the 11 women and 5 men was 52 years (range 37–80). Fourteen patients demonstrated single lesions, while the other two

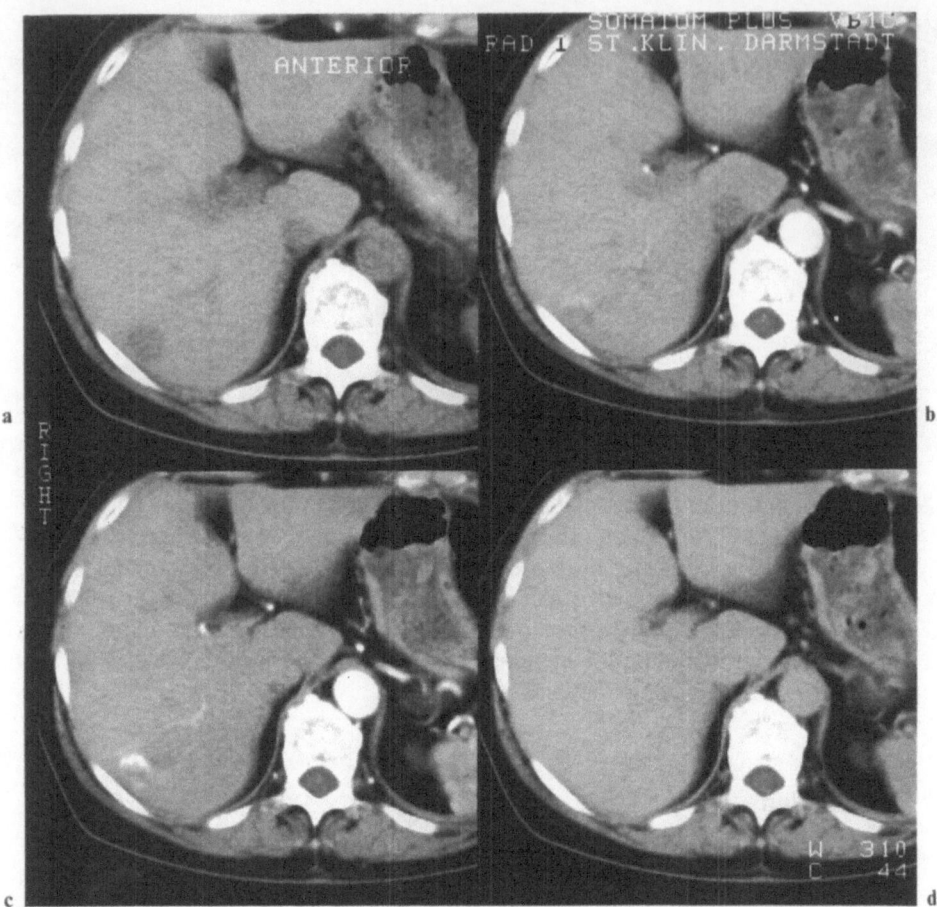

Fig. 1a-d. Hemangioma (1.5 cm in diameter) located posteriorly in the right liver lobe (**a**, precontrast). Evidence of an intense, peripheral "nodular" contrast medium enhancement during the early arterial (**b**) and arterial (**c**) phases. The focus is isodense to the remaining liver parenchyma 90 seconds after contrast medium administration (**d**)

patients revealed 2 or 4 foci each. Six patients had a known underlying malignant disease – 2 mammary carcinomas, 1 collum carcinoma, 1 bronchial carcinoma, 1 non-Hodgkin lymphoma, and 1 hypernephroma. The diagnosis of hemangioma was verified by fine needle biopsy, angiographically or nuclear medicine. Two foci (8 and 10 mm diameter, respectively) showed unchanged size in the follow-up examinations after 8 and 11 months and were classified as hemangiomas with CT.

Dynamic sequenced studies were performed with a computer tomograph of the newest generation (SOMATOM PLUS). The slice thickness and slice distance of 10 mm each were chosen after the precontrast examination of the liver. The plane of the focus was established and a dynamic bolus-CT with a scan time of 1 second was performed at this position. All patients were examined in expiration in order to retain the selected plane exactly in position. A peripheral, manual bolus injec-

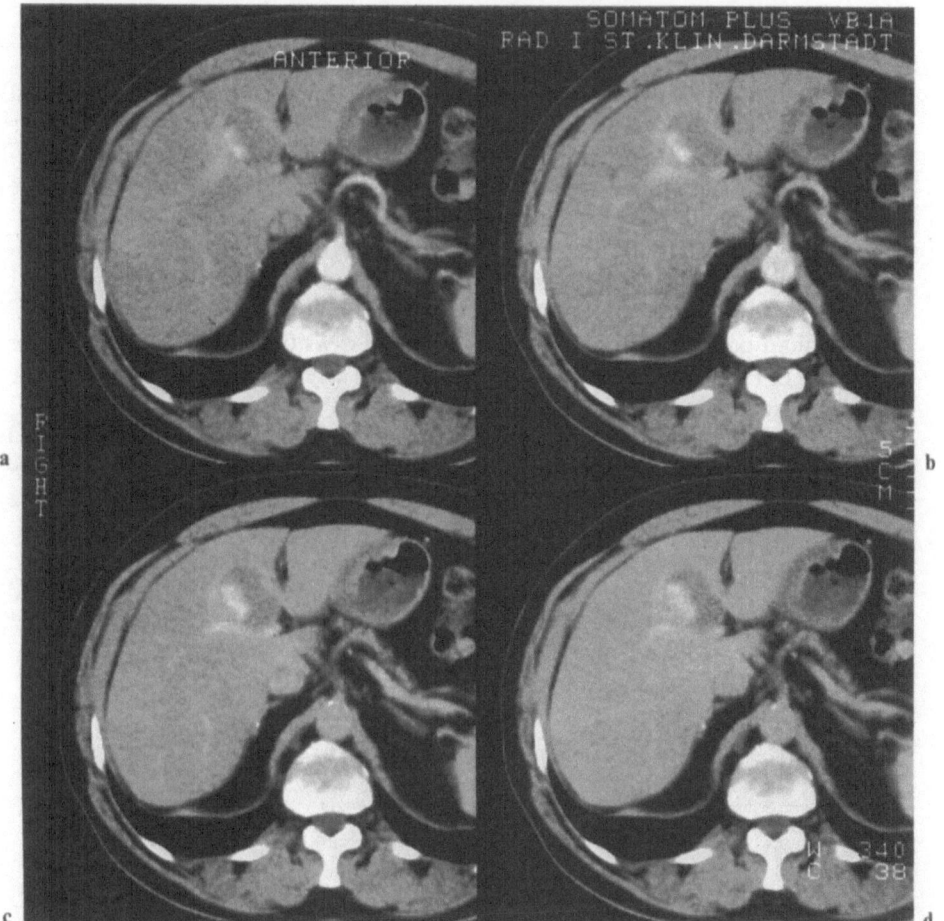

Fig. 2a-d. Hemangioma (4 cm in diameter) at the level of the portal fissure. The sequential CT series demonstrates an intense, peripheral "nodular" density increase during the arterial phase (**a** and **b**). A slow, centripetally directed increase in size of nodular regions with persistent contrast medium pooling is found in the early (**c**) and late (**d**) portal phases

tion of nonionic contrast medium (Solutrast 300, 1 ml/kg body weight) was administered i. v. within 5 to 7 seconds via an 18 gauge cannula. Ten scans were completed in the first 35 seconds, ten seconds after beginning contrast medium administration, at a scan time of 1 second. This was followed by six further scans during the 2nd to 5th minute. Subsequently, 1 scan/minute was performed until the end of the examination after a maximum of 30 minutes.

Results

Each of the twenty hemangiomas was seen to be hypodense in the precontrast scan with a mean density value of 44 HU (range 38–51). Seventeen hemangiomas between 1.5 and 12 cm in diameter (mean, 4 cm) already demonstrated a characteristic and especially intensive, "nodular" enhancement of an exactly localizable peripheral region during the early arterial phase. This enhancement was of a similarly high density as found in afferent, arterial hepatic vessels (Fig. 1). The maximum density value (157 HU) in the nodular region was reached 3.5 seconds after the highest density in the aorta (297 HU). It was characterized by a persistent contrast medium pooling with only a slow decline in density of 44 HU to an average value of 113 HU after 21 seconds. A centripetally directed increase in size of the nodular regions was observed simultaneously (Fig. 2).

This characteristic pattern was not observed in three cases: A thrombosed hemangioma of 4 cm diameter demonstrated a minimal, inhomogeneous enhancement in the arterial phase with no evidence of nodular regions. It continued to be hypodense to the surrounding hepatic tissue, even 30 minutes after contrast medium administration. Two lesions (8 and 10 mm in diameter) already demonstrated an intense, homogeneous, hyperdense enhancement in the early arterial phase and were still isodense 28 seconds after contrast medium administration.

The tpyical "iris-diaphram phenomenon" and a total isodensity to the remaining hepatic tissue was only found in 13 hemangiomas.

Discussion

The hemangioma is the most frequent benign, non-epithelial hepatoma generally identified sonographically. Further extensive and non-invasive examination methods are required, since the morphological differentiation between benign and malignant hepatomas with sonography is difficult. This is especially important if malignant underlying disease is present. Dynamic computed tomography with densitometric analysis can lead to the simple verification of a lesion as well as to a specific differential diagnosis (Araki et al. 1980, Itai et al. 1981). The specificity of this method for the diagnosis of hemangioma varies from 55 to 90%. This is dependent on computer tomographic criteria and the quite different examination conditions and system constellations (Ashida et al. 1987, Freeny and Marks 1986).

Earlier papers described an "iris diaphragm shaped" contrast medium enhancement and a partial or total isodensity in later scans compared to the normal liver parenchyma as obligatory signs, typical for hemangioma. The development of modern CT units makes the performance of even faster scan sequences possible so that the perfusion stage of a lesion can be evaluated better. The following specific criteria are necessary for the diagnosis of hemangioma. They conform to such angiographic signs for hemangioma as the early display of a hypervascularized tumor region and a persistent stasis of contrast medium in the form of mottled contrast medium depots easy to differentiate from the normal liver parenchyma:

a) Evidence of an intense, nodular enhancement in the focal periphery during the early arterial phase, the density of which is nearly equal to that of afferent liver vessels.
b) Sharply outlined nodular region.
c) An increasing propagation of nodular enhancement in every direction for longer than 20 seconds.

Seventeen of the twenty hemangiomas (85%) could be classified correctly based upon these criteria. Further signs mentioned in the literature provided no additional diagnostic advantage and were not taken into consideration (e. g. hypodensity of the lesion in the precontrast scan and a partial or complete "fill-in" in late scans). Comparative examinations on 23 patients with liver metastases from colorectal tumors and mammary carcinomas permitted a reliable differentiation to hemangiomas with the use of these criteria (Gaa and Deininger 1990). Our own results are in accordance with those of Itai, who demonstrated only one false-positive finding from 110 hemangiomas with the use of similar criteria (Itai and Teraoka 1989). Here, a very rare angiosarcoma of the liver was present which could not be differentiated from a hemangioma with CT, angiography, or MR tomography. The CT diagnosis of thrombosed hemangiomas continues to be a problem since they often demonstrate reduced enhancement. Another problem can be found in foci of 1 cm and less in diameter as these may show a homogeneous, hyperdense enhancement in the arterial phase. Therefore, they cannot be reliably differentiated from hypervascularized metastases of hypernephromas, malignant insulomas, pheochromocytomas or carcinoids (Bressler et al. 1987).

In summary, we believe that nonthrombosed hemangiomas larger than 1.5 cm in diameter demonstrate a nearly pathognomic, computer tomographic behavior from the early arterial to the venoportal phase. Therefore, they can be diagnosed reliably based on these specific criteria. An additional advantage is that late scans up to 30 minutes after contrast medium administration are no longer necessary, resulting in a substantial saving of time in routine diagnostics.

References

1. Araki T, Itai Y, Furui S, Tasaka A (1980) Dynamic CT densitometry of hepatic tumors. AJR 135: 1037–1043
2. Ashida C, Fishman EK, Zerhouni EA, Herlong FH, Siegelman SS (1987) Computed tomography of hepatic cavernous hemangioma. J Comput Assist Tomogr 11: 455–460
3. Bressler EL, Alpern MB, Glazer GM, Francis IR, Ensminger WD (1987) Hypervascular hepatic metastases: CT evaluation. Radiology 162: 49–51
4. Foley WD (1989) Dynamic hepatic CT. Radiology 170: 617–622
5. Freeny PC, Marks WM (1986) Patterns of contrast enhancement of benign and malignant hepatic neoplasms during bolus dynamic and delayed CT. Radiology 160: 613–618
6. Freeny PC, Marks WM (1986) Hepatic hemangioma: dynamic bolus CT. AJR 147: 711–719
7. Gaa J, Deininger HK (1990) Differenzierung benigner und maligner Leberläsionen mit einer schnellen, dynamischen Computertomographie. In print
8. Itai Y, Araki T, Furui S, Tasaka A (1981) Differential diagnosis of hepatic masses on computed tomography, with particular reference to hepatocellular carcinoma. J Comput Assist Tomogr 5: 834–842
9. Itai Y, Teraoka T (1989) Angiosarcoma of the liver mimicking cavernous hemangioma on dynamic CT. J Comput Assist Tomogr 13: 910–912

Dynamic Screening for Therapeutic Diagnosis and Radiation Therapy for Oncological Patients

M. Herbst, J. Drexler, P. Weber, K. Maatsch

Introduction

Anatomical and topographical tumor extension may be determined with a variety of imaging systems. In addition to their functions as diagnostic devices for the examination of tumors, Ultrasound, Computer Tomography, and Magnetic Resonance are used either in combination with a therapy simulator or as therapy simulators. The use of Ultrasound for therapy simulation is limited. Although compound ultrasound scanners provide body contours (contour representation is not on a 1:1 scale), measurements of tumor extension tend to be inaccurate or require optimal conditions such as tumor localization in the abdomen. Ultrasound is contraindicated for treatment planning of intrathoracic processes. Sonography should only be used to monitor treatment.

Magnetic Resonance provides excellent sagittal, coronal and transverse slices. However, due to technical reasons these slices are used only indirectly for the purpose of therapy simulation. It is Computer Tomography which excels as a method for determining the target volume by means of body contours, the size of tumors and their relationship to adjacent structures.

Methodology

The newest development in Computer Tomography incorporating a continuously rotating tube and detectors eliminates the delay between tomograms with a minimal effect on image quality. The results are instant images of surveys and high-speed organ scans. This technology opens up new possibilities in the area of pretherapeutic diagnostics and radiation therapy for patients severely incapacitated by their illness. The two most important factors for these patients are the short time spent on the patient table and uninterrupted shallow breathing, that is, the patient is not asked to hold his/her breath during expiration or inspiration. The short examination time is especially beneficial for patients suffering from severe pain caused by extensive bone metastases or for somnolent patients suffering from cerebral compression caused by primary brain tumors or metastases. The benefit of uninterrupted shallow breathing applies in particular to patients with obstructive or restrictive changes in the lungs.

Additional indications result for the above patients during the course of treatment monitoring.

If speed is not essential, the target volume and/or irradiation fields set with the therapy simulator should be verified in the course of treatment for patients not impaired by their pathology. The fields should be corrected or the target volume reduced as required. This indication gains in importance from the view point of high-speed organ or tumor surveys including the boundaries of the irradiation fields with simultaneous data transfer for physical therapy planning.

The value of dynamic screening will be demonstrated by way of three examples:

First case history

Sixty-three year old patient. Carcinoma of the rectum diagnosed in 1984. Dukes B. status after resection. In 1986 local recurrence including infiltration of the sacral cavity and the os sacrum. 1987 shows the status after radiotherapy with 60 Gy.

At present:

Metastases of the liver, large recurrence along the upper part of the ilium (left) which continues into the sacrum. Osteolysis is present throughout the sacrum. In addition, the left upper part of the ilium shows tumorous invasion.

The patient is experiencing severe pain in the sacral region, which radiates down into the thighs. The patient cannot walk by himself and suffers from unbearable pain when lying down.

Screening with SOMATOM PLUS (Fig. 1–6):

The tomographic examination involved 25 scans and was completed after 2:09 minutes. The scan cycle time was 5.1 seconds plus a time interval of 2 minutes between the topogram and dynamic screening. The total examination time including patient positioning and application of the contrast agent infusion (Omnipaque 300/100 ml) required between 10 and 15 minutes.

Results:

Despite the short examination and patient positioning time, it was possible to perform a complete examination of the pelvic without any loss in information. The time required for the examination approximated the tolerance level of the patient.

Second case history

Forty-one year old female patient with large tumor in the anterior mediastinum and simultaneous compression of approx. ⅓ of the left lung and approx. ⅔ of the right lung restricting the bronchial system in the bifurcation region. Histologically we were dealing with a Morbus Hodgkin of the nodular sclerosing type.

The patient suffered from increasing dyspnoea at rest which was further exacerbated when in the supine position, which made lying down nearly unbearable.

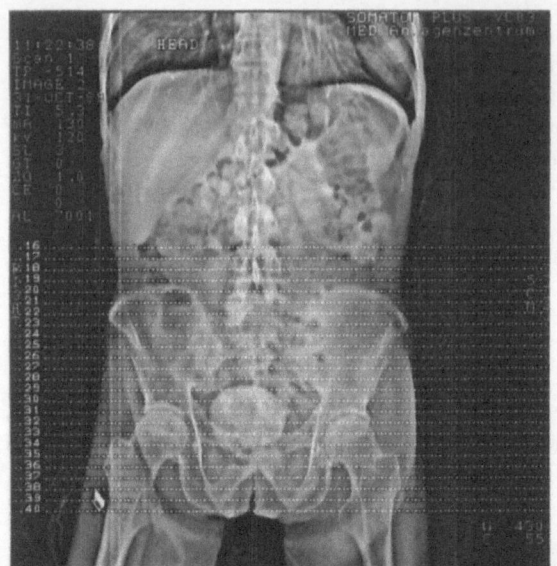

Fig. 1

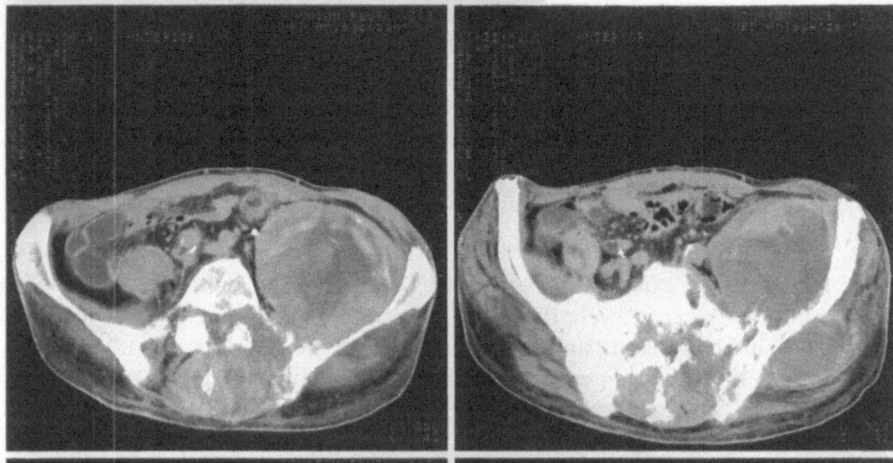

Fig. 2

Fig. 3

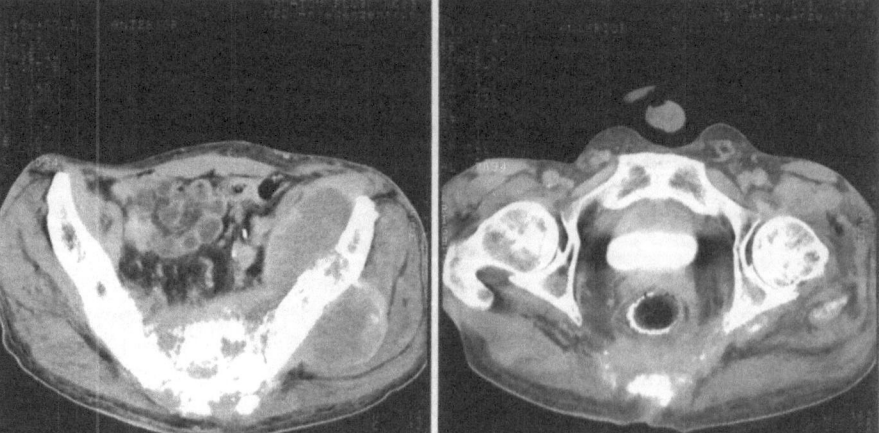

Fig. 4

Fig. 5

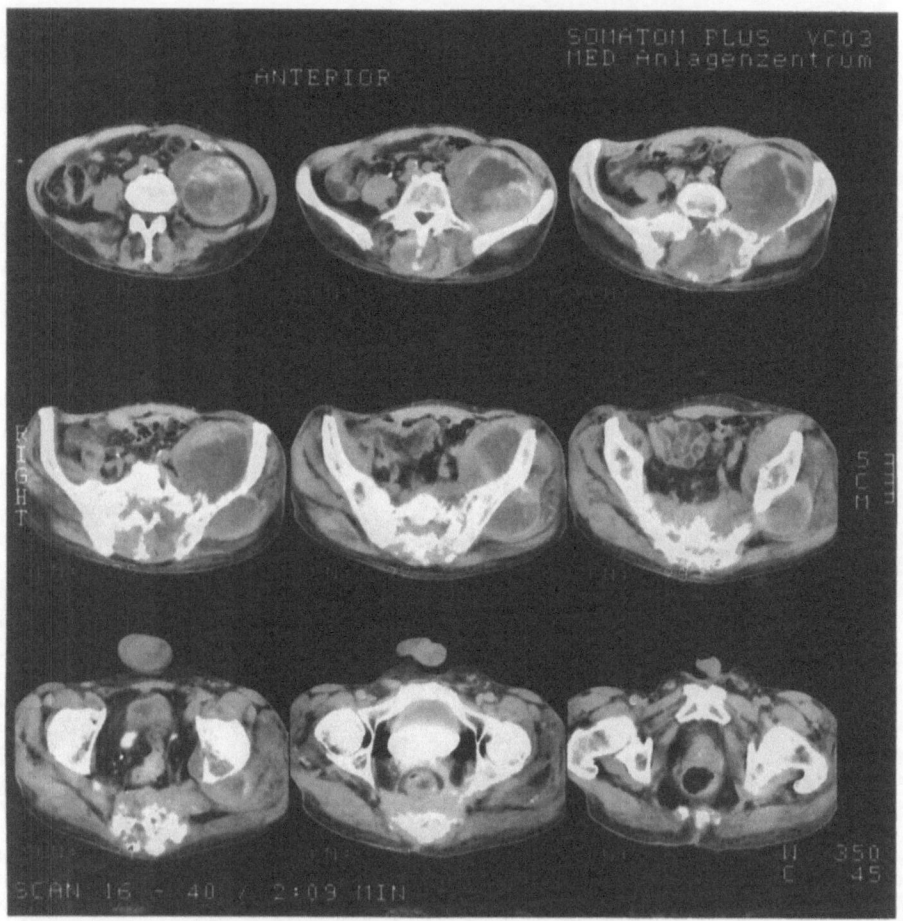

Fig. 6

Figs. 1-6. Screening tomograms (25 scans in 2:09 minutes) of a sixty-three year old patient suffering from a carcinoma of the rectum with large osteolytic and soft tissue metastases in the pelvic area. The tomograms were taken during a follow-up examination

Screening with SOMATOM PLUS (Figs. 7–14):

Patient was examined while in supine position. Contrast agent infusion was applied (100 ml Omnipaque 300). CT screening involved 44 scans and was completed in 3:45 minutes. Total examination time was approximately 10 minutes.

Results:

The patient was able to suppress movement during the relatively short examination time. She did not have to sit up to compensate for her dyspnoea at rest. Since the examination did not have to be terminated prematurely, a complete overview of the tumor extension was generated within a short time and without loss in image quality. The images were stored on magnetic tape for transfer to the treatment

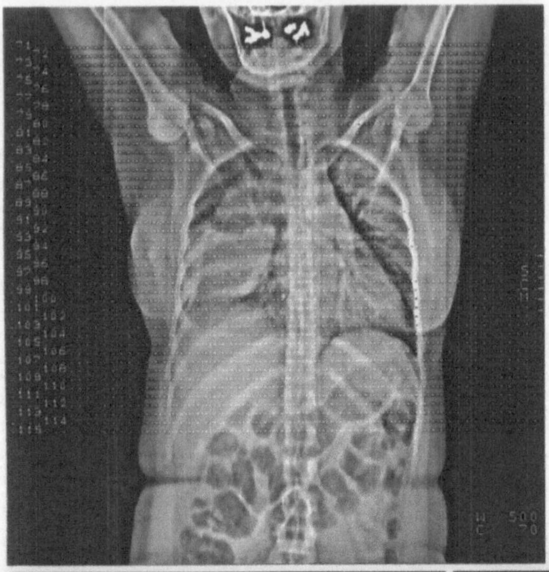

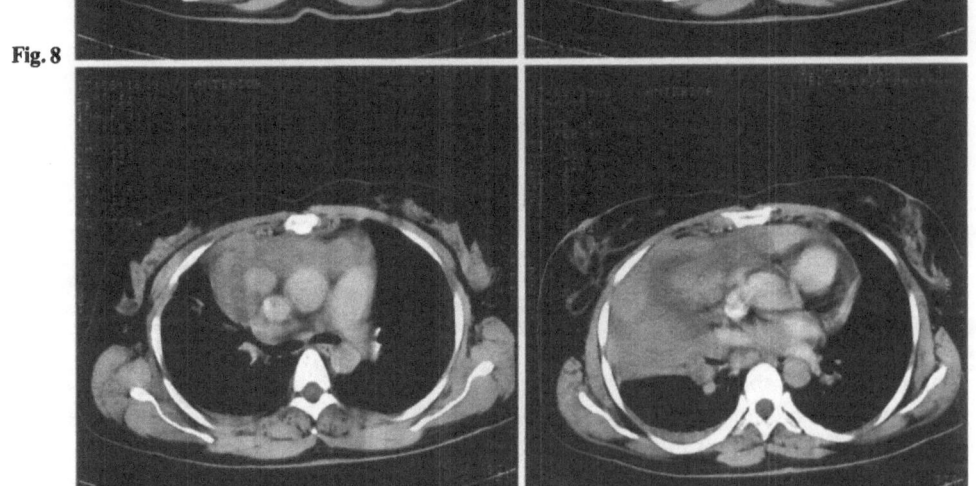

Fig. 7

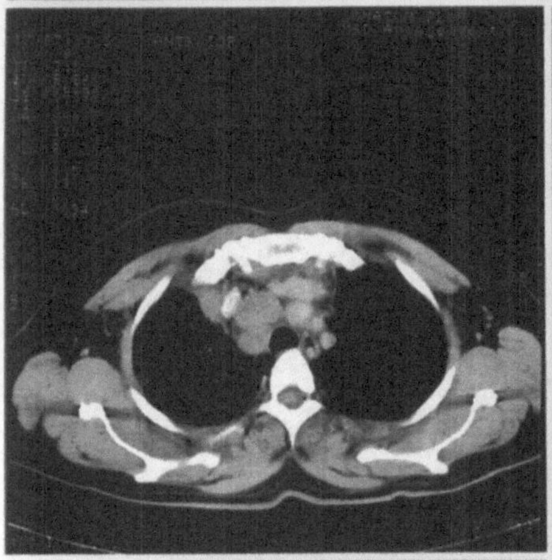

Fig. 8

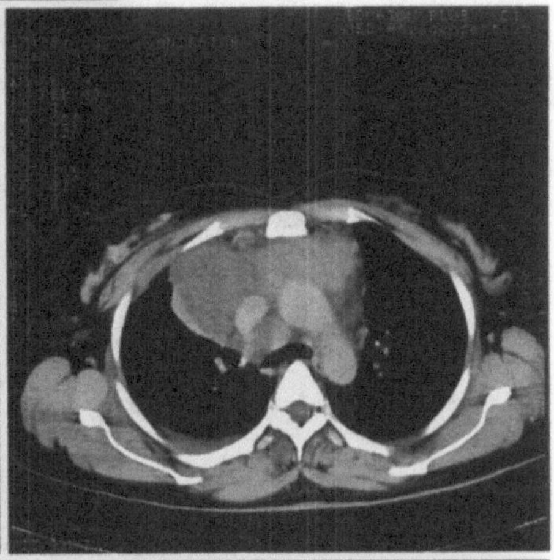

Fig. 9

Fig. 10

Fig. 11

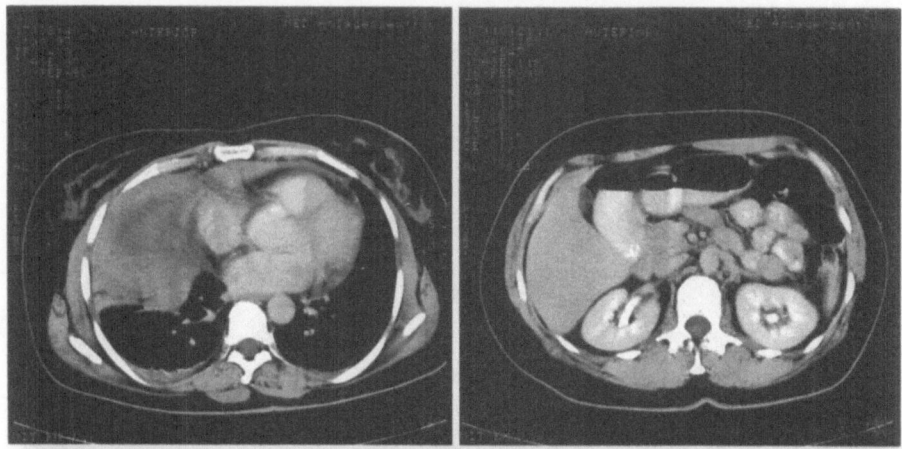

Fig. 12

Fig. 13

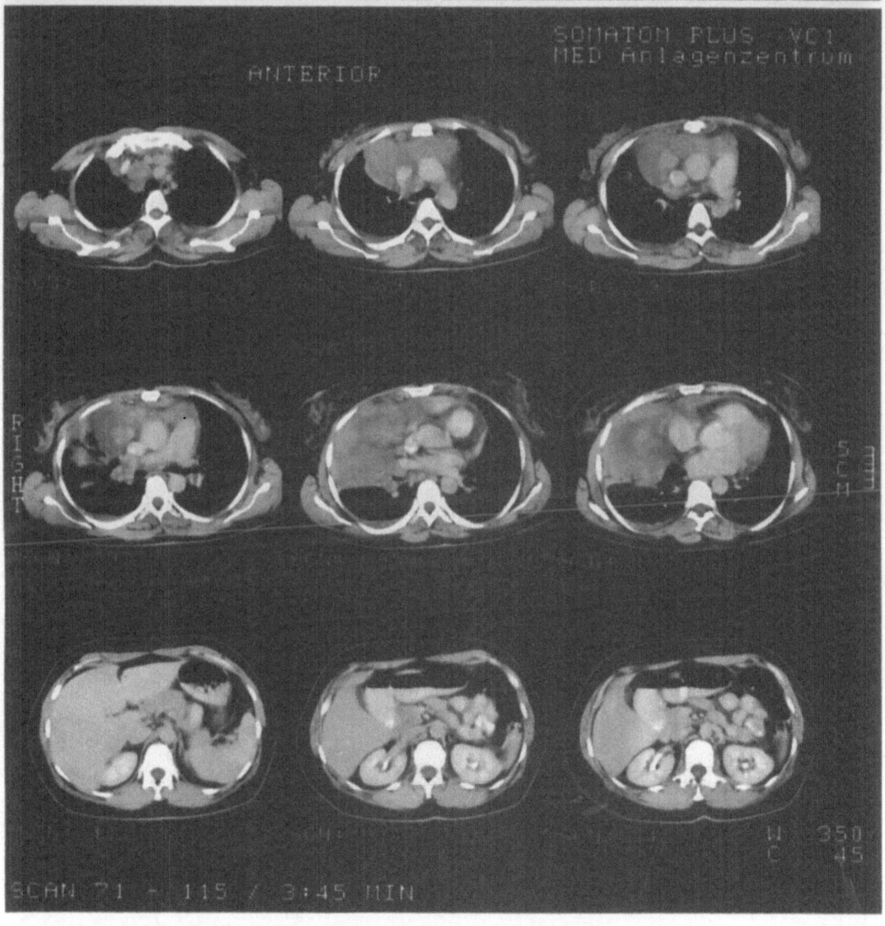

Fig. 14

Figs. 7–14. Pre-therapeutic screening tomogram (44 scans in 3:45 minutes) of a forty-one year old patient with extensive Morbus Hodgkin of the anterior mediastinum

Fig. 15

SOMATOM PLUS VC1
MED Anlagenzentrum
ANTERIOR
RIGHT
W 350
C 40
SCAN 43 - 73 / 2:28 MIN

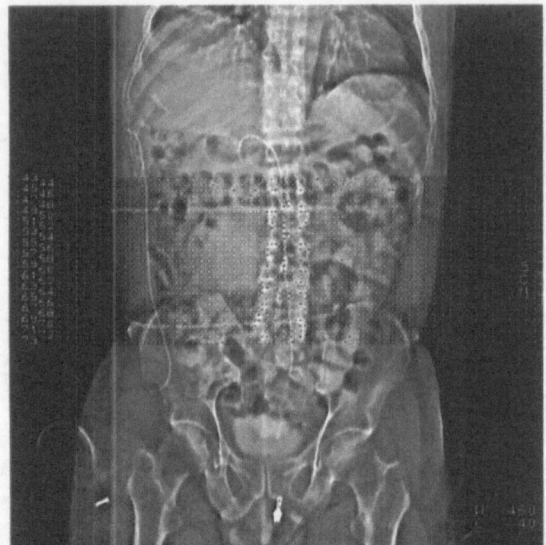

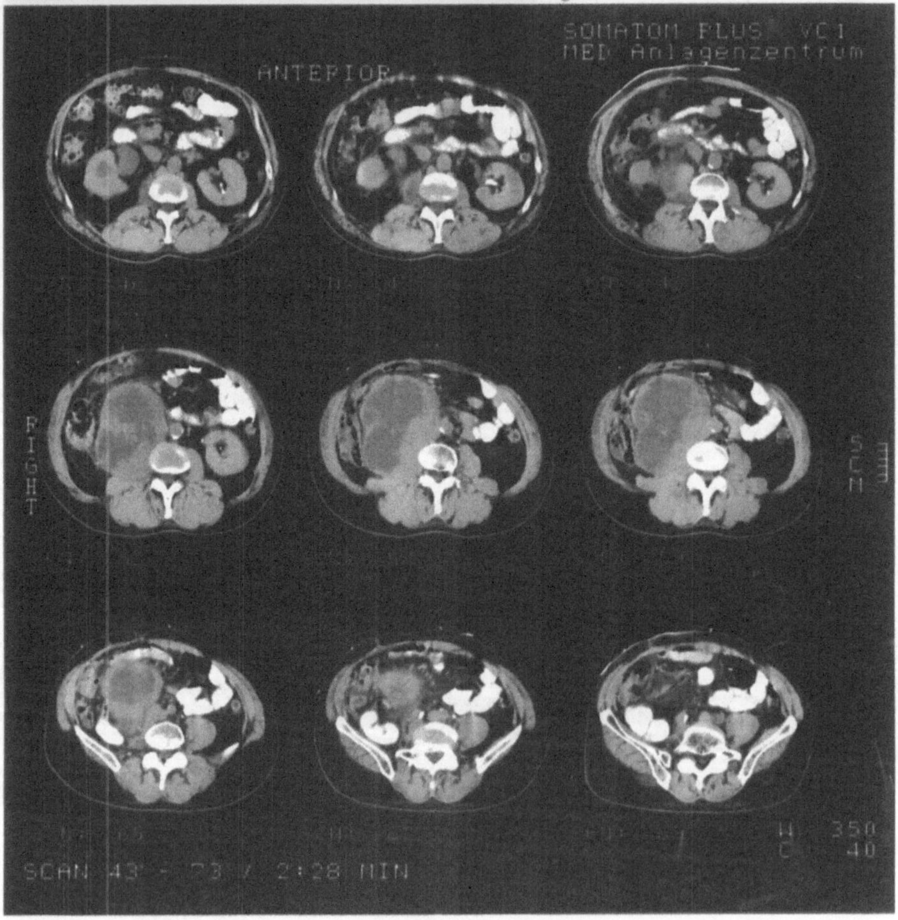

Fig. 16

planning system. This allowed us to simultaneously meet two objectives, namely the acquisition of data determining tumor extension and location as well as the acquisition of basic data for radiation therapy.

Third case history

Fifty-six year old patient. In 1985, resection of a malignant fibrous, class II histiocyte from the psoas of the right thigh. Resection was performed close in normal tissue. In 1987, second operation necessitated by tumor recurrence. Patient is in recovery phase including post-operative radiotherapy with 66 Gy.

At present:

In January 1990, massive edema in the right leg with extension into the right groin, the lower abdomen and the mons pubis. Large tumor in the right mesogastrium.

The therapy fields for this patient were simulated at the therapy simulator and monitored with Computed Tomography. Subsequent to radiotherapy, final verification was performed with the screening mode at the SOMATOM PLUS by marking the irradiation fields (Figs. 15, 16): The results showed that the target volume in the cranial direction was too small. In addition, new growth was detected which had changed the solid formation of the tumor into a cystic one. The screening method provided for quick and accurate tumor location with respect to the irradiation fields. In this case, the method also provided new information regarding tumor consistency. As a consequence of this examination, it was determined that the tumor in the right mesogastrium must be surgically removed.

Discussion

Computed Tomography constitutes an undeniable asset for therapeutic diagnostics and radiotherapy planning. The therapy simulator is used for primary localization of the tumor and target volume on the basis of diagnostic CT scans. After three-dimensional computation the tumor volume from the CT images is transferred via the therapy simulator to the patient so that the boundaries of the irradiation fields may be drawn on the skin of the patient.

According to Dobbs et al., localization was either incorrect or the treatment plan had to be changed in 105 out of 320 cases (33%) when the marked field

---

Figs. 15, 16. Screening tomogram of a fifty-six year old patient suffering from a malignant fibrous histiocyte and metastases of the lymph nodes. The tomogram was taken after resection of a second local recurrence in the right thigh. Volume screening verified the irradiation fields for a tumor of cystic degeneration which grew during treatment. Screening tomogram (30 scans in 2:28 minutes). Total examination time was approximately 9 minutes

boundaries were checked with Computer Tomography. The study of Goitein et al. showed that 52% of all cases required correction (40/77 patients). Errors do not only occur in the form of incorrect localization, they also appear as incorrect body contours. According to Bentel et al. 7% of the Co60 dose calculations and 4% of the 16 MV photon radiation for a field size of 10 × 10 cm were incorrect when the contour was offset by 1 cm. This error is removed completely with physical treatment planning using CT data.

The combination screening method/SOMATOM PLUS created a new high-speed method for examining sections of the body with automatic table feed. This technology is especially important in the area of radiation oncology for the following two reasons: It allows for an easy as well as compassionate examination of patients who suffer from bone metastases and concomitant disabling pain which no longer allows them to lie down for more than a short time. The same applies to patients with somnolence due to cerebral compression caused by primary brain tumors or metastases as well as to patients with pronounced dyspnea at rest due to obstructive or restrictive changes in the lungs. Most patients are able to endure their pain for the duration of the tomographic examination of the entire thorax so that the examination which lasts between 6-7 minutes (67 scans in 340 seconds) does not have to be terminated prematurely. Also, these examinations can be repeated in the course of therapy for these patients.

The second reason in support of the use of Computer Tomography in radiation oncology is the verification of the field boundaries in relationship to the tumor volume. The screening method allows for a quick and easy display of the areas of the body to be irradiated and the relationship of the tumor to adjacent structures. Also, by marking the irradiation fields, their position is determined correctly. An examination using the screening method is completed after 10-15 minutes including patient positioning and the application of contrast agent. This constitutes a time span which allows the physician to perform several examinations within a short time to increase the quality of radiotherapy. When comparing the examination times for the screening method with the SOMATOM PLUS to tomography with the SOMATOM H, Q or the DRH, a ratio of 1:2 and/or of almost 1:4 results. These values prove the suitability of the screening method as a high-speed image series with automatic table feed (volume scan technique) for use in radiation oncology when examining tumor patients who suffer from physical or respiratory disorders. The screening method also proved valuable in verifying the irradiation fields in relation to the tumor volumes to obtain a qualitative optimization of the radiation therapy.

References

1. Bentel GH, Nelson EC, Noell KT (1982) Treatment planning and dose calculation in radiation oncology, 3rd ed Pergamon Press, New York
2. Hobbs HJ, Parker RP, Hodson NJ, Hobday P, Hussband JE (1983) The use of CT in radiotherapy treatment planning. Radiotherapy and Oncology 1: 133-144
3. Goitein M (1979) The utility of computed tomography in radiation therapy: An estimate of out come. Int J Rad Oncol Biol Phys 5: 1799-1807

Advantage of "Dynamic Screening" in Major Trauma Victims and Critical Care Patients

J. Gmeinwieser, P. Gerhardt, K. Mühlbauer, M. Strotzer

Abstract

The use of "dynamic screening" has two great advantages in CT examination of major trauma victims and critical care patients. Data acquisition with one second scan time minimizes artifacts caused by uncontrolable respiration or motion. The scan rate of 12 images per minute allowes extensive scan series within a few minutes without significant loss of image quality. "Dynamic screening" makes CT of major trauma victims and critical care patients faster, easier and safer.

Introduction

Computed tomography has proved to be an indispensable diagnostic tool for the evaluation of major trauma victims and of many critical care patients (Mc Cort 1987). In critical care patients the indications for CT predominantly are unconsciousness and other neurological disorders, follow-up of pancreatitis and search of abscesses or bleeding in the abdomen.

In trauma victims CT surpasses other imaging methods in examination for craniocerebral, facial, abdominal, spinal and pelvic injuries (Heller and Jend 1984, Mc Cort 1987). Morbidity and mortality of craniocerebral traumas could be dramatically reduced by the immediate use of computed tomography (French and Dublin 1977, Zimmerman and Bilaniuk 1978). In abdominal trauma CT examination supports nonoperative management of hemodynamically stable patients (Friedman and Mödder 1982, Peitzman et al. 1986, Trunkey and Federle 1986). In spinal, pelvic and facial injuries, CT provides diagnostic information not available with conventional radiography, thus improving the therapeutic results (Brant-Zawadski et al. 1981, Dunn et al. 1983, Zilhka 1982)

Examination of critically ill patients by computed tomography rises several problems. While the patients are positioned in the gantry, it is difficult to observe them closely and to react quickly if reanimation is required (Sherck et al. 1984). In patients suffering on compensated cardiovascular or respiratory insufficiency the horizontal position during the CT examination may cause acute deterioration. Acute sub- or extradural hematoma and thoracoabdominal trauma often require immediate surgical intervention. Under these aspects CT examinations of critically ill trauma victims or intensive care patients have to be performed under pressure of time (Insel et al. 1986, Mc Cort 1987).

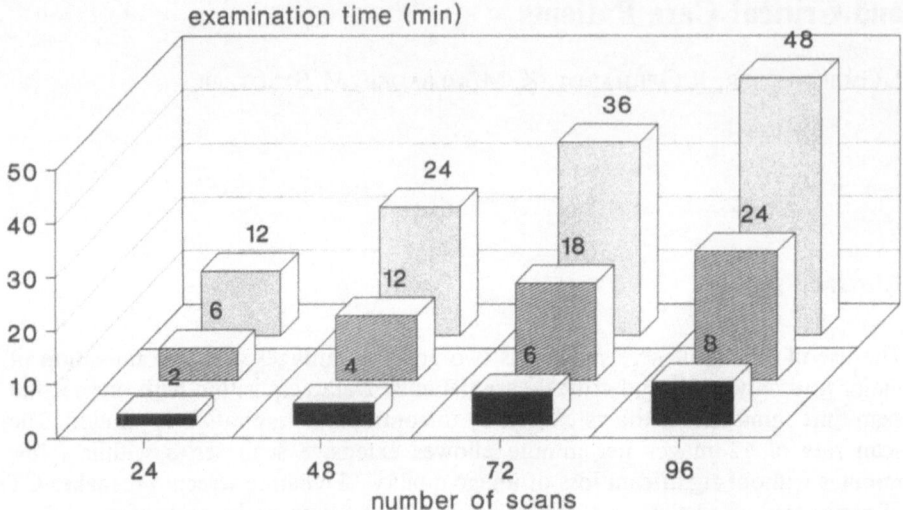

Fig. 1. Comparison of examination times with 2, 4 and 12 scans per minute. ■ dynamic screening, ▨ 4 scans/min., ▭ 2 scans/min.

Another problem is, that the diagnostic information of the CT-scans is often limited by artifacts due to uncontrolable respiration or patient movement (Trunkey 1986). The extent of these artifacts decreases with scan time (Schultz and Fisher 1982). Therefore CT examinations of major trauma victims and intensive care patients require fast acquisition of extensive scan series and short scan times. Both conditions are met by SOMATOM PLUS.

Version C of the "dynamic screening" mode allows to obtain an unlimited number of scans with a 5 second cycle time with instant image display and a 1 second scan time. We investigated the suitability of "dynamic screening" for the examination of major trauma victims and intensive care patients.

Patients and Method

During a period of 4 weeks we performed 4 cranial, 12 abdominal, 4 thoracic, 5 spinal and 2 pelvic CT exams in 6 patients with multiple injuries and in 14 critical care patients. 7 of these patients were artificially ventilated. All examinations were done with "dynamic screening" with 12 scans per minute and one second scan time. The number of scans varied between 28 and 102 per patient. For evaluation of image quality some identical scans were obtained with the "tomo" mode in 10 patients.

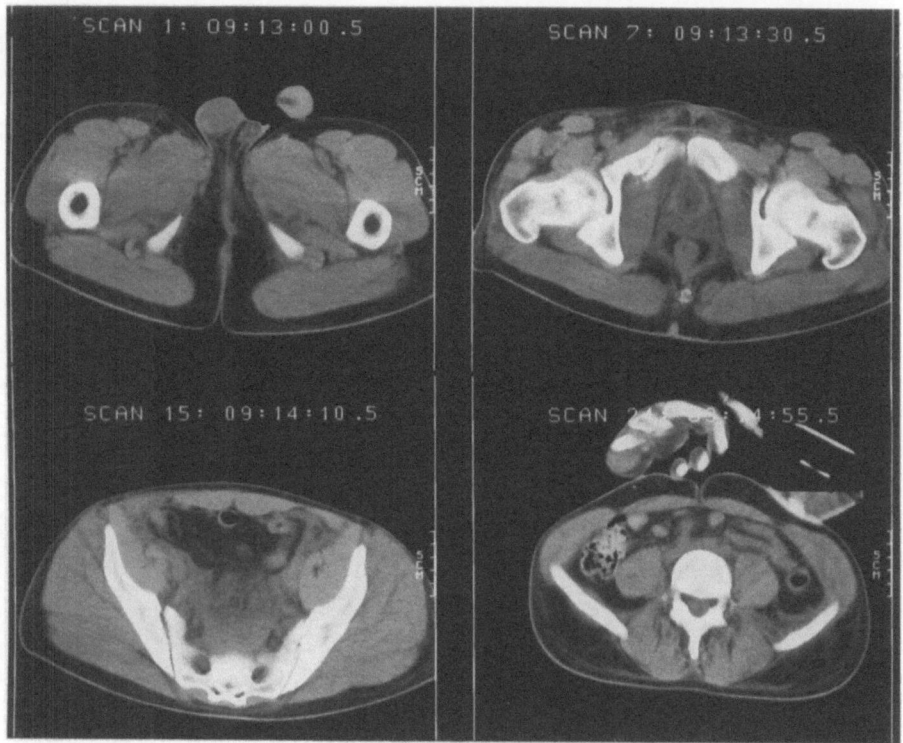

Fig. 2. Fracture of the right pubis and slight diastasis of the right sacroiliac joint. Examination time (24 scans): two minutes

Results

Using "dynamic screening" the acquisition of the scan series was three times faster in comparison to the "tomo" mode. If CT was done without topogramm this meant a saving of examination time of 66% or compared to scanners with 2 images per minute a saving of 83% (Fig. 1). Even in extensive scan series there were no wait times due to tube cooling. In examinations with 80 or more scans up to 20 minutes could be saved. For example a complete examination of the pelvis, abdomen and thorax can be done in 7 minutes.

Images of the pelvis, abdomen and thorax showed no significant difference in image quality between "dynamic screening" and "tomo" mode. "Dynamic screening" scans demonstrated a minimal unsharpness, that never limited diagnostic information (Fig. 2). In comparison to images of scanners of the last generation they were assessed to be excellent. Examinations of the cerebrum and spine showed a slight loss of detail and contrast if compared with the "tomo" mode. Inspite of that, evaluation of craniocerebral and spinal trauma was possible without problems (fig. 3, 4).

Because of the one second scan time examinations of the thorax and abdomen showed no or minimal artifacts during shallow respiration. Deep respiration or

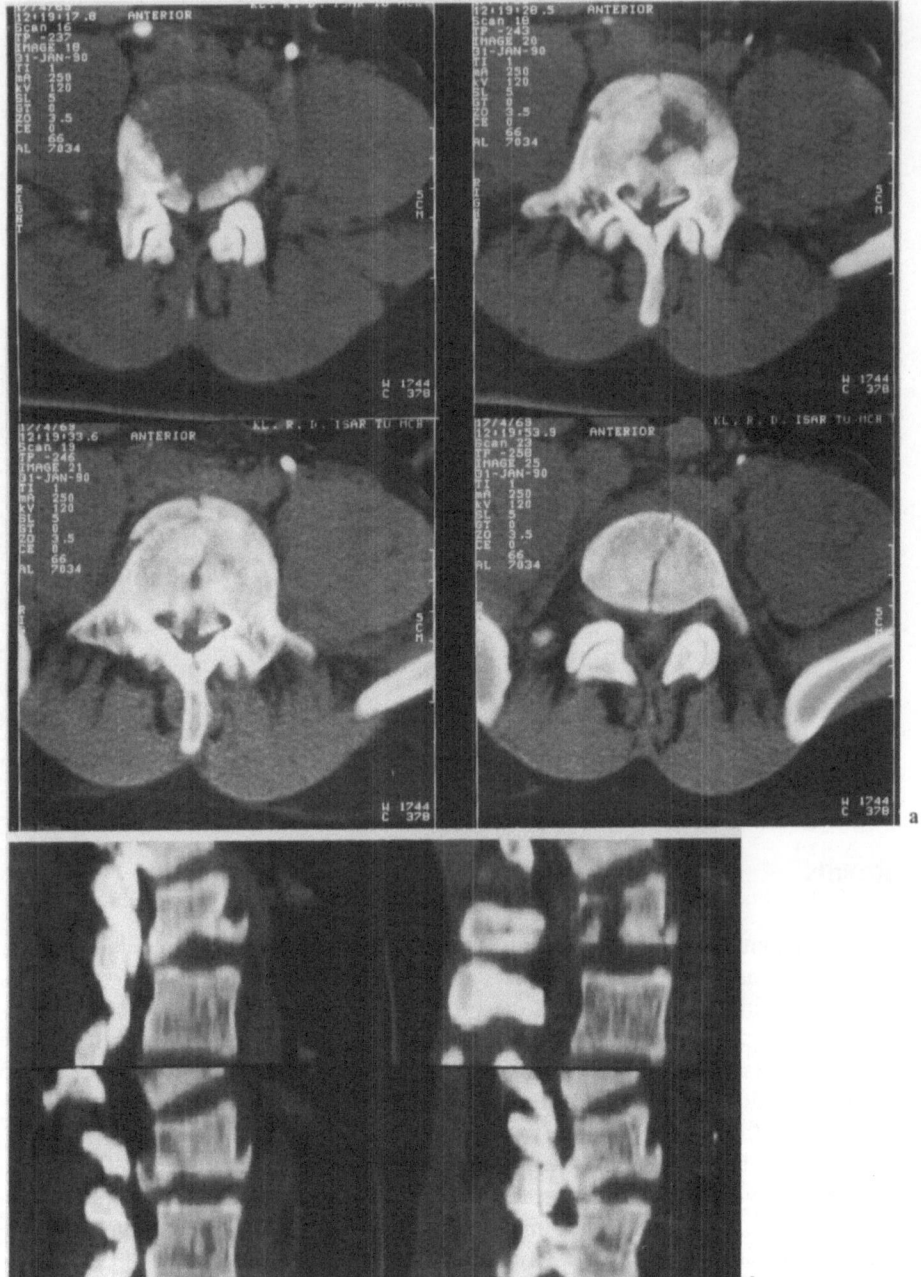

Fig. 3a, b. Compression fracture of L5 vertebral body with marked compromise of neural canal. Examination time (32 scans): 2 minutes and 40 seconds

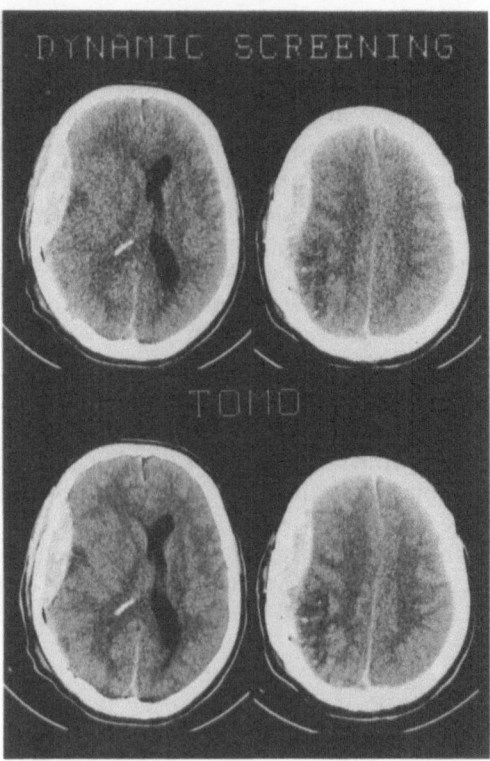

Fig. 4. Extradural hematoma and contusion bleedings. "Tomo" scans show slightly better image quality in comparison to "dynamic screening" scans

patient movement caused a deterioration of image quality that impaired diagnostic information. In patients, who were intubated, we therefore tried to scan in respiratory arrest. This proved to be possible without problems by performing manual ventilation simultaneously to the cycle time of 5 seconds.

Discussion

CT examinations of trauma victims and critical care patients often have to be done under pressure of time (Mc Cort 1987, Insel et al. 1986). Scan times longer than 2 seconds cause artifacts due to uncontrolable respiration and movement, that are limiting the diagnostic information.

Optimum examination of critically ill patients requires scan times of one second or shorter and short cycle times with instant image display. Both requirements are met by "dynamic screening". The continuous rotation of the tube-detector system of the SOMATOM PLUS allows an unlimited number of scans with 5 second cycle time and one second scan time. By the use of "dynamic screening" the critical time period during that the patient is positioned in the gantry could be dramatically reduced. The advantage of "dynamic screening" increases with the extent of the examinations, that have to be performed.

The image quality that can be achieved in the abdomen or thorax proved to be excellent. Only scans of the cerebrum and spine showed a slight loss of detail and contrast in comparison to the tomo mode, what was without significance in head and spine injuries. In our opinion the use of dynamic screening is indicated in major trauma victims and intensive care patients, when examinations with more than 20 scans have to be done, or when the cardiovascular or respiratory situation is instable. To obtain optimal image quality, scans of the abdomen and thorax shoud be performed in respiratory arrest. With manual ventilation of intubated patients this proved to be possible parallel to the scan rate of 12 scans per minute. In patients with shallow respiration artifacts could be significantly reduced in comparison to longer scan times.

A problem is the time-consuming documentation of the scans with a laser imager. This lasts about three times longer than scanning. Automated fast documentation is an absolute must for the future.

For further improvement of "dynamic screening" special organ programs for the spine and extremities and automated patient instruction with a 5 second cycle time should be developed.

In all, the use of dynamic screening made CT examinations of major trauma victims and intensive care patients faster, easier and safer.

References

1. Brant-Zawadski M, Miller EM, Federle MP (1981) CT in the evaluation of spinal trauma. AJR 136: 369–375
2. Dunn EL, Berry PH, Conally JD (1983) Computed tomography of the pelvis in patients with multiple injuries. J Trauma 23: 378–382
3. French BN, Dublin AB (1977) The value of computerized tomography in the management of 1000 consecutive head injuries. Surg Neurol 7: 141–143
4. Friedmann G, Mödder U (1982) Computertomographie bei Bauchtraumen. Radiologe 22: 112–116
5. Heller M, Jend H-H (1984) Computertomographie in der Traumatologie. Thieme, Stuttgart New York
6. Insel J, Weissmann C, Kemper M, Askanazi J, Hyman AJ (1986) Cardiovascular changes during transport of critically ill and postoperative patients. Crit Care Med 14: 539–542
7. Mc Cort JJ (1987) Caring for the major trauma victim: the role for Radiology. Radiology 163: 1–9
8. Peitzman AB, Makaroun MS, Slasky S, Ritter P (1986) Prospective study of computed tomography in initial management of blunt abdominal trauma. J Trauma 26: 585–591
9. Sherck JP, Mc Cort JJ, Oakes DD (1984) Computed tomography in thoracoabdominal trauma. J Trauma 24: 1015–1020
10. Schultz E, Fischer P (1982) Meßungenauigkeiten und Artefakte bei der Computertomographie. Fortschr Röntgenstr 137: 466–472
11. Trunkey D, Federle MP (1986) Computed tomography in perspective. J Trauma 29: 660–663
12. Zilhka A (1982) Computed tomography in facial trauma. Radiology 144: 545–548
13. Zimmerman RA, Bilaniuk LT (1978) Cranial computed tomography in the diagnosis and management of acute head trauma. AJR 131: 27–34

Discussion

A. K. Dixon, Cambridge: The SOMATOM PLUS in the Mediastinum: Preliminary Observations

Oudkerk, Rotterdam:
In dissecting aneurisms the intimal flaps are fast moving in the ascending aorta and are thus difficult to visualize. Sometimes the dissection is identified alone within the two lumina. Dynamic scanning on one level should improve the diagnostic capability of CT.

Dixon, Cambridge:
By staying on the same level, the differential pattern of enhancement in the two lumina is well identified.

Fuchs:
Sonography which is performed as a routine primary investigation is a very valuable tool to demonstrate the intimal flap in the dissection of the ascending aorta. We occasionally come across discrepancies between the ultrasound findings performing the CT scanning. The two methods combined will eliminate most of the cases where a false-negative diagnosis is made by CT.

zur Nedden, Innsbruck:
Using dynamic scanning with SOMATOM PLUS the patency of aortocoronary bypasses is readily evaluated. We compare the time – density relation in the bypass with that in the aorta and in the pulmonary arteries.

Struyven, Brussels:
I do not consider it feasible to assess the functioning of an aorto-coronary bypass by CT.

K. Engelhard, Nürnberg: New Clinical Perspectives in CT: Initial Results of Dynamic Contrast Medium Studies with Continuous Rotation Scanning of the Heart, Liver, Pancreas and Kidney

Vock, Bern:
Did you apply the cine mode for heart studies? Is it possible to display heart movements with a scan time of 0.7 seconds? Did you compare CT studies to MR studies?

Engelhard:
We performed studies in cases of myocardial infarction, left ventricular aneurysms, epicardial lesions and aorto-coronary bypass.

van Engelshoven:
Intraarterial CT-angiography by putting a catheter into the supermesentric artery or the hepatic artery is now an unnecessary procedure to demonstrate malignant liver tumors.

Oudkerk, Rotterdam:
Multiscan studies at different levels of the liver with a 1 centimeter slice thickness and an incremental of 1 centimeter may visualize an increased number of metastases.

Kloswijk, Rotterdam:
Intraarterial portography may demonstrate additional liver metastases thus changing the operative indications.

Adam, London:
The demonstration of the topographical relationship of lesions to the hepatic blood vessels by arterial portography is very important.

R. Rienmüller, Munich: Dynamic CT in Transplanted Hearts

Fuchs:
Could you specify the indications for angio-CT in heart transplant patients?

Rienmüller:
Dynamic angio-CT is indicated in patients with clinical symptoms, acute rejection and pacemakers which cannot be investigated by magnetic resonance imaging. Myocardial wall thickness and left ventricular volumes are then measured.

Struyven:
Electrocardiography, cardiac ultrasound and myocardial biopsy are the primary methods to evaluate transplant rejection.

Rienmüller:
Myocardial biopsy does not provide an overall estimation of myocardial pathology - imaging by CT or Magnetic Resonance may demonstrate functional aspects.

C. Zwicker, Berlin: Dynamic CT of Malignant Liver Tumors and Liver Transplants

Adam:
We started doing dynamic CT, but then abandoned this technique again because of the difference in quality between images obtained by routine and dynamic CT.

Zwicker:
The best method for the detection of liver metastases is dynamic intraarterial CT-portography. The performing of delayed scans is a time consuming procedure.

J. Gaa, Darmstadt: Diagnosis of Hepatic Hemangiomas Using Rapid Dynamic CT

Dixon, Cambridge:
How often can metastases give a peripheral enhancement?

Kloswijk, Rotterdam:
We rely on ultrasound to diagnose hemangiomas and when there are doubts biopsy is performed.

Zwicker:
In small hemangiomas we perform MRI. In large hemangiomas blood pool scintigraphy is indicated.

Adam, London:
For small hemangiomas we rely on ultrasound, for middle sized hemangiomas CT seems to be the method of choice. Large hemangiomas may mimick malignant liver tumors because of central fibrosis.

v. Engelshoven:
Lesions situated at the diaphragm may be very difficult to visualize when the patient is breathing.

Zwicker:
Single breathhold spiral volumetric computed tomography may certainly be the best method.

M. Herbst, Erlangen: Advantage of Dynamic Screening in Oncology Patients

Fuchs:
When it comes to therapy treatment and planning, what about the development of an integrated therapy planning system with 3-dimensional reconstruction?

Krumme, Erlangen:
At the moment there are no specific answers to that problem.

Zwicker:
In therapy planning we need floppies to convert the data from the CT scanner to the therapy planning unit.

Dixon:
A system has been developed by Siemens and has been installed in our unit.

Oudkerk:
Direct connection between the CT imaging system and the therapy planning unit is easily achieved by a computer net work system. The technical problem is the compatibility of various industrial products.

J. Gmeinwieser, Munich: Early Experience with Dynamic Screening in Polytraumatic and Intensive Care Patients

v. Engelshoven:
The total examination time is based on patient handling and on scanning time. The patient handling time with SOMATOM PLUS is much longer than the patient scanning time. The patient handling time is too long. A trolley system is mandatory. The patients are positioned on a trolley inside the intensive care room and are brought to the scanner room.

Alexander, Siemens Erlangen:
A trauma stretcher similar to a trolley will be available on which the trauma patient may easily be positioned in the CT unit.

Closing Remarks

Fuchs:
Well, dear Colleagues, Ladies and Gentlemen, it was certainly a pleasure to organize this SOMATOM User Meeting on behalf of Siemens Erlangen. Nine countries of Europe were represented in the audience, more than 50 participants, we enjoyed the 22 scientific presentations. Among the highlights were volume scanning, the spiral volumetric computed tomography, 3D reconstruction and dynamic computed tomography. The discussions were very important to all users of the SOMATOM PLUS. SOMATOM PLUS means quality and speed.

Subject Index